MEDICATION MADNESS

PROFESSIONAL BOOKS BY PETER R. BREGGIN, M.D.

College Students in a Mental Hospital: Contributions to the Social Rehabilitation of the Mentally Ill, jointly authored (1962)

Electroshock: Its Brain-Disabling Effects (1979)

The Psychology of Freedom: Liberty and Love as a Way of Life (1980)

Psychiatric Drugs: Hazards to the Brain (1983)

Toxic Psychiatry: Why Therapy, Empathy and Love Must Replace the Drugs, Electroshock, and Biochemical Theories of the "New Psychiatry" (1991)

Beyond Conflict: From Self-Help and Psychotherapy to Peacemaking (1992)

Talking Back to Prozac, with coauthor Ginger Breggin (1994)

The War Against Children, with coauthor Ginger Breggin (1994)

Psychosocial Approaches to Deeply Disturbed Persons, with coeditor E. Mark Stern (1996)

Brain-Disabling Treatments in Psychiatry: Drugs, Electroshock, and the Role of the FDA (1997)

The Heart of Being Helpful: Empathy and the Creation of a Healing Presence (1997)

The War Against Children of Color: Psychiatry Targets Inner City Children, with coauthor Ginger Breggin (1998). Revision of *The War Against Children* (1994)

Reclaiming Our Children: A Healing Solution to a Nation in Crisis (2000)

Talking Back to Ritalin, revised edition (2001)

The Antidepressant Fact Book (2001)

Dimensions of Empathic Therapy, with coeditors Ginger Breggin and Fred Bemak (2002)

The Ritalin Fact Book (2002)

Your Drug May Be Your Problem: How and Why to Stop Taking Psychiatric Medications, revised and updated, with coauthor David Cohen (2007)

Brain-Disabling Treatments in Psychiatry: Drugs, Electroshock, and the Psychopharmaceutical Complex, revised edition (2008)

2995B
2009/02

MEDICATION
Madness

A Psychiatrist

Exposes the Dangers

of Mood-Altering

Medications

PETER R. BREGGIN, M.D.

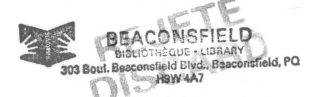

BEACONSFIELD
BIBLIOTHÈQUE · LIBRARY
303 Boul. Beaconsfield Blvd., Beaconsfield, PQ
H9W 4A7

ST. MARTIN'S PRESS NEW YORK

WARNING

Psychiatric drugs can be *spellbinding*, insidiously compromising your mind and emotions before you realize what is happening to you. They can make you feel sad, agitated, or fearful. They can make you think you're doing better when you're doing worse. In the extreme, some can drive you toward mania or depression, and compel you to act in violent or self-destructive ways that would ordinarily appall you.

It can be both dangerous to start psychiatric drugs and dangerous to stop them. Medication withdrawal should be done gradually with the support of friends and family, and with experienced clinical supervision.

No book can substitute for individualized medical or psychological care, and this book cannot be used as a treatment handbook.

MEDICATION MADNESS Copyright © 2008 by Peter R. Breggin, M.D. All rights reserved. Printed in the United States of America. For information, address St. Martin's Press, 175 Fifth Avenue, New York, N.Y. 10010.

www.stmartins.com

Design by Patrice Sheridan

LIBRARY OF CONGRESS CATALOGING-IN-PUBLICATION DATA

Breggin, Peter Roger, 1936–
    Medication madness : a psychiatrist exposes the dangers of mood-altering medications / Peter R. Breggin.— 1st ed.
        p. ; cm.
    Includes bibliographical references.
    ISBN-13: 978-0-312-36338-3
    ISBN-10: 0-312-36338-9
  1. Psychotropic drugs—Side effects. 2. Brain—Effect of drugs on. 3. Forensic psychiatry—United States. 4. Liability for emotional distress—United States. I. Title.
    [DNLM: 1. Psychotropic Drugs—adverse effects—United States. 2. Homicide—United States. 3. Jurisprudence—United States. 4. Mood Disorders—etiology—United States. 5. Suicide—United States. QV 77.2 B833m 2008]
    RC483.B728 2008
    616.86—dc22   2008001477

First Edition: July 2008

10 9 8 7 6 5 4 3 2 1

For my wife, Ginger
Her mother, Jean
Our daughter, Aly
Her husband, Chris
And their new son, Cole.
Love you!

Contents

Acknowledgments

For at least a decade, my wife, Ginger, has wanted me to write this book with all its real-life stories from my practice. It always seemed too daunting a task and with the passing years and the mounting number of cases, it became still more intimidating. However, with her encouragement, I have finally done it. I cannot separate Ginger's influence from anything that I accomplish in this life; she helps everything good to happen and makes everything better. Ginger's marvelous mother, Jean, generously spent hours on detailed editing.

My research assistant, Ian Goddard, has worked with me for many years, searching scientific literature and obtaining articles for me, and often coming up with original insights of his own. Ian also accompanied me on an important three-day site visit to examine documents in a drug company's headquarters, and once again came up with important documents and analyses. Most important to this book, Ian read almost the entire manuscript, once again making numerous insightful observations, some of which are acknowledged in the text as well.

Alaskan lawyer and heroic psychiatric reformer Jim Gottstein is president of the Law Project for Psychiatric Rights (www.PsychRights.org), whose mission is to mount a strategic litigation campaign around the United States against forced psychiatric drugging and electroshock. He is a board member of the International Center for the Study of Psychiatry and Psychology (www. icspp.org). Along with many other reformers and attorneys mentioned in this book, Jim can usually be heard at the organization's annual conferences. Recently, he has been fighting to make Eli Lilly, a drug company you'll hear too much about in this book, reveal its secrets about how its drug Zyprexa can cause diabetes, pancreatitis, and other potentially fatal diseases. Amid everything else going on in his career and life right now, Jim was also kind enough to read this manuscript with great care and to offer many helpful suggestions.

Derek Braslow of Pogust & Braslow, LLC, in Conshohocken, Pennsylvania, is one of the busiest and most experienced attorneys in the field of litigation involving antidepressant medication, including product-liability lawsuits against pharmaceutical companies. He is knowledgeable, dedicated, and a genuinely nice human being. He answered specific questions for me in regard to the book and zealously edited a number of the chapters in a most helpful fashion.

Andy Vickery of Houston, Texas, is one of the nation's premier attorneys in antidepressant litigation, including criminal defense cases and product-liability cases against drug companies. Andy was kind enough to review a few specific sections of the manuscript for me. Another attorney, Don Farber of San Rafael, California, is second to none in antidepressant drug litigation, especially product liability. He also volunteered time to review specific sections of the book. In addition, I want to acknowledge attorney Michael Mosher of Paris, Texas. Although he did not help with the manuscript, over the years he has shared with me his voluminous knowledge about psychiatric drugs, which always exceeds that of the medical "experts" hired to go against him. John Friedberg, MD, a Berkeley, California, neurologist who has courageously opposed electroshock treatment, also reviewed a few sections.

One of our friends, Jay, an engineer and an arctic explorer brave enough to face down polar bears, read the manuscript from start to finish, finding errors that had escaped everyone else's attention, and made important suggestions. I appreciate his and his wife Suzanne's encouragement.

Richard Curtis, my agent and old friend—we go back to high school together—is ultimately responsible for this book's very existence. When we got together again at our fiftieth(!) high-school reunion, he suggested seeking a revision of one of my earlier books with St. Martin's Press. The publisher agreed but eventually that project was postponed as it morphed into this brand-new book. If it hadn't been for the reunion with Richard, I don't know if this book ever would have come about. I also want to thank my editor at St. Martin's, Sheila Curry Oakes, especially for having the flexibility to switch projects midstream, for agreeing to publish *Medication Madness* as a hardcover, and also for her wise editing.

Even after my generous editors had done their work, I continued to edit and to add to the manuscript, and I take responsibility for any remaining errors.

MEDICATION MADNESS

These Are True Stories

NOTHING LIKE THIS BOOK has ever before been written. I have evaluated *hundreds* of cases of drug-induced mental and emotional disturbances, some in my clinical practice as a psychiatrist treating patients, some as a consultant to patients injured by drugs, and many in my role as medical expert in criminal cases, in malpractice suits against doctors and hospitals, and in product-liability suits against drug companies. The stories in this book are about children and adults who have been emotionally injured and sometimes driven mad by psychiatric medications, many committing horrific crimes. Psychiatric drugs can and do transform the lives of otherwise well-meaning, ethical people, sometimes causing them to act in ways they would ordinarily find reprehensible.

Although I have studied and written about these adverse drug effects for several decades, only in the last year have I grasped and described the unifying concept of the *spellbinding* effects of psychiatric drugs. Many people who take the drugs become desperately depressed and suicidal, violently aggressive, or wildly out of control without realizing that their medication is causing them to think, to feel, and to act in unusual and otherwise abhorrent ways.

There are no secondhand stories in this book. I have *personally* evaluated each and every one of the dozens of detailed cases, as well as the many additional cases that are scattered throughout the book. The stories in this book are accurate down to the details. I have not taken dramatic license with any of them. Nothing has been "fictionalized" to make them more interesting; the truth is dramatic enough. Although the book is written for the public, health professionals can rely on the stories as valid case studies of medication-induced adverse effects on the brain, mind, and behavior.

In those cases where the victims of medication madness have survived their adverse drug effects, I have personally interviewed each one at length, usually on more than one occasion. In nearly every instance, I have interviewed other surviving participants in the tragedies described here. Often, I have gathered additional information from friends, family, and coworkers. In all cases, I have sought and nearly always obtained any relevant medical, police, educational, and employment records. Sometimes, I have visited the crime scene and I have always had access to any coroner's reports, autopsy findings, and toxicology results. I have often read depositions given under oath by doctors and by others involved in the case. For most of the cases, I have written lengthy medical-legal reports, and on many occasions I have testified in depositions, hearings, and trials.

Some of the cases were high profile and generated considerable publicity; in those cases—such as Eric Harris, one of the Columbine shooters—I have used real names, since they could not be adequately disguised. I have *not* changed the names of any of the lawyers with whom I have worked on these cases.

I have chosen to provide names, mostly pseudonyms, to the more detailed cases in the book. Additional shorter cases scattered throughout the book remain unnamed. For the reader's convenience, the named cases can be located in the index. An appendix provides tables listing the various psychiatric drugs by category, including antidepressants, stimulants, tranquilizer/sleeping pills, antipsychotic agents, and mood stabilizers. Another appendix provides a description of the International Center for the Study of Psychiatry and Psychology (icspp.org), a psychiatric reform organization open to professionals and nonprofessionals alike, which promotes ethical and human service-oriented approaches.

This book is much more about bad drugs than about bad doctors. Although some of the cases do involve gross medical negligence, *Medication Madness* is not meant to be an indictment of incompetent doctors. It's about the harmful, spellbinding effects of psychiatric drugs, even when prescribed at approved doses by well-intentioned, seemingly informed doctors. As some cases illustrate, even sophisticated physicians, including psychiatrists, can be driven mad by psychiatric medications that have been prescribed to them.

After reading this book, you will possess more knowledge about medication-induced abnormal mental and behavioral reactions than almost any psychiatrist you are likely to encounter—including those who call themselves experts and who give lectures and write papers about medication for other psychiatrists. Although knowledge gained from a book cannot substitute for medical training and clinical experience, or for a visit to a genuinely good medical doctor, *Medication Madness* will make you better informed in these critical areas than the overwhelming majority of doctors who routinely prescribe psychiatric drugs.

In the nearly thirty years since I published my first medical book in 1979, awareness of the dangers of psychiatric drugs and electroshock treatment has not grown as much as I might have hoped. Yes, there is now much more science to substantiate my views. For example, the Food and Drug Administration (FDA) has recently issued warnings about antidepressants that corroborate much of what I've been saying for many years in numerous books and scientific articles. But most of my colleagues in medicine and psychiatry continue to practice without sufficient regard for the dangers of medication madness or, for that matter, electroshock treatment. The public—and not the medical or psychiatric profession—will have to stem the tide of cavalier prescription practices and the widespread use of mind-altering drugs that often do more harm than good.

I hope the many stories in this book—plus the accompanying scientific explanations—will make the dangers of psychiatric drugs unmistakably clear. I also hope they will add to our knowledge about how drugs act upon human beings and about human nature itself.

Chapter 1

Killing the Pain—and Almost the Cop

IF HARRY HENDERSON had been able to reflect on his behavior at the time, his mission would have seemed tragically and senselessly absurd—something no man in his right mind would consider carrying out. Nothing in Harry's thirty-eight years suggested that he was capable of such a horrendous act. Yet he would become an extreme example of the havoc caused by medication madness.

Everything was going well with Harry's wife and family. After the catastrophe, many family and friends confirmed to me that Harry's marriage was a model for others; in his brother's words, "the best in the family." Meanwhile, it was Harry's most successful year financially. He owned a small business and expected to continue making a comfortable living. He was known for his meticulous work and his scrupulous honesty. Since he and his wife Cindy did most of the work, he had limited expenses, and he was generous to the relatives he employed.

Harry was an elder of his church with considerable responsibility for administration and teaching. He and Cindy had no children; their family was the church and the community surrounding it.

When Harry's mother- and father-in-law needed a place to live, he encouraged them to buy the duplex adjoining his own house, and then he went to work renovating it free of charge. His wife hadn't pushed him into it. That's the way Harry was: he saw a need and he tried to take care of it.

In my many years of forensic work as a psychiatrist and medical expert, I have rarely conducted so many wholeheartedly positive face-to-face interviews and read so many laudatory testimonial letters about an individual. So many people were eager to tell me about his good qualities, I had to meet with them as a group in Harry and Cindy's kitchen. Harry wasn't there because he was languishing in jail.

Did Harry need to be in jail? Was he violence prone? As far as I could ascertain, the only time Harry ever displayed aggression was at age fifteen: A classmate called his girlfriend a "bitch" while she was standing beside him and Harry hit the boy without inflicting serious injury.

Harry had to rise above an abusive childhood. His alcoholic father and beleaguered mother barely took care of him and his brothers and sisters. If Harry were the self-congratulatory sort, he could have exuded pride at being a self-made man. Instead, his childhood left him with a Lincoln-esque sadness. He had accepted these "blue" feelings as "just the way I am," and no one who knew him described him as depressed.

Not viewing himself as depressed, Harry never considered seeking treatment until he happened to visit his family doctor for an annoying gastrointestinal problem. The problem eventually went away but something else happened that day in the doctor's waiting room—something that would forever change his life and the lives around him. Harry noticed a flyer about depression and its treatment. Couched as an "educational" brochure and prominently displayed in the doctor's office, it was really an advertising pamphlet for a pharmaceutical product. For the first time in his life, Harry thought, "Maybe I'm depressed."

Harry was dealing with two stressors in his life: in-laws who were making excessive demands on him, and his own mother who was dying of Alzheimer's disease. In his criminal case, I wrote to the court, "It is no exaggeration to say that all of these problems were related to his sense of altruism and responsibility; none of them were selfish or self-centered in nature."

Following his physical, which revealed nothing to be worried about, Harry talked briefly to the physician's assistant about feeling "blue" on and off for much of his life. Although Harry does not recall being at all suicidal or reporting such feelings to the doctor, the medical record states that he had some suicidal feelings in recent times. But never in his life had Harry experienced anything remotely like the compulsive drive toward violence that would soon overcome him.

Harry walked out of the medical office with a prescription for Paxil 20 mg per day. Paxil is one of the commonly used Prozac copycats that also include Celexa, Lexapro, Luvox, and Zoloft (see table I in appendix A). All are selective serotonin reuptake inhibitors (SSRIs) that block the normal removal of the neurotransmitter serotonin from its active site in between neurons in the brain. Among them, in my clinical experience, Paxil is the antidepressant most often implicated in acts of violence and suicide.

One month later, Harry's prescription was increased to 30 mg and then 40 mg per day over a one-week period, well within the suggested dose range for treating depression. However, most negative psychiatric reactions to antidepressants occur within the routine dosages, often when the dose has been recently changed, either up or down.

HARRY ON PAXIL

AT THE TIME, Harry's wife Cindy did not connect the changes in her husband with his starting Paxil, but in retrospect it became clear. Usually, he was very gentle and considerate, a model husband, but now he sometimes became irritable. On one occasion he shocked Cindy by gesturing obscenely at a driver who had cut him off. Again, out of character for him, Harry cried uncontrollably while visiting his ailing mother and on another occasion burst unaccountably into tears on a weekend vacation. He also showed a maniclike lack of judgment, buying worthless or extravagant items at auctions, including a car the family didn't need. Again, this was not typical behavior for Harry Henderson.

Antidepressants frequently cause overstimulation of the brain and mind, ranging from insomnia and mild agitation to psychotic levels of mania. They can also drive compulsive behaviors. Harry would display all of these behaviors while taking Paxil.

Harry ran out of Paxil for one day and "crashed," sleeping for two days, but he had no idea this was a drug-withdrawal reaction. His doctor had failed to warn him about that eventuality and Harry did not check other sources of drug information. Of all the side effects Harry experienced, sexual dysfunction was the only one his doctor had mentioned to him and was, therefore, the only one Harry could identify as drug-related.

One friend who saw Harry several days a week at church activities noticed that Harry was "nervous and agitated," "fidgety," "forgetful," and "like a radio turned to all channels." But in general, Harry managed to keep his inner turmoil from almost everyone who knew him.

Eight months after starting on Paxil, Harry's dose was again increased, this time to 60 mg per day, somewhat above the recommended maximum of 50 mg per day for depression, but well within medical practice habits. Harry's mental state drastically worsened. He felt a growing, compulsive desire to put a stop to the strange pain inside his head, one of the most agonizing and difficult-to-describe adverse effects of the newer antidepressants like Paxil, Zoloft, Prozac, and Celexa.

Harry began to think that his wife would also be better off dying, because "it wasn't right" to leave her behind to feel guilty and to suffer. Killing her and then killing himself was the morally correct thing to do. But the idea of harming her became so intolerable that he focused instead on destroying himself.

These impulses came out of the blue. Harry had none of the risk factors commonly found in people who become desperately suicidal. He was not abusing drugs or alcohol; he was not elderly; he did not suffer from a debilitating physical illness; he had not experienced a severe loss, trauma, or death of a loved one; and his business and finances were sound. Although Harry may have told his doctor that he had experienced suicidal feelings in the past, he never made suicidal threats or attempts. He was feeling pressured by his in-laws to work on their house and his mother was dying of Alzheimer's but everyone who knew him agreed that Harry had been handling these stresses without displaying unusual strain. Over the years, his depressed feelings had been relatively mild and at no time debilitating.

Harry began to search for a way to obtain a gun to kill himself. After failing in his attempts to purchase a pistol, he imagined finding a police officer on a bicycle. He could push over the officer's bike and seize his gun to kill himself. Harry drove around the city but could not find any cops on bikes. Besides, he felt no animosity toward the police and had donated money to the local police department. His brother-in-law was a fireman, a job that Harry associated in a positive way with the police force.

Then, Harry got a new idea. It made perfect sense at the time because it would pose no risk to others. He would break into a police car to get a shotgun; that way he wouldn't have to hurt anyone else. So he began driving toward the town police station where he knew he could find parked patrol cars. He was determined to get a gun without doing any harm to a policeman.

When interviewing Harry in jail, I inquired about his knowledge of guns. He had never handled one and had no idea about differences between automatic shotguns and pump guns, or what might be required to fire them. He had no idea if he could manipulate a long gun barrel into position to shoot himself. He was equally ignorant about handguns. He had no notion about safety catches. He didn't know that he would have to slide back a chamber to cock an automatic handgun. He was a man possessed with a mission; details or practical considerations didn't clutter Harry's mind. Fixated on his goal, nothing could stand in his way. Meanwhile, Harry had no idea that the drug was driving his wholly out-of-character behavior.

Before turning onto the street toward the police station, Harry happened to spot a patrol car parked by the side of the road down the block. A policeman sat in the car, apparently writing a traffic ticket for a driver he had pulled over to the curb ahead of him. Now a new impulse took over Harry. He stealthily drove his car into a parking area near the police car.

The policeman sat in his car with the turret lights flashing, ignorant of the fact that a man was planning to assault him most violently. Meanwhile, Harry's compulsion had completely seized him. In his own words he had "tunnel vision." He felt mesmerized: "All I could see was the red lights flashing like I was zonked out. All I could think was I can't stand this anymore—I got to do this."

Harry sat waiting in his car with the engine idling until the policeman began to open the door to his cruiser. Perhaps fifteen or twenty feet separated them. The moment the man's feet hit the pavement, Harry went into action. Keeping his left foot pressed on the brake for an instant, he pumped down hard on the gas pedal to rev up the engine. As the policeman turned wide-eyed in his direction, Harry burned rubber and drove his car into the officer, knocking him flat to the ground, and bashing in the side of his patrol car.

Next, Harry backed his car off of the prostrate man, leaped out, and heard the officer calling out, "He's trying to kill me." Harry bent over and tried to reassure him, "I just want your gun. I just want your gun." He wanted the cop to know that he wished him no harm.

Harry's memory is mostly blank for the next minute or two. He remembers someone restraining his arm as he tried to grapple for the officer's gun. He heard someone saying, "Oh, he's going for his gun." He envisioned getting the gun, pushing it into his own body, and pulling the trigger. He next remembers someone holding him down. Two men had intervened to drag him off the policeman.

The policeman was badly injured. He was cut, bruised, and shocked. One of his legs was broken. But with the help of good Samaritans, he fought off the crazed stranger who was trying to grab his gun from his holster.

During this horrendously violent assault on the officer, Harry—a man known for his gentle, caring nature—had given no thought to the harm he was inflicting on another human being. "I wasn't thinking about anything but dying. I obviously didn't think about consequences for anyone else." He had no plan for escaping or he wouldn't have run his own car into the cruiser. He felt compelled to end his life on the spot, then and there, at any cost.

After the assault was over, Harry failed to grasp the enormity of what he had done, nearly crippling or killing an innocent person, an officer of the law whose position he ordinarily held in respect. Later, after the Paxil effects began to wear off, Harry grew dismayed and remorseful. He became Harry Henderson again—and yet his life would never be the same. The man who had suffered from excessive feelings of responsibility for others throughout most of his life now had something really dreadful to feel guilty about. He entered into a period of deep depression.

Unexpectedly, the policeman Harry had assaulted came to Harry's legal rescue. After reading my detailed scientific evaluation of Paxil's capacity to cause compulsive, violent suicide, and my clinical analysis of Harry's particular case, the policeman decided that Harry was the victim of medication madness and should be dealt with leniently.

In mid-2002, when Harry Henderson drove his car into the policeman, there was hardly another psychiatrist in America who would have taken his case. Nearly all were in denial, and most remain in denial, about the capacity of antidepressants to drive people over the edge. Even today, after the FDA has acknowledged that the newer antidepressants like Paxil and Prozac cause suicidality, there are only very few psychiatrists with the combination of expertise and determination required to take a stand in court against powerful drug-company interests. If I hadn't intervened in Harry Henderson's case, he might have spent much of the rest of his life in jail. Instead, my analysis of his case led the prosecution and the judge, as well as the injured policeman, to rethink their attitudes regarding their originally tough stance toward Harry. He was allowed to plead to a lesser charge that resulted in his release from jail after a relatively short stay.

Several months after the resolution of his case, Harry drove a considerable distance with his wife to see me to get help in dealing with the emotional aftermath of what had happened to him. The law had forgiven him more readily than he could forgive himself. With additional help from a local counselor and from his wife, it took Harry more than a year to begin his recovery from disabling guilt over what he had done. I am hopeful that some day he will feel fully recovered from the emotional aftereffects of his bout with medication madness, but it will take time.

SPELLBOUND BY PAXIL

MEDICATION SPELLBINDING occurs along a continuum from mild to severe, and Harry was driven into extreme madness. His reactions on Paxil displayed all four aspects of spellbinding by medication:

- His mental condition deteriorated without his appreciating it.
- He had no idea that his psychiatric drug had anything to do with what was happening to him.
- Although he was getting worse, he at times thought he was doing better than ever, especially when he became euphoric and went on spending sprees.
- Ultimately, he developed compulsive, destructive behaviors that took over and ruined his life.

DID HARRY "GET AWAY WITH IT?"

HARRY HIMSELF FOUND it hard to believe that a drug could have made him do such terrible things, and he did not advocate well for his cause. For example, while in jail, Harry had written numerous letters of encouragement to friends and fellow parishioners, confirming his generous and caring nature, but I only learned about these letters from other people. In his interviews with me, Harry made no claim to being insane or psychotic at the time of the crime. Like most people who are spellbound by medication, he had so little memory or appreciation for how disturbed he had become on Paxil that most of the information about his emotional deterioration had to come from other people.

Harry could not explain this obsessive desire to die that ran roughshod over his normal moral restraints but he made no effort to attribute his actions to the drug. Until I shared it with him, he had no idea that there was a large body of scientific literature documenting obsessive suicidality and madness produced by Paxil and similar antidepressants such as Prozac, Zoloft, and Celexa.

Harry was fortunate in working with Pennsylvania criminal attorney George Matangos who believed that his client was a good man driven mad by Paxil and he was eager to utilize my expertise. In the conclusion to my hefty 11,000-word report to the court about the criminal charges against Harry, I summarized the reasoning process that goes into determining if a drug has caused or contributed to an act of violence—the same reasoning I have described more elaborately in my scientific papers and books.[1]

CRITERIA FOR EVALUATING MEDICATION MADNESS

HERE ARE SEVERAL CRITERIA that can be used to determine if a medication has caused or contributed to an individual's abnormal behavior:

- A recent change (up or down) in the dose of the medication;
- A relatively sudden onset and rapid escalation of abnormal thoughts and behavior;
- Escalating symptoms of drug toxicity, such as insomnia, agitation, memory dysfunction, hallucinations, or other abnormal behaviors leading up to the event;
- An unusually violent, irrational, bizarre, or self-defeating quality to the behavior;
- An obsessive, compelling, and unrelenting quality to the behavior;
- A prior history indicating that the abnormal behaviors were uncharacteristic and unprecedented before exposure to the drug;
- The individual's subjective feeling that the drug-induced emotions and actions are alien, inexplicable, and ethically repugnant;
- Gradual disappearance of the abnormal mental state after stopping the medication (although some residual effects may last much longer).

In addition to these criteria that are specific to the individual case, there should be scientific evidence that the drug can alter brain function, causing abnormal mental and behavioral states.

Not every case of medication madness meets all of these criteria, but Harry Henderson's did.

In medical terms, at the time Harry assaulted the policeman he was suffering from a "Substance-Induced Mood Disorder with a mixture of Depressive and Manic Features." The substance, of course, was Paxil. We will find that every class of psychiatric medication can produce mood disorders.

Substance-induced mood disorder is an official diagnosis (292.84) in the American Psychiatric Association's *Diagnostic and Statistical Manual of Mental Disorders (DSM-IV-TR)* in 2000. As I wrote in my report to the court, "This is a genuine central nervous system neurological disorder caused by drug-induced disruption of neurotransmitter systems." Consistent with this, and typical of almost all my cases, Harry's mood and outlook improved when the Paxil was stopped. This improvement in his emotional state occurred even though Harry was in jail facing trial for his actions while undergoing enormous remorse over what he had done to the policeman, and despite the fact that his life and the life of his family had been drastically transformed for the worse.

INVOLUNTARY INTOXICATION:
A NEUROLOGICAL DISORDER

I PURPOSELY EMPHASIZED that Harry was suffering from a "genuine central nervous system neurological disorder" rather than a vague and ill-defined "mental illness." Psychoactive drugs like Paxil have a physical impact on the brain. Instead of claiming that Harry was not guilty by reason of insanity, my analysis in this and similar cases leads to a conclusion of involuntary intoxication caused by a drug-induced neurological impairment.

With good reason, most of us want to hold drug abusers and alcoholics responsible for their actions. We believe that they should have anticipated the potential negative consequences of using intoxicating agents and taken responsibility for themselves. Similarly, the law offers little or no relief to someone who knowingly drinks or takes illegal drugs, and then commits a crime. The law treats drunkenness as a voluntary, rather than involuntary, intoxication.

The legal system looks more sympathetically on people who become intoxicated against their will or without foreknowledge of the drug's potential to cause them to behave badly. This is considered an involuntary intoxication. I explained in my report:

> Because Harry was unaware of the potential for this medication to produce abnormal thought processes and behavior, and because it was medically prescribed to him, Harry's condition qualifies as an *involuntary intoxication*.
>
> As a result of this medication-induced physical disorder of the brain, Harry was (1) unable to exercise his customary moral judgment, (2) unable to control his violent impulses, (3) unable to appreciate the consequences of his violent actions, and (4) unable to appreciate right and wrong in regard to what he was doing, including the wrongness of striking the policeman with his car.

If I had developed the concept at the time, I could have added that Harry was a classic example of a man *spellbound* by medication in that he did not realize how mentally impaired he had become, did not attribute his dramatic transformation to the drug, and felt compelled to take actions that would ordinarily have appalled him. The more disturbed Harry became, the more his thoughts and actions seemed sensible and his actions inevitable to him. At the moment of violence, he was compulsively and inexorably focused on the act as if he had no choice at all.

Harry not only displayed obsessive violence on Paxil, his depression worsened and he eventually began to show some maniclike symptoms. In Harry's story, the more subtle manic aspects included his increased irritability, mood swings, and extravagant purchases. In other cases we'll see people who suffer from more grossly apparent manic episodes caused by psychiatric drugs.

WHAT WAS THE PAIN INSIDE HARRY'S HEAD?

HARRY DESCRIBED his destructive actions as an attempt to stop the "pain" inside his head.[2] When taking SSRI antidepressants such as Prozac, Zoloft, Paxil, and Celexa—and more commonly during withdrawal from the drugs—individuals frequently cite indescribable mental and physical pain inside their heads as their greatest source of unendurable distress. Because most of these antidepressants are relatively short acting, more than half the drug is eliminated from the body in less than a day, so that people can go into withdrawal between doses. Harry's painful feelings inside his head could have resulted from direct toxic-drug effects, from interdose withdrawal effects, or from a combination of both.

Typically, the pain is both physical and emotional, making the individual feel tortured from the inside out. Sometimes the unbearable sensations are compared to "shocks" and "electricity" or to "impulses," often localized inside the head but sometimes spreading throughout the body. Two days after one of my patients began tapering off her last small dose of Paxil, she endured several days of throbbing headaches like "knives stabbing into my brain," as well as dizziness and depression with fits of inexplicable, uncontrollable weeping.

When patients attempt to describe the "weird feelings" caused by antidepressants, frustration often sets in. There is no adequate vocabulary to communicate the bizarre internal experience. Unsympathetic or uninformed physicians often fail to realize that the prescribed medication is causing this torture. Instead, the doctors blame the patient's "craziness" and increase the dose of the offending agent, too often with tragic consequences. Or, the misinformed doctors attribute the mental deterioration to an "unmasking" of the patient's supposedly underlying mental illness, and then add yet another mind-altering drug to the treatment regimen.

AKATHISIA: A PAINFUL DANCE OF DEATH

SOME OF THESE BIZARRE SENSATIONS MEET the diagnostic criteria for akathisia, a drug-induced neurological disorder that is known to drive people to suicide and violence, and to madness. Akathisia means the inability to sit still and the syndrome is usually but not always associated with a compulsive need to move about in a futile attempt to stop the torment. Several people observed that Harry was agitated and restless in the days before he assaulted the policeman. Because the Paxil had caused such obvious agitation and maniclike behavior in Harry, in my initial evaluation and report I did not focus on this more subtle clinical syndrome—but his case nonetheless provides an example.

Several years earlier, when I gained access to sealed company records in a product-liability suit against GlaxoSmithKline, the manufacturer of Paxil, I investigated the relationship between akathisia and suicidal or violent behavior. Although the drug company systematically tried to avoid diagnosing patients with the dread disorder akathisia, a number of cases turned up in their European database. Working with my research assistant Ian Goddard, we found many correlations between akathisia and suicidal behavior, including completed suicides.[3]

The official American Psychiatric Association's *Diagnostic and Statistical Manual of Mental Disorders,* fourth edition (*DSM-IV*), is the diagnostic bible of psychiatry. It discusses akathisia at length in both of the two most recent editions (1994 and 2000). This conservative, establishment textbook specifically warns, "Akathisia may be associated with dysphoria, irritability, aggression, or suicide attempts." Dysphoria is painful emotion; irritability is overreacting with anger or hostility; aggression and suicide speak for themselves.

This heavily relied-upon diagnostic authority further warns that akathisia can lead to "worsening of psychotic symptoms or behavioral dyscontrol." Behavioral dyscontrol means loss of impulse control. Almost the entire description applies to Harry Henderson, as well as to many other cases in *Medication Madness.*

After describing the horrific symptoms of akathisia, the diagnostic manual makes a key observation: that the newer SSRI antidepressants can cause akathisia with all its associated adverse effects.[4]

You might assume that such a dreadful and potentially deadly adverse drug reaction must be relatively rare. To the contrary, we have known for nearly two decades that akathisia is commonly associated with the newer antidepressants, like Paxil, Prozac, Zoloft, and Celexa. The watershed year was

1989, when investigators reported on five cases of akathisia caused by Prozac.[5] They reviewed the scientific literature, found rates of 9.7 to 25 percent for Prozac-induced akathisia, and concluded that Prozac "and perhaps other anti-depressant drugs as well, may produce the side effect of akathisia fairly frequently." In 1990, the Public Citizen Health Research Group followed up with an estimated rate of 15 to 25 percent for Prozac-induced akathisia. While studies of SSRI-induced akathisia vary greatly in the frequency with which this disorder is observed, the weight of evidence confirms that it is common.

Soon after the introduction of Prozac in 1989, the connection between antidepressant-induced akathisia and suicide was documented in the scientific literature. For example, in 1991, a report was published on three cases of suicidality in patients suffering from Prozac-induced akathisia.[6] Each case of compulsively suicidal feelings developed on Prozac and resolved when the drug was stopped. The self-destructive feelings returned when the drug was started a second time and then went away once more when the drug was again stopped.

The above process of starting and stopping drugs, and observing the patient's reactions, is called *challenge* (the drug is given, causing the symptom), *dechallenge* (the drug is withdrawn, stopping the symptom), and *rechallenge* (the drug is restarted, reinitiating the symptom). During rechallenge each of the patients developed akathisia and reported that this feeling had driven them to become suicidal each time. The challenge, dechallenge, and rechallenge results clearly confirmed a cause-effect relationship between the drug and the adverse effect of suicidal impulses.

In 1992, another group of researchers reported on five more cases of a Prozac-induced akathisia with suicidality.[7] In all five cases, the akathisia and the suicidality disappeared when the drug was stopped or reduced in dosage. In one case, a rechallenge with an increased dose of Prozac reproduced the syndrome. The researchers concluded, "Our cases appear to confirm that certain subjects experience akathisia while taking fluoxetine [Prozac] and that this effect is dose-related in the individual patient." They declared that akathisia "can apparently be associated with suicidal ideation, sometimes of a ruminative intensity."

From Prozac to the newer drugs like Celexa and Lexapro, this group of SSRI-antidepressants share common characteristics, and indeed they now all carry the same black-box warning in their labels about causing suicidality in children and young adults. They all carry a string of warnings about a variety of abnormal behaviors including mania that we'll examine in more detail. However, in my clinical experience Paxil seems to be among the worst offenders, perhaps because it is more potent and shorter acting, giving it a strong, sudden impact.

THE PERPETRATOR PROFILE

IN *BEYOND CONFLICT* (1992), I developed a profile of the characteristics of perpetrators of violence. Based on the criteria in my book, here is my comparison between the perpetrator profile and Harry Henderson's profile:[8]

Perpetrators deny or minimize the damage they are doing to others. After recovering from the Paxil, Harry never lost sight of the harm his actions had done to the policeman, as well as to his wife and family, and to his church.

Perpetrators tend to rationalize the harm they are doing. Harry blamed himself and hesitated to attribute anything to the drug.

Perpetrators tend to blame the victim. Harry never blamed the unfortunate policeman, his doctor, or anyone else, for what he had done.

Perpetrators suppress their own feelings of empathy. Harry felt very badly about what he had done, wrote letters to try to make things right while he was in jail, and continued to feel remorseful after he was let out of jail.

Perpetrators tend to dehumanize their victims. Harry saw the policeman as a person whom he had badly injured.

Perpetrators tend to feel empowered through their perpetrations, gaining a sense of potency from injuring and controlling others. Harry felt completely demoralized by his actions.

Perpetrators seek to win conflicts through exercising authority, power, and domination. Harry tended to be conciliatory and even overly compliant.

Perpetrators tend to become grandiose and self-centered. Harry felt the opposite: helpless and preoccupied with the harm he had done to others.

Perpetrators become alienated from their genuine basic needs, especially those related to love. Harry did feel withdrawn. Gradually, he began to recover, to relate to his needs more fully again, and to reach out to his family.

Hardly any of the dozens of cases in this book fit the perpetrator profile before they became spellbound by medication. That is in part due to how I screen my cases before taking them but even more so it is due to the nature of medication madness—it can strike innocent, good people who harbor no tendencies to perpetrate violence against others.

Chapter 2

What Is Medication Spellbinding?

MEDICATION SPELLBINDING describes how drugs mask or hide their harmful mental and emotional effects from the people who are taking them. Under the influence of drugs, many people feel better when in reality they are doing worse. Some become desperately depressed or violently aggressive without realizing that their medication is causing it.

Every psychiatric drug impairs brain function and can, therefore, cause spellbinding. The cases in this book cover the entire spectrum of psychiatric drugs: antidepressants, stimulants, tranquilizers, antipsychotic drugs, and mood stabilizers.

Starting in 2004 the FDA began at long last to acknowledge some of the more devastating effects of psychiatric drugs, including its recent confirmation that antidepressants cause increased suicidality (suicidal thinking and behavior) in children and young adults. Nonetheless, the agency continues to minimize the mental devastation and behavioral abnormalities caused by every class of psychiatric drug, for example, by not recognizing that antidepressants cause suicidal behavior in *all* ages of adults. Drug companies often conceal from the FDA, the medical profession, and the public the harmful psychological or emotional psychiatric reactions caused by their products. Misled by the FDA and the drug companies, most physicians who prescribe psychiatric drugs vastly underestimate the frequency and severity of medication-induced suicide as well as other potentially life-destroying adverse effects such as violence, mania, and psychosis caused especially by antidepressants, stimulants, and tranquilizers.

Medical spellbinding in technical language is *intoxication anosognosia*—the inability when intoxicated by drugs to recognize the mental and emotional impairment caused by the intoxication. Medication madness is an extreme expression of medication spellbinding, leading people to behave in ways that they would otherwise reject as hazardous or wrong. Some feel falsely empowered as they compulsively pursue bizarre, dangerous, and even violent actions. Others feel overwhelmed and inexorably compelled toward despair and suicide. Typically, these victims of spellbinding are acting in ways that would ordinarily terrify and appall them. Throughout, they remain unaware that they are drug impaired and display little or no awareness of the disastrous consequences that lie in store for themselves and others.

Most of the many cases in this book illustrate extreme adverse drug reactions, sometimes involving psychotic reactions with horrendous acts of violence. However, medication spellbinding takes place along a continuum from mild to severe. Millions of cases are relatively mild and the reactions never get attributed to prescribed medications, but they nonetheless impair or ruin the person's quality of life. Some people are driven toward more maniclike behavior: individuals destroy their marriages, ruin friendships, abuse their children, lose their jobs, or get caught fudging expense accounts or shoplifting. Among those whose drug reactions drive them more toward depression and apathy, countless lives spellbound by psychiatric drugs plod along in lackluster ways: a man loses interest in his wife, a mother withdraws from her children, an artist loses her creativity, or a young boy loses his sense of humor and the twinkle in his eye.

Many medication spellbound people become more irritable, less optimistic, or more emotionally shallow, without realizing that they have changed. In the more extreme cases, these spellbound individuals will fail to grasp the role of drugs in changing their personalities or the degree to which their lives have become transformed for the worse.

Most, but not all, acts of drug-induced violence or suicide have warning signs that are more likely to be perceived by friends, family, or coworkers than by the spellbound victim. The individual can become apathetic and indifferent, yet more irritable and easily angered. He or she may seem less focused or attentive, and more distant, preoccupied, or withdrawn. Anxiety or depression may develop or worsen for no apparent reason. If the drug is causing overstimulation, the individual may lose weight, have trouble sleeping, pace compulsively, or act in an impulsive manner. Commonly, the individual seems "different" with a subtle change for the worse in personality and in behavior. Due to medication spellbinding, if an individual is confronted about any of these adverse effects, he or she will most likely deny them or blame them on someone or something else other than the medication.

Potentially serious drug-induced changes commonly occur soon after a medication is started or after the dose is increased, as well as during or after withdrawal from the medication. The addition of other medications can also precipitate a dramatic worsening. In some cases, however, the drug-induced changes do not become apparent until the individual has been taking the medication for many months or longer.

As this book illustrates time and again, medication spellbinding takes an enormous toll not only on the medicated individual but also on families, innocent strangers, and whole communities. Cases in the book document how medication has driven otherwise loving mothers and fathers to murder their children. We'll see that far too little attention has been given to the fact these seemingly unlikely murderers were taking psychiatric drugs that are scientifically documented to cause mania, a disorder with considerable potential for violence. Society needs to face the huge human toll in prescribing mind-altering drugs to millions of people, and we all need to be alert to the early warning signs of medication madness. A better understanding of spellbinding and medication madness may make us more skeptical about the rampant use of psychiatric drugs and may avert future tragedies.

The concept of medication spellbinding helps to explain medication-induced mayhem, murder, and suicide, and also why so many people take psychiatric drugs that are doing them more harm than good.

A CLOSER LOOK AT MEDICATION SPELLBINDING

BECAUSE HUMAN BEINGS are complex with varying reactions to drugs, no two cases of spellbinding are alike. They can vary in intensity and not all will display every characteristic.

First, spellbound individuals fail to perceive the degree of mental or emotional impairment that the drugs are inflicting on them.

Second, spellbound individuals tend to rationalize and to justify their drug-induced mental distress, typically blaming negative feelings on themselves or on something else, potentially leading to violence against themselves or others.

Third, spellbound individuals often feel as if they are doing better than ever, when in reality they are doing worse.

Fourth, extreme spellbinding produces medication madness in which the individual feels driven or compelled to behave in out-of-character and potentially disastrous ways, for example, to murder a loved one, to commit suicide, or to pull a series of senseless robberies. The spellbound actions are typically carried out without realizing that he or she is drug impaired and without stopping to consider or grasp the disastrous consequences.

The four principles of spellbinding can be illustrated by applying them to how individuals act when intoxicated with alcohol. Typically, drunks don't realize how impaired they are: when they feel badly, they typically blame themselves or others in an exaggerated, irrational manner; often they feel better than ever when they are in reality behaving badly; finally, they can do stupid things and even perpetrate violence that is wholly out of character for them when sober. However, we shall find that there is a critical difference between intoxication with alcohol and intoxication with psychiatric drugs. Because the individual drinking alcohol should be aware that alcohol impairs mental function and behavior, he or she should be held responsible for any resultant bad behavior. By contrast, in every case in this book the individual had little or no idea that psychiatric medication impairs mental function and behavior with the potential for destructive actions.

Medication spellbinding also impairs the individual's perception of his or her emotional or real-life problems. For varying periods of time, drug-induced emotional anesthesia (apathy and indifference) or a drug-induced emotional high (euphoria) can mask the person's personal conflicts and emotional suffering. All psychoactive drugs share this combined capacity to hide their adverse effects from the individual while also masking or burying the individual's awareness of personal problems, including nagging responsibilities and painful emotional conflicts. The individual's *overall* capacity for self-observation or self-awareness is impaired. This is well illustrated by the familiar figure of the individual intoxicated with alcohol who fails to perceive the degree of his intoxication while simultaneously "forgetting about his troubles."

MEDICATION MADNESS CAUSED BY NONPSYCHIATRIC DRUGS

THERE'S AN UNDERSTANDABLE TENDENCY to blame medication madness on the individual rather than on the drug. After all, many of these people have mental problems or they wouldn't be taking psychiatric drugs. The truth is these drugs often drive people crazy who previously seemed normal or healthy. Examining how nonpsychiatric drugs and medications can spellbind people can clarify that this is not a phenomenon limited to "psychiatric patients."

Medication Madness Caused by "Recreational" Drugs

In the 1950s, the U.S. government experimented on unwitting people by giving them the powerful hallucinogenic drug, LSD. At least one of the experimental subjects, army officer Eric Olson, committed suicide by leaping out the window of an office building in which he was confined for the experiment. Eric didn't know he was the subject of an experiment and therefore had no idea that he was being driven mad by a drug.[1] But even someone who intentionally takes LSD for "recreational purposes" can end up on a "bad trip"—so spellbound that he loses track of ever having taken the drug. With no idea what hit him, the drug user descends into a nightmarish psychotic state.

Antibiotic Madness

Hardly anyone thinks of antibiotics as potentially dangerous psychoactive drug but many of them are. Pennsylvania attorney Derek Braslow told me about the case of a thirty-nine-year-old police officer with no history of mental disturbances who became psychotic while taking Levaquin for a cold. Within days of starting the drug he became paranoid and manic, and entered his neighbor's home where he held three children hostage at gunpoint while under the delusional belief that they were involved in gang activity. Thinking he was doing the right thing, the deluded policeman even called the police to report what was going on. This otherwise upstanding citizen had become the victim of antibiotic-induced psychosis with paranoid and manic features. As a result, he was sent to jail and he lost his career in law enforcement.

Levaquin is a member of the quinolones family of antibiotics, a group that is known to cause severe emotional reactions. The WARNINGS section of the label for Levaquin, as reprinted in the 2008 *Physicians' Desk Reference (PDR)*, states that convulsions, increased pressure in the brain, and toxic psychosis have been reported in patients taking these antibiotics. It more specifically warns about "central nervous system stimulation which may lead to tremors, restlessness, anxiety, lightheadedness, confusion, hallucinations, paranoia, depression, nightmares, insomnia, and rarely, suicidal thoughts and acts. These reactions may occur following the first dose." That little string of words reflects untold numbers of nightmarish personal experiences. These reactions are consistent with the overstimulation of the brain and the mind that appear in many of our cases of medication madness.

If something as seemingly innocuous as an antibiotic can cause spellbinding medication madness, how much are psychiatric drugs more likely to cause similar emotional disasters that are even more frequent and more intensive?

Accutane Depression

The acne treatment Accutane (isotretinoin) contains a strong warning about its capacity to cause suicide and other psychiatric disturbances. Directly under the WARNINGS headline, the FDA-approved label reads.[2]

WARNINGS

Psychiatric Disorders

Accutane may cause depression, psychosis and, rarely, suicidal ideation, suicide attempts, suicide, and aggressive and/or violent behaviors.

The WARNINGS section goes on to elaborate in detail upon these risks.

Tamiflu Madness

The antiviral drug Tamiflu (oseltamivir) is approved for treatment of the flu and has gained public attention because of the speculative hope that it might prove useful in the advent of a worldwide bird flu epidemic. The Japanese label for Tamiflu already warns that the drug can cause disturbances in consciousness, abnormal behavior, delirium, hallucinations, delusions, and convulsions.[3] Belatedly, on November 14, 2006, the FDA and drug manufacturer Roche announced the need for an added warning in regard to Tamiflu inducing confusion and self-injury.[4]

Rebetron Suicide

Rebetron, a combination of the antiviral agents ribavirin and interferon, has proven very hazardous to the brain and mind. Under the WARNINGS section, the FDA-approved label for Rebetron contains the following bold-letter statement:[5]

Psychiatric

Severe psychiatric adverse events, including depression, psychoses, aggressive behavior, hallucinations, violent behavior (suicidal ideation, suicidal attempts, suicides), and rare instances of homicidal ideation have occurred during combination REBETOL/INTRON A therapy, both in patients with and without a previous psychiatric disorder.

I have been consulted in suicide cases involving prisoners who were given this drug for experimental research.

Keppra Rage

The anticonvulsant drug Keppra (levetiracetam) was approved by the FDA in late 1999, and has enjoyed widespread use, despite displaying an impressive array of psychiatric adverse effects. The FDA-approved Keppra label in the 2007 *Physicians' Desk Reference* issues serious warnings about three categories of neurological and psychiatric side effects including somnolence and fatigue, coordination difficulties, and "behavioral abnormalities." Most striking, 13.3 percent of Keppra-treated patients in controlled clinical trials experienced behavioral symptoms "reported as aggression, agitation, anger, anxiety, apathy, depersonalization, depression, emotional lability, hostility, irritability, etc." In addition, 0.7 percent of patients became psychotic and 0.5 percent became suicidal with one completed suicide. That's a grand total of 14.5 percent of patients with psychiatric adverse events that were probably caused by the drug.

This array of symptoms will come up repeatedly in this book and is worth reviewing again: "aggression, agitation, anger, anxiety, apathy, depersonalization, depression, emotional lability, hostility, irritability, etc.," as well as psychosis and suicide. It could be used to describe the psychiatric adverse effects of antidepressants, stimulants, and tranquilizer/sleeping pills.

Due to spellbinding, most patients will not report to the doctor that they have had increased emotional lability (instability) or outbursts of anger. One experienced neurologist explained to me that none of his Keppra patients spontaneously told him that the drug was making them irritable and angry, but when specifically asked, *most* of them reported an increase in these symptoms.

Undoubtedly, the drug company would have elicited even greater numbers of Keppra-rage reports if their investigators had actively sought out the information. Furthermore, if more than 14 percent of patients are reacting this way in controlled clinical trials, the rate will be much higher in real-life clinical practice where patients aren't screened or monitored as carefully, and where multiple drugs are often given at once.

Steroid Psychosis

Steroids such as prednisone cause a broad spectrum of emotional reactions that can mimic the diagnosis of bipolar disorder with its extreme highs and lows. In describing the risks associated with the steroid class of drugs, *Drug Facts and Comparisons* warns about "delirious or toxic psychosis," including clouding of the mind as well as "euphoria, insomnia, mood swings, personality changes, and severe depression."[6]

Is steroid psychosis the result of giving these drugs to psychiatrically disturbed people? The pharmacology textbook in effect answers "no" when it observes, "A patient history of psychiatric problems does not correlate well with predisposition to steroid-induced psychosis." In other words, prior psychiatric problems haven't predisposed these people to becoming psychotic on steroids.

When the body produces too much steroid, the results are similar to an adverse drug reaction to steroid medication. One of the most bizarre and tragic cases I have evaluated involved a previously robust young man, Ernesto Younger, who developed an obvious Cushing's syndrome in his twenties. Cushing's disease causes excess steroid production and can cause the same symptoms of mood instability and in the extreme, psychosis. Physical examinations disclosed typical signs of the disorder, including a buffalo hump fat distribution, a round face, and purple stripes on his abdomen. Along with his physical symptoms of Cushing's, Ernesto also developed emotional ups and downs, and he became more irritable and easily angered.

Unfortunately, Ernesto's family doctor became so focused on his patient's psychiatric symptoms that he mistakenly diagnosed him as suffering from bipolar disorder, and therefore missed the obvious diagnosis of Cushing's. After Ernesto was initially misdiagnosed as suffering from a primary psychological problem rather than a hormonal disorder, a string of other doctors, including endocrinologists, overlooked or ignored his grossly apparent physical symptoms, such as the purple stripes on his bloated abdomen. Instead of diagnosing and treating Ernesto's real biological hormonal imbalance, his psychiatrists treated his mythical biochemical imbalance, giving him multiple drugs and eventually electroshock to cure his "bipolar disorder."

Unlike patients who are spellbound by drugs, Ernesto knew there was something physically wrong with him and he tried to convince his doctors that he wasn't crazy. Nonetheless, he progressively lost his judgment and his ability to control his behavior, and mentally collapsed under the combined influences of his hormonal disorder and then psychiatric drugs and shock treatment. Ultimately, Ernesto's life was ruined by the combination of his untreated Cushing's disease and his abusive psychiatric treatments.

The capacity of excessive internally produced hormones and hormonal treatments to cause spellbinding emotional disturbances is impressive. It makes more readily acceptable the notion that psychiatric drugs can cause similar unfortunate results.

A wide variety of other physical disorders routinely cause mood disturbances that can reach the intensity of madness. One review of medical disorders associated with depression listed more than twenty-five causes including Cushing's, thyroid disorders, AIDS, diabetes, hepatitis, influenza, brain tumors, heart attack, Parkinson's disease, lupus, and viral pneumonia.[7]

Beyond drugs, anything that impairs brain function can become spellbinding. Many individuals with debilitating disorders, such as even relatively minor cases of the flu, often fail to perceive how ill and in need of help they are, and have to be encouraged to eat, drink, and otherwise take care of themselves.

A Six-Year-Old Hallucinates Bleeding Hands

A six-year-old child was a bed wetter and her pediatrician prescribed a widely used drug, Ditropan (oxybutynin), for her "overactive bladder." A few weeks later, she started seeing bugs and insects that were not there and ultimately saw her hands bleeding. She became very "hyper," and then frankly agitated and paranoid, accusing her mother of being out to get her.[8]

Although the label for Ditropan already warned about drug-induced hallucinations, nervousness, confusion, and convulsion, the FDA received so many additional reports of the drug causing hallucinations in children that it decided in April 2007 to emphasize the special vulnerability of youngsters to Ditropan madness.[9]

MANY DEPRESSING DRUGS

THERE ARE A SEEMINGLY endless number of prescription drugs, psychiatric and nonpsychiatric, that have been reported to cause depression. Doctors who work with the elderly are especially aware of this hazard. A 2004 report in *American Family Physician* reviews more than sixty drugs in multiple categories that cause depression.[10] It lists almost all the groups of drugs that we'll examine in *Medication Madness,* including antipsychotic drugs, stimulants, sedatives and antianxiety drugs, and anticonvulsants. It also lists numerous cardiovascular drugs, antiinflammatory and antiinfective agents, hormones, chemotherapy drugs, and miscellaneous others. Yet, as thorough as the article is, it leaves out antidepressants as a cause of depression, confirming how slow the profession has been to identify these culprits.

HOW THE CONCEPT OF SPELLBINDING CAME ABOUT

WHEN I BEGAN WORKING on *Medication Madness,* no one had as yet put together this package of effects that I am calling medication spellbinding. The concept occurred to me while I was reviewing dozens of cases for inclusion in the book. Instead of waiting for the book to be published, I decided to write about medication spellbinding for the scientific community and designated it by the more technical term *intoxication anosognosia.*[11] The term anosognosia means "ignorance of the presence of disease."[12] More simply, it means not recognizing something obvious that is physically wrong with you, such as a paralyzed limb or a poorly functioning memory.

The concept of medication spellbinding is an extension of theories I first published in my 1983 medical book, *Psychiatric Drugs,* and further elaborated in its most recent revision entitled *Brain-Disabling Treatments in Psychiatry* (2008). The brain-disabling principle states that all the physical treatments in psychiatry—medication, electroshock, and lobotomy—have their primary or "therapeutic" effect by causing malfunctions in the brain and the mind that are then misidentified as "improvements." Spellbinding more specifically builds on a brain-disabling corollary, which states that patients receiving medications and other mind-altering treatments "often display poor judgment about the positive and negative effect of the treatment on their functioning."*

As illustrations of the overall brain-disabling principle, the apathy or euphoria created by antidepressants is misinterpreted as an improvement in depression—the blunting of all emotions and self-awareness caused by antipsychotic

---

*In 2007 British psychiatrist Joanna Moncrieff authored a scientific analysis and elaboration of my brain-disabling theory in an issue of *Ethical Human Psychology and Psychiatry* celebrating my work, and further applies the principle in her 2008 book, *The Myth of the Chemical Cure.*

drugs is seen as an improvement in the psychosis; and the generalized sedation and suppression of brain function caused by antianxiety drugs is viewed as a treatment for anxiety. In reality, no specific improvements have occurred in the underlying depression, psychosis, or anxiety. Instead, the brain has been partially disabled, artificially changing the individual's mood and rendering the patients less able to feel, to perceive, or to express their underlying mental condition or outlook.

Psychoactive drugs, including psychiatric medications, not only impair the individual's ability to perceive their adverse effects but also impair the individual's ability to perceive his or her emotional problems. Under the influence of psychiatric drugs, the individual lacks awareness of both drug-induced mental dysfunction and his or her psychological problems. This dual impact is one of the main reasons why people persist in taking psychoactive agents, including prescription psychiatric drugs. In an extreme example, during routine electroshock "treatment," the individual often dutifully submits to continued shocks over a period of many days while the trauma to the brain produces so much brain dysfunction that the befuddled victim has no idea what has happened to him.

Do psychiatric drugs ever "help" people? As I describe in scientific detail in *Brain-Disabling Treatments in Psychiatry* (2008), this depends on how the brain-disabling effects are perceived by the patient, the patient's family, and the doctor. For example, sometimes the patient will feel helped by drug-induced emotional anesthesia or euphoria. The doctor and the family may also see this as an improvement. At other times, the patient may resent the mind-numbing effects of a drug, but the doctor and the family may feel relieved to have the patient "under control." But drugs cannot provide genuine help in improving brain function or in enhancing mental function; they always impair the activities of the brain and mind.

A Spellbound Family Devastated

The fate of Patrick Cunningham's family demonstrates how multiple prescribed drugs could spellbind a mother, a father, and a son without any of them realizing what had befallen them. This story chronicles the actions of a very reckless doctor, but, as I wrote earlier, this book is not about bad doctoring, it's about harmful drugs. While keeping in sight that even carefully prescribed psychiatric drugs can cause mayhem, murder, and suicide, the Cunningham family story is useful because it shows what can happen when outrageously bad doctoring causes several extreme cases of medication spellbinding in the same family.

Patrick Cunningham was practically carried into my office by several relatives who had come to town for the funeral of his wife. Mrs. Cunningham had suddenly and unexpectedly died only a few days earlier. She was in her early forties.

The family was frightened and puzzled by Patrick's condition. He was crushed mentally and physically but he didn't seem to be reacting to his wife's death. He was locked inside a very dark world of his own. His zombielike condition led his relatives to phone me for an emergency consultation.

Within moments of Patrick entering my office, I knew that I was facing a medical emergency. As I attempted to communicate with him, I could see that this case was not about grief; there was something physically wrong with him. The man was like a dark, smoldering hulk, and the fire was going out.

Then, Patrick's family showed me the medication bottles that they had gathered from his house. I was astounded. The prescription bottles, now partly used up, had originally contained 720 tablets of the tranquilizer Xanax, 225 tablets of the antidepressant Celexa, 90 tablets of the antidepressant Effexor, and 180 tablets of the antiseizure (mood stabilizer) Lamictal. He was also prescribed the stimulant Provigil.

Xanax is so addictive that no responsible physician prescribes 720 tablets at once. It's an invitation to accidentally overuse or to abuse. Also, the Xanax dose of 8 mg (milligrams) per day was itself relatively high, especially for long-term use. The Celexa dose of 200 mg per day was *five times* the recommended maximum amount. The Lamictal, Effexor, and Provigil doses were prescribed within the recommended range, but in combination with one another and the Xanax and the Celexa, they contributed to a poisonous witch's brew of five drugs. Patrick's body and brain were cooking a deadly experiment in synergy, the tendency of drug combinations to produce more than a simple additive degree of toxicity. No wonder he looked so physically ill, almost moribund.

With his wife gone and his own mind so clouded, Patrick had lost track of his medication, putting him into a potentially life-threatening state of combined toxicity and withdrawal. After a brief few minutes, I arranged for him to be seen without delay at a nearby hospital emergency room. I wanted the ER to be looking for him when he arrived. Instead of waiting for an ambulance, I asked the family to drive him the short distance to the hospital. The doctors in the ER took a quick look at Patrick and admitted him to the detoxification unit.

Several months later, Patrick Cunningham came to see me again, this time for family psychotherapy for himself and his two sons. He was no longer taking any medication but had only the most vague recollection of his initial visit to my office. His brain had been so chemically disrupted by the multiple drugs that it

had been unable to store memories for that period of time, and he could remember nothing of the office itself or anything we talked about. Probably due
in large part to the more lasting memory dysfunction caused by large doses of
Xanax, his memory remained full of holes for the past two years but he was now
sufficiently recovered to begin to piece together some of what had happened.

Patrick, a man in his early forties, had been a brilliant engineer earning
one hundred thousand dollars per year in a government post. Then, a rapid
emotional and intellectual decline occurred, rendering him unable to perform
at work. He was granted total disability from the government because of psychiatric impairments, including very poor memory and depression.

In reality, Patrick hadn't been psychiatrically impaired: he had been intoxicated and spellbound by medication. At the time he was declared disabled, his
doctor was prescribing him Xanax, Lamictal, Effexor, and Celexa, as well as the
stimulant Provigil to help keep him awake. As I've already observed, the dose
of Celexa by itself would have been enough to disable most people.

How did Patrick Cunningham become so spellbound and toxic? It began
four years earlier when his eight-year-old son was hospitalized for a painful
physical disorder and came under treatment with one of the best-known psychiatrists in Washington, D.C., a professor at a local medical center. Shortly
thereafter, his wife came under the same doctor's care. Both mother and son
were soon much too heavily medicated. As their mental conditions deteriorated, stress grew in the family, and soon Patrick sought help from the same
doctor. As three of the four family members deteriorated from drug toxicity,
the other son ran emotionally aground. He was caught in the maelstrom of his
family's descent into emotional hell. The doctor was destroying four people at
once—and many others as it later turned out—but none of these victims had
an inkling of what was happening.

This scenario is an extraordinary confirmation of the spellbinding effect
of psychiatric drugs. An entire family—a highly educated and intelligent
one—was caught in the grips of drug toxicity without any one of them realizing what was afflicting them. Only the death of Patrick's wife and the intervention of his family brought an end to it.

When Patrick's wife died in her home, most probably from cardiac arrest
caused by drug toxicity, the psychiatrist did something extraordinarily outside the
rules of medical practice: He came to the house and wrote the death certificate. As
a psychiatrist he wasn't qualified to write a death certificate for an unknown
physical cause, but he did so—never mentioning that Mrs. Cunningham was intoxicated by his prescribed medications and almost certainly died of their effects.

Now, several months later and in my office for the second time, Patrick had not fully recovered. His memory and ability to concentrate remained flawed, which in itself was an enormous loss for this man who prided himself on his mind and his professionalism. He was now sufficiently clearheaded to mourn his wife and responsible enough to feel the weight of single parent-hood for his two youngsters. He looked fatigued and he felt sad and fearful, but he was determined to be a good father.

Patrick was also left with a particularly nagging and disabling physical symptom—a neuritis (a painful nerve inflammation) that tortured his legs and feet. The pain made it difficult for him to sustain any activity. Although I could not find any scientific literature describing this drug-induced disorder, I have seen persistent and painful peripheral neuritis develop in several patients after prolonged exposure to Xanax.

Despite his disability, Patrick took over the raising of his two children, ages twelve and thirteen. Twelve-year-old Arthur had spent four years on psychi-atric drugs when his father and I now began withdrawing him from his cur-rent Luvox and Risperdal. Fortunately, he developed none of the persistent abnormal movements commonly caused by Risperdal, and over many months he would gradually recover his mental quickness and the ability to discipline his behavior.

Patrick put extraordinary effort into his new role of full-time father. He was naturally open and loving, and benefited from guidance in developing consistent ways of disciplining his distressed boys. His children had been trau-matized by their mother's death, by their father's incapacity, and, in Arthur's case, by psychiatric drugs. Patrick proved to be a most responsible and effective parent and both of his children made remarkable recoveries. As we worked to-gether, I grew in respect and affection for him.

After suggesting that Patrick bring a malpractice suit against the doctor, I referred him to Michael Mosher, a lawyer from the small town of Paris, Texas, who knows more about psychiatric drugs than most psychiatrists. The multiple psychiatric drugs involved in this case would test even Mosher's broad expert-ise. Attorney Mosher contacted local Virginia lawyers to work with him and a lawsuit was brought against the errant psychiatrist.

Already Patrick's treating physician, I now became a consultant to his lawyers. Eventually, the case was settled, without admitting liability, for close to the limits of the doctor's policy. Patrick and his children received enough money to provide for their futures. Meanwhile, they have continued to do bet-ter and better, although Patrick remains permanently unable to work.

MEDICATION SPELLBINDING, FAITH, AND AUTHORITY

MEDICATION SPELLBINDING is a biological effect that promotes drug taking by disguising the harmful effect of the drug, as well as by masking the individual's underlying psychological or real-life problems. But medication spellbinding is by no means the only reason why people persist in taking drugs that do more harm than good. Especially in regard to psychiatric drugs, patients take them because they have faith in "science" and faith in their doctor. They may get some relief from emotional anesthesia caused by the blunting effects of many drugs, or they may get a brief mood elevation from drug-induced euphoria. The mood-elevating effects are almost always short-lived but they encourage the individual to keep hoping that one or another drug will finally provide sustained relief from suffering.

Many people receive a placebo effect, especially early in their first treatment. In studies comparing placebo and antidepressants, the placebos tend to do almost as well in relieving depression in six- to eight-week-long trials.[13] If the placebo produces side effects such as dry mouth or blurred vision, mimicking a potent medicine, the placebo becomes as effective as an antidepressant. A very important review examined all the controlled clinical trials submitted to the FDA for the approval of the newer antidepressants. When all the studies were evaluated, it turned out the antidepressants were no more effective than the sugar pill.[14] Put simply, there is little evidence that antidepressants work, other than as placebos.

Increasingly, social and family pressure is brought upon patients to take prescribed drugs. Patients can be forced by the courts to take medication as a condition for staying out of jail. In many states, if a mental patient refuses to take medication, he can be involuntarily committed as an outpatient. Mental-health workers can actually invade the individual's home to force long-acting injections of highly toxic drugs into his or her body. These oppressive laws are highly favored by the American Psychiatric Association and by groups that lobby on behalf of the psychiatric authorities such as the National Alliance on Mentally Illness (NAMI).[15]

CAUSATION AND FREE WILL

IN THE COURTROOM when an expert testifies that a drug caused an adverse event "within a reasonable degree of medical certainty," he merely means that the drug "more likely than not" caused the effect. When I use the term "causation" in this book, I intend to indicate an even stronger association. I mean that in my medical opinion the preponderance of evidence available to me confirms a direct causal link between the drug and the adverse event.

Of course, not everyone who takes a psychiatric drug will have a dramatic or dangerous reaction; but the existence of these life-threatening, destructive adverse effects is important, especially when millions of individuals are exposed to the drugs. While many of these more serious drug reactions are relatively uncommon, such as homicidal assaults, we will find that others are more common, such as antidepressant-induced suicidality and mania.

The fact that an individual becomes violent, suicidal, or disinhibited while taking a psychiatric drug does not in itself prove that the drug caused the reaction. Often, a variety of influences are driving the abnormal behavior, including stresses in the person's life or a previously existing psychological tendency. I have excluded most of my cases in which causation was overly complicated or uncertain. In the vast majority of cases selected for presentation in *Medication Madness,* in my opinion the drug played a predominant role in causing or contributing to the abnormal behavior.

All of the drug-induced psychiatric side effects described in this book can be documented in the scientific literature, and the Food and Drug Administration has now confirmed most of them, including antidepressant-induced suicide and mania. Several sections in *Medication Madness,* including chapter 1, will describe and discuss the criteria necessary for determining whether a drug played a causative role in producing a harmful outcome. Additional scientific data and analysis are presented in my recent medical book, *Brain-Disabling Treatments in Psychiatry* (2008), and in several dozen of my scientific articles.

The capacity of drugs to modify feelings and even behavior challenges concepts and values that many of us cherish, including free will, rationality, personal responsibility, and self-determination. I explore these questions in more depth later in the book, but it's useful to underscore the issues at the onset. While different people will react in different ways to the same psychiatric drug, one fact remains incontrovertible: In double-blind controlled clinical trials where patients and observers are kept in the dark about who is getting a psychiatric drug and who is getting an inactive sugar pill, individuals receiving the psychiatric drug will experience more frequent and intense emotional and behavioral disturbances than the same or similar individuals given a sugar pill. Even when these drugs are given to "normal volunteers," they will experience the same kinds of adverse emotional reactions as patients with psychiatric diagnoses. Put simply, psychiatric drugs are proven to cause bizarre, unwanted, and dangerous mental states.

In addition, we shall find that many psychiatric drugs produce apathy and indifference, greatly impairing the capacity to make choices and to take actions of any kind. As examples, stimulants given to children often reduce all spontaneous behavior, and the antipsychotic drugs given to children and to adults can utterly crush free will. These scientific facts should not be surprising. Free will and rational-choice making require an intact brain, and psychiatric drugs, one and all, *always* cause brain dysfunction. That's how they work.

Varying Degrees of Adverse Effects

Psychiatric drugs do not spellbind everyone. In fact, many people sense when a drug is impairing them and they stop taking it. Despite the exceptions, all psychoactive drugs have beguiling characteristics that ensnare many unfortunates. My clinical experience suggests that most people who continue taking psychiatric drugs for lengthy periods of time are suffering from spellbinding, most commonly the dulling of their emotions and self-awareness, and their sensitivity to others.

Drug side effects almost always occur along a continuum. For example, drug-induced rashes can vary from mild to severe and even life-threatening. This is also true in regard to the emotional or mental adverse effects. Most of them are mild, producing only minor glitches in the individual's mental life, but some become very severe and even lethal.

For every severe case of medication madness there are many times more examples of milder or subtler cases. Vast numbers of people experience lesser degrees of the same or similar drug-induced problems, often greatly to the detriment of themselves and their friends, family, and colleagues. They, too, are likely to be medication spellbound—that is, they are unaware that the drug is causing their more illusive mental or emotional problems.

Rather than becoming outright manic, these individuals show lesser signs of overstimulation, becoming a little agitated or "hyper," and have trouble sitting still or sleeping. Instead of becoming violent, they become a little irritable, grouchy, or touchy. Instead of becoming suicidal, they feel a "little blue," losing their sparkle. They become listless and apathetic with diminished interest in their own lives and in the lives of people around them.

Most drug-induced tragedies are mistaken for the vicissitudes of normal life. A man loses interest in his wife as a result of the dulling effect of antidepressants, stimulants, or tranquilizers. The marriage falters and dies. A woman becomes manic on one of the same drugs, decides her previously beloved husband is a "jerk," has affairs, and gets divorced—ultimately to realize much too late that she destroyed "the best thing in her life." These cases of medication spellbinding rarely come to a doctor's attention or land in court but they nonetheless ruin lives.

SOCIETY REINFORCES THE SPELLBINDING EFFECT

THE SPELLBINDING EFFECT of psychiatric drugs is enhanced by the psychopharmaceutical complex—combined powers of drug companies, psychiatry, organized medicine, the FDA, and other federal agencies, all of whom generate an enormous amount of propaganda to convince people to overcome their natural and healthy skepticism about taking psychiatric medications.[16] Often the attempts are orchestrated with the drug companies giving financial support to the National Institute of Mental Health (NIMH) or the American Psychiatric Association in their "educational efforts" to alert the public to the need for psychiatric drugs.

However, spellbinding can occur even when people are fully informed about the hazards of drugs. Spellbinding is not caused by an individual's ignorance of drug effects or prevented by an individual's knowledge about drug effects. We will see how psychiatric drugs can spellbind sophisticated physicians. Furthermore, our citizenry abuses innumerable drugs, becoming spellbound by alcohol, nicotine, methamphetamine, and other drugs despite extensive public education and legal efforts aimed at curtailing these hazardous habits. How much more readily will prescribed drugs spellbind people when they enjoy the sponsorship of the government, organized medicine and psychiatry, the insurance industry, and the drug companies?

The only certain way to avoid medication madness is to avoid taking drugs that impact on the brain and the mind. Informing people about the risks in advance can be helpful but it by no means eliminates the risk. Because of medication spellbinding, individuals who are fully informed ahead of time about the dangers can nonetheless lapse into mental and emotional dysfunction without realizing what is happening to them. On a broader societal level, medication spellbinding helps to explain why so many people take psychiatric drugs, as well as other psychoactive agents, long after the chemicals have begun to do more harm than good.

Chapter 3

The Toothless Watchdog Growls

DURING THE TIME that most of the men, women, and children in this book were having their lives ruined and sometimes destroyed by antidepressant drugs, what position was being taken by the pharmaceutical companies, organized psychiatry, the National Institute of Mental Health (NIMH), and legions of so-called medication experts? Despite mountains of evidence, they were avidly denying that antidepressants can cause mayhem, murder, and suicide.

From the moment Prozac burst on the scene in 1989, to the start of the FDA hearings on antidepressants in 2004, many stories of antidepressant-induced violence and suicide had been reported in the press. Hundreds more had been sent to the FDA and had even been published in the scientific literature concerning antidepressant-induced "harm to self and others." But the interest groups in the psychopharmaceutical complex continued to reject the idea that psychiatric drugs and antidepressants in particular could cause destructive adverse drug reactions.[1]

Meanwhile, the FDA, an increasingly toothless watchdog, hadn't even growled. When the agency finally took action beginning in 2004, it would struggle to tread lightly on pharmaceutical interests that, to this day, spend more energy covering their tracks than admitting to the dangers posed by their chemical products. Put simply, individual health professionals and the psychopharmaceutical complex have yet to awaken to the facts documented in *Medication Madness.*

THE DRUG LABEL

THE FDA APPROVAL process revolves around the development and approval of the *label* for the drug. The label, commonly known as the "package insert," contains basic information on the efficacy and safety of the drug. The company generates drafts of the label and then, in a lengthy and intensive process, negotiates with the FDA over its final contents. As a medical expert in product liability suits, I have had the opportunity to review this entire process for numerous psychiatric drugs. Inevitably, the drug company tries to make its product look more efficacious and safer than it really is, and with equal inevitability, the FDA repeatedly compromises its original critical concerns and caves in to drug-company interests.

FDA regulations specify the basic form of the label, including everything from the size of the print to the specific headings and subheadings, such as "Warnings," "Precautions," "Adverse Reactions," "Indications," and "Dosage and Administration." Black-box warnings are used at times to describe problems of particular urgency, such as the potential for medication-induced abuse and dependence, suicidality, or death.

Drug companies almost always publish their approved labels in the *Physicians' Desk Reference* (PDR), a voluminous book that is mailed free to healthcare providers around the country. The *PDR* can be found in most medical offices, on hospitals wards, in clinics, and in emergency departments, where it is often the first resort for professionals seeking information about drugs, their therapeutic effects, and their adverse effects.

Drug advertisements in professional journals and in publications for the general public must provide an additional page of information based on a summary of the FDA-approved label. Pharmacy handouts are supposed to review the most important safety information from the drug label. Most professional publications about drugs, especially in the initial years after drug approval, draw extensively from the label.

Overall, the drug label or "package insert" is the single most important document in communicating the therapeutic and adverse effects of the drug to both professionals and consumers. When the FDA makes a significant change in a label, such as requiring a black-box warning for antidepressant-induced suicidality, it is big news in both professional publications and the public media.

CONFIRMATION FROM THE COURTS

THE AMERICAN COURT SYSTEM usually resists allowing evidence into trial that's inconsistent with FDA-approved drug labeling and drug-company research. As slow as the courts are to accept frontier science, they nonetheless have been a decade or more ahead of the FDA in permitting experts like me to testify about antidepressant-induced violence and suicide. As early as 1994, in *Michigan v. Stephen Leith,* I testified in a criminal trial that Prozac caused a manic episode in a schoolteacher, leading him to shoot two men, a close friend and colleague, as well as the school superintendent. In part because my conclusions were too far ahead of their time and in part because the assaults were so violent, the jury found Mr. Leith guilty. (I have written letters on his behalf to the parole board but he remains incarcerated.) In the same year, in a product-liability suit against Eli Lilly, Judge John W. Potter approved me to testify that Prozac had caused or contributed to Joseph Wesbecker's mass murders and suicide in Kentucky.* Although I would continue to testify in criminal and malpractice cases, after the Wesbecker case none of the antidepressant drug manufacturers have chosen to take any of my other cases to trial, instead often settling to the satisfaction of the plaintiffs. The drug companies are not only afraid of losing in court, they are probably more afraid of allowing sealed (secret) in-house documents with their smoking guns to see the light of day during public trials.

Finally, in 2001, in a Wyoming case, attorney Andy Vickery of Houston, Texas, went to trial against GlaxoSmithKline (GSK) in a Paxil product-liability lawsuit in which I was not involved.[2] Sixty-year-old Donald Schell suffered from an episode of depression but had never before been violent or suicidal. After taking only two doses of Paxil, Donald went on a murderous rampage, killing his wife, his daughter, and his granddaughter before killing himself. The judge found sufficient scientific basis for permitting expert testimony implicating Paxil in murder and suicide, and the jury returned a 6.4-million-dollar verdict against GlaxoSmithKline. Because the drug companies have avoided going to court in the vast majority of cases, including all of mine since 1994, Vickery's case remains the first and only victory in an antidepressant product-liability trial.

How did GlaxoSmithKline react to the jury verdict? Did the company remove Paxil from the market? GSK didn't blink. It didn't even put a warning in

---

*For details of the bizarre outcome of the Wesbecker case, see chapter 18.

its label and instead went on with business as usual, selling more and more Paxil to the public, while quietly settling additional cases as they came along. More recently, as we'll see, GSK felt compelled to issue a "Dear Healthcare Provider" letter warning that Paxil causes suicidality in children and adults. Yet, in a recent deposition in which I was testifying against GSK in a Paxil suicide case, company lawyers continued to spin their way out of admitting what the company itself had declared in the letter.

Meanwhile, the FDA continued to lag behind and to this day the most powerful psychiatric and pharmaceutical interest groups continue to reject the reality of antidepressant-induced violence and suicide.

SOUNDING A WARNING IN 1991

FOR A LONG TIME, I was an isolated, lone voice in the medical community, the media, and the courtroom in my insistence that antidepressants were driving people to commit suicide and horrendous acts of violence. While occasional confirmatory reports appeared in the scientific literature, no one else put the entire picture together and took a strong stand in books and in articles. Although the reality of antidepressant-induced suicidality has now been confirmed by the FDA and grudgingly accepted by many professionals, organized psychiatry and the media continue to reject the broader array of antidepressant-induced madness and violence. Nonetheless, there is at least as much evidence for antidepressant-induced violence as for antidepressant-induced suicidality, and the two phenomena—violence and suicide—are very closely related to each other.

I first drew attention to the spectrum of antidepressant madness in 1991 in *Toxic Psychiatry,* when I warned that Prozac was causing a constellation of stimulating adverse effects that could cause violence, suicide, and mania. Basing my conclusions on clinical experience, research reports, and documents obtained from the FDA through the Freedom of Information Act (FOIA), I described in the book how Prozac can cause "murderous and suicidal behavior" by means of overstimulation. The following excerpt from that book illustrates how there was already sufficient data in 1991 for me to come to conclusions that would evade the FDA for more than a decade:

> Prozac often affects individuals as if they were taking stimulants, such as amphetamine, cocaine, or PCP. . . . Like amphetamine or cocaine, Prozac can produce the whole array of stimulant effects, such as sleeplessness, increased

energy, jumpiness, anxiety, artificial highs, and mania. Some patients taking Prozac do indeed look "hyper" or "tense," and even aggressive, without even realizing it. . . . Indeed, the FDA's internal review of Prozac side effects by psychiatrist Richard Kapit twice mentions the drug's "stimulant" effects, but these important observations were not included in the final labeling requirements.[3]

Dr. Kapit, the FDA's medical officer in charge of evaluating Prozac's adverse effects, had warned the agency in memos and reports that Prozac's stimulating effects were dangerously worsening depression in some patients.[4] He explicitly declared that Prozac "causes a set of adverse effects which resemble those caused by amphetamine." He wanted the Prozac label to definitively describe how the drug causes stimulation or activation but that never occurred.[5] The FDA and Eli Lilly chose to disregard Dr. Kapit's findings. This occurred inside the FDA in the mid-1980s, almost *twenty years* before the agency finally began to acknowledge the problem of antidepressant madness.

After writing *Toxic Psychiatry,* I continued to warn about antidepressant activation or stimulation as a cause of violence and suicide in books like *Talking Back to Prozac* (1994), the first edition of *Brain-Disabling Treatments in Psychiatry* (1997), and *The Antidepressant Fact Book* (2001). In a scientific paper published in 2003, entitled "Suicidality, Violence and Mania Caused by Selective Serotonin Reuptake Inhibitors (SSRIs)," I compiled and analyzed all available research, verifying that the newer antidepressants cause overstimulation, akathisia, and mania, often resulting in obsessive suicidality and violence. I also warned about other clinical syndromes linked to antidepressant madness including obsessive suicidality and indifference toward others.

Shortly after my paper's publication, at my request the FDA distributed a copy to each of the members of the FDA advisory committee at the agency's two hearings in 2004, concerning antidepressant-induced suicidality. The FDA advisory committee members are appointed by the agency and consist mostly of "experts" in the field of psychopharmacology. All, or nearly all, of these experts are closely affiliated with the drug companies as consultants, as members of their speakers' bureaus, or as recipients of grants.[6] Even when they are not personally involved with the drug companies, they are likely to have indirect ties, for example, through drug-company support of their professional associations, their universities, or the journals that they edit and contribute to. The ties are so intimate that the FDA always issues a series of letters before each hearing in which the agency lists these conflicts of interest and then exonerates each committee member from any legal liability for these conflicts. The role of these committees is advisory, but they have considerable influence over FDA decisions.

At the time Prozac was passing through the FDA, it typically took ten years or more to get a drug approved. This had little or nothing to do with the conduct of the required clinical trials, which typically last only a few weeks in duration; it had everything to do with the useless bureaucratic hoops imposed on the companies by the FDA. In recent years, Congress has arranged for the FDA to receive funding directly from the drug companies to expedite the approval process, and the length of the approval process has been greatly shortened. Although speeding up the process is a worthy aim—a decade is much too long to wait for a new medicine—involving drug companies in paying for the expedited process would inevitably give them even more influence over the agency's decisions.

THE FDA BEGINS TO REACT

AS A RESULT OF DECISIONS made by the British drug-regulatory agency in 2003 associating antidepressants with increased suicidality in children, the FDA at long last felt compelled to look into the problem. In 2004, the agency held two public hearings on the risk of suicide in children associated with the newer antidepressants. At the second public hearing, the FDA presented reevaluations of antidepressant clinical trials for children documenting that the suicide risk was *doubled* in children taking antidepressants compared to similar or the same children taking a sugar pill. The FDA-sponsored study examined all available controlled clinical trials involving the newer antidepressants and children. The agency also reported that only three of the fifteen (20 percent) controlled clinical trials demonstrated any efficacy for antidepressants in children and youth under age eighteen.[7] In short, antidepressants turned out to be ineffective in children and teenagers—and explosively dangerous—conclusions I had been documenting for years.

THE FDA ADVISORY COMMITTEE AWAKENS TO THE BROADER DANGERS

ALTHOUGH THE HEARINGS were focused on antidepressant-induced suicidality in children, many outraged citizens showed up to testify about a broad array of dangerous reactions, including murder and psychosis involving adults as well as children while under the influence of antidepressants.

In addition to submitting my paper, I made presentations to the FDA's advisory committee at both public hearings in February and September 2004, and was the only expert to emphasize this broad spectrum of antidepressant-induced abnormal behaviors in children and adults, and to identify them as commonly caused by activation or stimulation. After fifteen years of frustration, I assumed that I was still talking to deaf ears, but to my surprise and gratification, the theme of stimulation or activation was picked up by the FDA committee members in their discussions and in their comments on the proceedings.

Immediately after February 2, 2004, the following information appeared on the nongovernmental Web site FDAAdvisoryCommittee.com:[8]

> Members of the FDA's advisory committee said that the panel should not only look at suicidal behavior but also evidence of "activation" in patients on the drugs. Indications of activation could include increased agitation, aggression, akathisia (uncontrollable limb and body movements), confusion, and violence toward others.

At the end of the second hearing, committee chairman Wayne K. Goodman, MD, thanked the public presenters who "poured out their hearts today."[9] Victims and their families had presented stories of lives ruined by antidepressants. Dr. Goodman confessed, "I, for one, feel exhausted not only because of the late hour but because of some of the heartrending stories that I have heard today." He spoke of the "public testimonials" as "passionate and plausible."

Dr. Goodman then suggested that there might be an emerging "pattern" of "behavioral toxicity" that often seems to occur early in treatment. He tentatively offered the same hypothesis that I had been presenting in books and articles, and testifying about in court, for more than a decade. Referring specifically to "activation" including "akathisia and insomnia," he suggested that "those symptoms or signs may represent a precursor to the symptom we most fear, that of suicide intent."

Chairman Goodman emphasized that the drugs were not only proving to be dangerous in children, they were also ineffective. He told the hearing:

> We learned that three out of the fifteen studies in pediatric major depression were positive so that the majority of the studies were either failed or

negative. So, in addition to adverse effects that were of concern, we had questions about the overall benefit of this class of agents . . .

Two myths came crashing down at once: that the antidepressants are safe in children and that they are effective. The FDA's belated observations once again took a page from my many books, including *Talking Back to Prozac* (1994), where I had reviewed the scientific literature concerning Prozac's lack of efficacy and marked capacity to cause violent and suicidal behavior in children. I had also warned, "It becomes apparent that these drugs should not be given to children and youth." With unfortunate prescience, I added, "A drug's lack of proven efficacy in children, however, has never discouraged psychiatrists or pediatricians from liberally prescribing it. Neither has the inherent danger of exposing the growing brain to toxic substances."[10]

The FDA should have come out with an unqualified warning not to prescribe the newer antidepressants to children. It could have required the labels to announce, "Contraindicated in Children and Youth"—meaning, never to be prescribed to children and youth. Although it did not dare go this far, what it did do exceeded expectations and shocked many drug advocates.

On March 22, 2004, about six weeks after the first public hearing, the agency issued a Public Health Advisory on "Cautions for the Use of Antidepressants in Adults and Children." In its accompanying press release, the agency declared that it is "known" that antidepressants are associated with "*anxiety, agitation, panic attacks, insomnia, irritability, hostility, impulsivity, akathisia (severe restlessness), hypomania, and mania.*"[11] The language is startling in its similarity to mine in the 2003 paper that I distributed to the FDA committee in which I described a stimulant syndrome that begins with "insomnia, nervousness, anxiety, hyperactivity, and irritability, and then progresses toward more severe agitation, aggression, and varying degrees of mania." I also went on to describe the hazards of akathisia. The underlying concept of activation is identical to what I call stimulation and the FDA's words often overlap with mine.

This array of adverse effects—including irritability, hostility, akathisia, impulsivity, and mania—is a prescription for violence, as well as suicide. This is the same stimulant syndrome that manifests itself in many of the cases in this book.

THE NEW BLACK BOX ABOUT ANTIDEPRESSANT-INDUCED SUICIDALITY IN CHILDREN

THE FINAL VERSION of the class label was approved and published by the FDA on January 26, 2005.[12] From then on, antidepressant labels had to contain a black-box warning with a bold heading, SUICIDALITY IN CHILDREN AND ADO-LESCENTS. The warning begins, "Antidepressants increased the risk of suicidal thinking and behavior (suicidality) in short-term studies in children and adolescents with Major Depressive Disorder (MDD) and other psychiatric disorders."

This current black-box warning is remarkably strong but the FDA deleted an even stronger declaration from its original proposed warning: "A causal role for antidepressants in inducing suicidality has been established in pediatric patients."[13] Although something of a fine point, the phrase "causal role" would have been especially damning to the drug companies in product-liability cases against them. When I am deposed or cross-examined in court, drug-company lawyers often repeat the mantra, "But the FDA didn't say that my company's medication *caused* the adverse effects, the FDA only said the drug was *associated* with adverse effect." By deleting the phrase "causal role," the FDA was serving the interests of the pharmaceutical industry. The data used by the FDA to make this determination of causality had been in the possession of the drug companies for many years. In most cases, the data had been generated years earlier during the original FDA approval process, but the companies had interpreted the data to their own favor. Therefore, the failure of drug companies to determine this causative role on their own years earlier was glaring.

In the wake of the label changes, Harvard psychiatrist Joseph Glenmullen protested the manner in which the FDA negotiated with drug companies before finalizing the label, challenging the agency with a series of poignant questions: "Why would they negotiate with industry? Why isn't the FDA just sticking with what they thought was best for the public health and safety? And if they are going to negotiate with industry, why wouldn't they also negotiate with their advisory board, consumer advocates, and the congressman who held hearings on this warning, to be more balanced?"[14]

Meanwhile, the FDA continued to protect the drug companies in its final analysis of antidepressant suicidality in children and youth. In March 2006, the agency published its findings and concluded, "Use of antidepressant drugs in pediatric patients is associated with a modestly increased risk of suicidality."[15] This is simply false. For the signal to show up in clinical trials, it had to be much more than modest. The report itself acknowledged that the signal from the clinical trials was "robust."[16] In addition, the risk the FDA assessed took place in closely monitored, highly selective, short-term clinical trials, and therefore will be much higher in routine clinical use.

The FDA was so eager to protect the drug companies that it failed to require them to mention the proven lack of efficacy of these drugs in treating childhood depression. Under heavy political influence, the agency has come increasingly prone to favor drug-company profits over consumer safety.

The president of the United States appoints the FDA commissioner, Congress directly supervises the agency, and both the president and the Congress are eager to stay in favor with the enormously wealthy and powerful pharmaceutical industry. Furthermore, when Prozac was going through the final approval process, the president and the vice president were especially responsive to the needs of the drug's manufacturer, Eli Lilly. In *Talking Back to Prozac* (1994), I pointed out that Prozac was approved under the first Bush administration and that George Bush had been a member of the board of directors of Eli Lilly, the manufacturer of Prozac. I also pointed out that Vice President Dan Quayle was from Indiana, the home state and international headquarters for Eli Lilly. At the time the FDA was approving Prozac, Quayle employed former Eli Lilly personnel on his own staff, and Quayle had considerable leverage over the FDA as the chair of a special committee that was investigating its operations. I questioned whether the FDA might have rejected Prozac and that the entire SSRI onslaught might never have gotten started if the president and vice president of the United States had not been so closely affiliated with Eli Lilly.

APPLYING THE SUICIDE WARNING TO ADULTS TAKING ANTIDEPRESSANTS

BENEATH THE BLACK BOX, the FDA mandated another new section entitled, "WARNINGS: Clinical Worsening and Suicide Risk," that applies to children and to *adults*. It observes, "There has been a long-standing concern that antidepressants may have a role in inducing worsening of depression and the emergence of suicidality in certain patients." After additional warnings about suicidality in children, it warns that adults "should be observed similarly for clinical worsening and suicidality, especially during the initial few months of a course of drug therapy, or at times of dose changes, either increases or decreases." Because this section warns about the association between suicidality and changes in drug dose for adults, it is tantamount to saying that antidepressants *cause* suicidality in children and adults—but this implication was lost upon the media and the professional community. Indeed, as I documented in *Brain-Disabling Treatments in Psychiatry* (2008), the American Psychiatric Association and other members of the psychopharmaceutical complex have been criticizing the FDA for mandating the black-box warning and have been trying to discourage doctors from taking its message seriously. Except for a small decline in prescribing these drugs to children, I have not as yet seen any significant change in the prescribing habits of physicians or in the warnings that they give to their patients.

The hearings and the data presentations that led to these warnings focused entirely on the newer antidepressants. The drugs under review at that time, according to the March 22, 2004, FDA Talk Paper, were bupropion (Wellbutrin), citalopram (Celexa), fluoxetine (Prozac, Serafem), fluvoxamine (Luvox), mirtazapine (Remeron), nefazodone (Serzone), paroxetine (Paxil), sertraline (Zoloft), escitalopram (Lexapro), and venlafaxine (Effexor). These were the drugs most often cited by the public at the two FDA hearings.[17] A more recent product, duloxetine (Cymbalta), shares similar risks.

CONFIRMING MEDICATION MADNESS, INCLUDING STIMULATION OR ACTIVATION

OF GREAT BUT OVERLOOKED SIGNIFICANCE, every antidepressant label must also warn in detail about the overall stimulation or activation problem for children and adults. This critical new addition to all antidepressant labels is found in the section entitled, "WARNINGS: Clinical Worsening and Suicide Risk." The label warning specifically refers not only to children but also to adults. It warns about "anxiety, agitation, panic attacks, insomnia, irritability, hostility, aggressiveness, impulsivity, akathisia (psychomotor restlessness), hypomania, and mania." This is medication madness! Except for suicidality, which is covered elsewhere in the label, this part of the warning applies to and describes one or another aspect of all the cases in this book.

There's a commonly held myth that these drug reactions have more to do with the psychiatric problems of the patients than with the drugs. The new FDA label challenges, indeed undermines, that commonly held belief by pointing out that these adverse effects can occur in patients treated for "nonpsychiatric" purposes.

A special section of the label tells doctors what information about antidepressants should be given to patients and their families. It mentions "clinical worsening and suicide" and again describes the risks of drug-induced "anxiety, agitation, panic attacks, insomnia, irritability, hostility, aggressiveness, impulsivity, akathisia (psychomotor restlessness), hypomania, mania, and other unusual changes in behavior, worsening of depression, and suicidal ideation." To its discredit, the agency fell short of specifically stating, "Beware of amphetaminelike overstimulation!" Instead, it repeats on several occasions the whole string of stimulating effects that are associated with amphetamine, methamphetamine, and cocaine—the core of adverse effects that often appears in our cases of medication madness.

The FDA also required a special booklet to be given to the parents of children placed on antidepressants. On November 3, 2004, the FDA published its "FDA Proposed Medication Guide: About Using Antidepressants in Children and Adults." The final version, published by the FDA in early 2005, can be found at the end of each label in the *Physicians' Desk Reference* beginning in 2006, and also on the FDA Web site. In a heading entitled "What to Watch Out For in Children or Teens Taking Antidepressants," it lists twelve psychiatric items with bullets. Almost all of them confirm antidepressant overstimulation, and several specifically mention manifestations of violence and suicidality:

- Thoughts about suicide or dying
- Attempts to commit suicide
- New or worse depression
- New or worse anxiety
- Feeling very agitated or restless
- Panic attacks
- Difficulty sleeping (insomnia)
- New or worse irritability
- Acting aggressive, being angry, or violent
- Acting on dangerous impulses
- An extreme increase in activity and talking
- Other unusual changes in behavior

After providing this ominous list, the FDA's required booklet vaguely warns about withdrawal reactions: "Stopping an antidepressant suddenly can cause other symptoms." The new booklet, like the label itself, describes what I am calling medication madness and confirms the underlying scientific basis for each of the cases in this book.

It was gratifying to witness this outcome after years and years of work, often in the face of professional outrage, judicial hostility, and media disbelief. For the millions of patients already exposed to these dangerous drugs, the warnings came much too late—and too often continue to be ignored with catastrophic results for patients and their families.

GSK CONFESSES: PAXIL CAUSES SUICIDAL BEHAVIOR IN ADULTS

FINALLY IN 2005 TO 2006, the FDA gave more specific public notice of its concern that the newer antidepressants might also be causing suicidality in adults. The agency asked the drug companies to carry out reanalyses of the data from their controlled clinical trials and specified the guidelines the companies must use to organize their data on suicidality.

GlaxoSmithKline (GSK) asked an experienced team at Columbia University to carry out the required reanalysis of the preexisting data from their controlled clinical trials. In May 2006, GSK published a "Dear Healthcare Professional" letter—sent to all physicians and many other health professionals—in which it admitted that Paxil increases the risk of suicidal behavior for adults of all ages who suffer from Major Depressive Disorder, as well as for younger adults who suffer from lesser depressive disorders and anxiety disorders.

Of importance, GSK specifically admitted that the risk of suicide *attempts* was elevated for all ages of adult patients who took Paxil in clinical trials for major depressive disorder. GSK described the incidence of events as "small." In fact, the Paxil suicide attempt rate is 6.4 times greater than the placebo suicide attempt rate (0.32 percent for Paxil divided by 0.05 percent for placebo). That's a truly enormous difference, the kind rarely found in short-term controlled clinical trials that are developed and conducted by drug companies on their own behalf. And keep in mind, the rates of suicidality in actual clinical practice will be much higher!

Paxil is not substantially different in its clinical effects from the other selective serotonin reuptake inhibitors (SSRIs) such as Prozac, Zoloft, Luvox, and Celexa, as well as other antidepressants such as Effexor and Wellbutrin. If Paxil causes suicidality in depressed adults of all ages, so do all the antidepressants that block the reuptake of serotonin or that tend to cause overstimulation. These two factors, blocking the removal of serotonin from the synapses (spaces between the cells) and causing stimulation, are both associated with the tendency of these drugs to cause a wide range of psychiatric adverse reactions from suicidality to violence and mania. Based on data gathered on all of the newer antidepressants, the FDA mandated identical new warnings for all of these drugs.

FDA ADVISORY COMMITTEE CONFIRMS ANTIDEPRESSANT-INDUCED SUICIDALITY IN ADULTS

FINALLY, ON DECEMBER 13, 2006, the FDA held hearings on a proposal to add a black box to warn about drug-induced adult suicidality into the antidepressant labels.[18] The FDA's panel ended up recommending a black-box warning about increased suicidality in the eighteen-to-twenty-four-year-old age group. Eventually the FDA decided to accept the nonbinding recommendation.

The FDA's parsing of a warning into various age brackets is quite unprecedented and panders to the drug companies' needs to obscure the reality that antidepressants cause suicide in children and adults. Data from short-term controlled clinical trials are simply too limited to make such fine distinctions as the age at which a serious adverse reaction might no longer be a risk. Furthermore, common sense indicates that if children and young adults are at risk for antidepressant-induced suicidality, so would somewhat older adults. In addition, GSK had already sent out its "Dear Healthcare Professional" letter confirming that Paxil caused increased suicide attempts in all ages of depressed patients. Beyond that, the FDA's own analysis of the data by staffers Marc Stone, MD, and M. Lisa Jones, MD, in late 2006 confirmed that Paxil caused increased suicidality in adults of all ages and in all diagnostic categories. The FDA ignored all of this when it decided to limit the warning to increased suicidality in children and young adults taking the newer antidepressants like Paxil.

An objective panel of experts—one not riddled with drug-company indebtedness[19]—would have recommended the black-box warning for all ages. Indeed, there is evidence that the elderly are at much greater risk of completed suicides—that is, actually killing themselves—when taking SSRI antidepressants compared to when taking older antidepressants. A study published a few months before the FDA hearings evaluated coroner's records, prescription data, physician billing claims, and hospitalization data for more than 1.2 million Ontario residents age sixty-six and older from 1992 to 2000.[20] After evaluating more than one thousand deaths by suicide, they found "SSRI antidepressants were associated with a nearly fivefold higher risk of completed suicide than other antidepressants." Consistent with what we find throughout this book, the increased rate of suicide on SSRIs occurred during the first month of treatment and "suicides of a violent nature were distinctly more common during SSRI therapy."

Members of the "public" were allowed to make three-minute presentations.[21] In my presentation, I politely told the FDA that it was playing with
junk when it tried to analyze the suicidality data produced by drug companies.
I emphasized that the drug companies cannot be trusted to deliver accurate
data from their clinical trials. As proof, I gave examples of how Eli Lilly hid
suicide data on Prozac and how GlaxoSmithKline distorted the presentation of
suicide data on Paxil.

Psychiatric and medical expert Joseph Glenmullen pointed out that the
FDA had previously demanded that Eli Lilly conduct an entirely new study
aimed at detecting Prozac-induced suicidality, and that the company had
agreed on the design but failed to carry through. Concerning the current FDA
studies, Dr. Glenmullen reminded the advisory committee that a strong signal
generated from such poor-quality data indicated a much more extensive and
more serious problem than the FDA was willing to admit.

Additional three-minute critiques were offered by several of the nation's
most experienced attorneys in suing drug companies including Derek Braslow,
Don Farber, and Andy Vickery—men I've known for years and worked with on
many cases. Two months earlier in October 2006, I had chaired a panel with all
three lawyers, along with Texas attorney Michael Mosher, at the annual public
meeting of the International Center for the Study of Psychiatry and Psychology
(www.icspp.org).

Medical experts and lawyers who routinely peer into the ugly insides of
the drug companies offered surgically precise critiques of the data, emphasiz-
ing that good data would have presented an even more disastrous picture. By
contrast, the FDA's advisory committee hemmed and hawed in its efforts to
find a way out of the embarrassing truth that all these years it has been routinely approving drugs that are far more likely to make people worse, and even
to kill them, than to make them better.

Dozens of patients and their surviving families gave vivid testimonials of
violence and suicide that resemble many of the stories in this book. Sometimes
speaking through tears, sometimes muffled by sadness, sometimes shouting in
outrage, they reminded the panel that that murderous and suicidal reactions afflict people well over the age of twenty-four. With the exception of Paxil,
drug-company–manipulated data might be insufficient to demonstrate statistically significant antidepressant suicidality for older age groups but in the real
world people are dying at every age as a result of antidepressant-induced suicidality. This book adds additional testimonials to that tragic fact.

CONTROLLED CLINICAL TRIALS PREVENT SUICIDE, REGARDLESS OF THE DRUG

THE FDA AND PRO-DRUG ADVISORY committee members at the hearing emphasized that there were no *completed* suicides in the antidepressant drug trials submitted to it by the drug companies. The FDA also promotes this misleading claim.[22] When confronted with the question during a deposition against GlaxoSmithKline in early 2007, I realized that there were no suicides in either the drug groups or the *sugar pill* groups. None of the depressed and vulnerable patients who participated in the trials committed suicide including those who were given placebo. Therefore, the lack of completed suicides had nothing to do with the antidepressants.

My conclusion? Putting a depressed patient in a controlled clinical trial by itself probably protects against suicide. Why? Because patients in controlled clinical trials are given the hope that they will be helped and for several weeks they are also given a great deal of weekly professional attention. *Hope* and *personal attention* are the two most important human factors in preventing suicide. Therapists routinely prevent suicide by offering hope and attention. The fact that so many antidepressant-treated patients attempted suicide in the trials indicates that even under these protected circumstances, antidepressants nonetheless made people suicidal.

LINING UP TO DEFEND THE DRUGS

AT THE FDA HEARING, professional apologists for organized psychiatry and the drug companies lined up behind the podium at the adult antidepressant hearings to warn the FDA not to "scare off" patients by requiring yet another suicide warning. What they really meant was, "Don't scare off all our business." These well-known leaders of American psychiatry argued that the black-box warning about suicidal behavior in children had—horror of horrors—resulted in a precipitous 20 percent drop in prescribing these useless toxic chemicals to children. Several other speakers replied to this fearmongering by reminding the FDA that its mandate was not to protect the public from the truth but to tell people the facts.

Representing the American Psychiatric Association, David Reiger lamented the chilling effect that the pediatric black-box warning was having on doctors who had cut back on prescribing antidepressants to children, and he pleaded with the FDA not to expand the warning to include adults. Once again, the psychiatric association was on the side of the devil, lamenting even a modicum of drug-company oversight by the FDA and promoting the use of antidepressants for children when they are known to be ineffective and highly dangerous to them.

As I documented in *Toxic Psychiatry* (1991), the American Psychiatric Association made a pact with the drug companies in the early 1970s when the association was in financial crisis. Despite one ethical dissenter, the board of directors of the association voted to start taking huge amounts of money from the drug companies in order to stave off bankruptcy, in return for which the association surrendered its soul to the pharmaceutical industry.

A representative from the National Mental Health Association, now Mental Health America—which takes money from drug companies—said she suffered from lifelong depression, needed antidepressants, and was glad there hadn't been a black box to scare her off. Without seeming to realize the implications, she described herself going through the worst depression of her life *after* she began taking her first antidepressant.

Dr. Carl Salzman represented the American College of Neuropsychopharmacology, a group that touts itself as the premier organization of specialists in the field of psychopharmacology. Coming toward the end of the day after seventy earlier witnesses, and having heard all the evidence, the well-known psychiatrist declared that no valid conclusion about drug-induced suicidality should be drawn from the day or the data, and he urged the panel to stand pat and to do nothing. If Salzman had described all of his group's ties to the drug industry, he would have needed three hours rather than three minutes.

After the advisory committee announced its conclusions, president-elect Carolyn Robinowitz of the American Psychiatric Association weighed in with the media. She decried the proposed black-box warning for young adults, and declared, "Black-box warnings give the impression to prospective patients that these are dangerous medications that can cause death."[23] But that's what all the research and the hearings were about. That's what all the people were saying in their heartrending testimonies. That was the reason for the black-box recommendation: to warn that the medications can cause death.

This kind of unscrupulous damage control by the newly elected leader of American psychiatry confirms the need for the public to take the necessary actions to curtail the use of dangerous psychiatric medications.

DO ANTIDEPRESSANTS WORK AT ALL?

AS ALREADY DOCUMENTED, the FDA admitted at its 2004 hearings that there is no substantial evidence supporting the usefulness of antidepressants in treating depression in children. What about the treatment of adults? Is it possible that the antidepressants aren't antidepressants at all?

In 1994, I first brought to light in *Talking Back to Prozac* the failure of Prozac to prove its effectiveness in the studies done for FDA approval. In 2002, a team led by psychologist Irving Kirsch at the University of Connecticut published an analysis of efficacy data submitted to the FDA between 1987 and 1999 for six of the most commonly prescribed antidepressants: Prozac, Paxil, Zoloft, Effexor, Serzone, and Celexa.[24] Each of the drugs had been approved based on a drug company submitting *two* positive studies to the FDA. But all of the companies conducted numerous additional studies before they were able to obtain the required two that seemed positive. So Kirsch and his colleagues looked at *all* the antidepressant studies—not just the ones submitted for approval.

Kirsch and his colleagues obtained forty-seven studies, an average of almost eight per drug, conducted as a part of the FDA approval process. After examining all the studies, they found that any beneficial or positive effects in comparison to placebo were "negligible."

How do psychiatry and the psychopharmaceutical complex react to the mounting evidence that antidepressants are not only dangerous but also useless for both adults and children? They ignore it. However, the Kirsch study has received positive recognition from those few professionals brave enough to face the facts, including Marcia Angell, the former editor of the *New England Journal of Medicine,* and Charles Medawar, the respected British researcher and public-safety advocate.[25]

In 2006, British psychiatrist Joanna Moncrieff and Kirsch published another review and analysis of antidepressant effectiveness in the *British Medical Journal (BMJ).* They focused on studies conducted on SSRIs such as Prozac, Zoloft, and Paxil, and concluded that these drugs "do not have a clinically meaningful advantage over placebo." As this book goes to press, a research team led by Kirsch (2008) has once again produced a meta-analysis of the scientific literature demonstrating the ineffectiveness of antidepressants.

It is a sad, ironic, and tragic tale: It's impossible to prove that antidepressants actually relieve depression but it's relatively easy to demonstrate that they can worsen depression and cause mania, murder, and suicide. If my colleagues wanted to be scientific about it, they would call them "depressants" rather than antidepressants, and take them off the market.

To compound the problem, these drugs can cause severe withdrawal problems, including a variety of neurological symptoms, agitation, and a worsening of depression.[26] A substantial portion of my psychiatric practice involves working with patients who suffered frightening and sometimes agonizing withdrawal symptoms before coming to me for help in stopping the drugs. Sometimes, these withdrawal symptoms persist for months or even years after stopping antidepressants.

It bears repeating that antidepressants are dangerous to start taking and dangerous to stop taking, as well as ineffective. The best advice is to stay away from them. In forty years of psychiatric practice, I have never started a patient on an antidepressant, although I do prescribe them during the withdrawal process or if the patient is unable to go through withdrawal. Although good fortune undoubtedly plays a role as well, I believe my refusal to start patients on these drugs has contributed to my success in never having a suicide in my practice.

NO LONGER ALONE

I'm no longer so alone in my criticism of the FDA's failure to address life-threatening adverse drug effects. On September 30, 2004, Merck withdrew the painkiller Vioxx from the market after it was linked to cardiovascular deaths, leading to congressional investigations. The FDA then came under fire from Congress for its handling of SSRI-induced suicidality, especially in children and youth.[27] Then in the September 23, 2006, headline on the front page of *The New York Times* reported criticism of the agency in general: STUDY CONDEMNS F.D.A.'S HANDLING OF DRUG SAFETY: SWEEPING CHANGES URGED.[28] The report was issued by the Institute of Medicine of the National Academy of Sciences, itself a government-sponsored organization. The Institute of Medicine suggested, for example, that the FDA review the safety of each drug every five years! This kind of recommendation underscores just how lax and even remiss the agency has been in regard to safety reviews. The report also suggested putting a few teeth back into the agency's gummy mouth by giving it authority to issue fines, injunctions, and drug withdrawals from the market "when the drug makers fail—as they often do—to complete required safety studies." That gives you more of an idea of what the FDA and the drug companies have not been doing all these years—safety studies and safety enforcement.

In response to this criticism, the FDA recently proposed a few relatively minor changes, including an experimental program to review the safety of two or three drugs each year after they have been on the market for eighteen months. The agency will also start an online newsletter that will publish the pilot-program safety reviews as they are completed. However, the FDA plans to continue its policy of withholding confidential, commercial data—that is, the sealed information necessary to determine if the companies are telling the truth about their commercial products. The savvy *Wall Street Journal* commented that this is "a move likely to please the drug industry."[29] Unfortunately, that pleasure will come at the expense of human lives.

More recently, a study commissioned by the FDA itself came out with similar conclusions to mine in March 2007.[30] It lamented the culture of conflict, avoidance, and waste inside the FDA when it comes to tracking adverse drug reactions.

Few of the FDA's critics squarely face the stark reality that the FDA culture has become more concerned about protecting the drug companies than protecting the public. An exception is Marcia Angell, former editor of the *New England Journal of Medicine* and now senior lecturer at Harvard Medical School. In a column entitled, "Taking back the FDA" in *The Boston Globe* on February 26, 2007, she observed:

> The FDA also refuses to release unfavorable research results in its possession without the sponsoring company's permission. . . . It's no wonder that serious safety concerns about drugs such as Vioxx, Paxil, and Zyprexa have emerged very late in the day—years after they were in widespread use.

Dr. Angell concluded that the FDA was becoming more dedicated to serving the drug companies than to serving the consumer of psychiatric drugs. Americans need to know that the FDA is not their friend. It's the friend of the pharmaceutical industry.

Chapter 4

Young Girl Murderers in the Making

THESE TWO STORIES are about young girls driven by Prozac into compulsive states of violence. The first story is about unblemished innocence, a teenager enjoying life in a comfortable and loving household. The second is more complicated, a child raised amid hardship and conflict.

MURDERING MOM

EMILY ASHTON was the least likely youngster to want to murder her mother. A petite blue-eyed blonde, Emily was in her junior year at a small private high school where she enjoyed herself and earned above-average grades. She had two or three close girlfriends and a boyfriend. She played soccer and liked to hang out at the beach and go to the movies. At sixteen, she was happy about getting her driver's license and was so responsible that her parents gave her easy access to the family car.

With her older brother away at college and doing well, sixteen-year-old Emily received as much attention as she wanted at home. Other than an occasional teenage drama over what to eat or what she should wear, she had no conflicts with her parents. She felt close to her mother and liked her stepfather whom she affectionately called "a good guy." Emily had known him her whole life.

Trouble began after a six-week school trip to India over Thanksgiving and Christmas. Soon after returning home from overseas, Emily started getting sick to her stomach, probably from an exotic gastrointestinal parasite that a raft of tests failed to identify. An operation on her gallbladder seemed to help for a few weeks but then the chronic nausea returned. The disorder did not interfere with her eating and she didn't have to vomit but being nauseous much of time wasn't fun. Even worse in some ways than the nausea, Emily had to submit to multiple blood tests, invasive GI studies, doctor visits, and pills.

Emily handled all this fairly well for a teen. Her mother recalls only one outburst of frustration. It was an adolescent temper tantrum over constantly feeling sick. "She wanted to have a normal life and didn't want to feel nauseous all the time. She felt like it was never going to end."

The following summer, Emily's family doctor could see that six months of intermittent nausea, as well as stressful medical tests and treatments, were getting to the teenager. Emily had no history of psychiatric problems and there were none in her family. She had never been suicidal or homicidal. She never experimented with illegal drugs. Her family viewed her as "an easygoing kid." Emily's doctor didn't think her problem was serious enough to refer her to a psychiatrist or psychologist, so he wrote her a prescription for Prozac.

Put on the market in January 1989, Prozac or fluoxetine was the first of the new group of antidepressants known as the SSRIs—selective serotonin reuptake inhibitors—because they block the removal of the neurotransmitter serotonin from the synapse, the submicroscopic location where these chemical messengers cause nerves to fire in the brain. By blocking the removal of the neurotransmitter, the drug is supposed to increase the amount of serotonin in the synapse, thereby increasing the rate at which these nerves fire.

Prozac was followed by several competing SSRIs, including Paxil, which Harry Henderson was taking when driven in an anguished, suicidal state. All of the SSRI antidepressants have very similar and often identical adverse effects, so that as of early January 2005, the FDA has required the identical black-box warning for all of them concerning drug-induced suicide and mental deterioration in children and youth age eighteen and younger, which was then expanded to include young adults (see chapter 3).

Did Emily know the potential risks involved in taking Prozac? Like almost every other victim of medication madness you will meet in this book, Emily had no idea that her prescription drug could make her crazy or push her toward doing something that would otherwise horrify her. She didn't even know it was an antidepressant. In retrospect, she remembers thinking it was just one more of the endless string of pills that her family doctor wanted her to take. No one in the family had as yet become aware of the controversy that was already brewing around Prozac in the early 1990s.

Within a week of starting Prozac, Emily began to become obsessed with killing her mother. Never before had thoughts like these entered her mind. She imagined taking the eight-inch chef's knife from the kitchen. She saw herself sneaking up on her mother at an unsuspecting moment—when her mother was bathing in the tub or asleep in bed—and plunging it into her back. Emily envisioned blood spurting but not the unbearable consequences beyond that image.

The drive to kill wasn't wrapped in any reasons, excuses, or rationalizations. Emily didn't feel upset with her mother. In her words, "It came out of nowhere." Typical of the spellbinding effect of psychiatric drugs on victims, Emily had no idea whatsoever that her medication had anything to do with her violent feelings. Again, characteristic of more extreme spellbinding, she felt compelled to act in a way that was wholly alien to her.

As her compulsion became increasingly overwhelming, Emily initially tried to resist it and then started to come apart emotionally. She had trouble sleeping—a common side effect of Prozac. She isolated herself from her friends and family and, as she told me, "I spent a lot of time alone in my room not doing much of anything." She began taking the family car out for rides by herself at night. Driving bolstered her flagging sense of self-control. At least she could make the car go where she wanted it to go. At home she would sit by herself huddled up in her bed. She explained, "I didn't think of help at all, of going to people. I definitely withdrew." Not knowing what was wrong—or even knowing with certainty that something was wrong—she hid inside herself. It was summer vacation and she wasn't in school, so there were fewer people around to notice the changes in her.

Emily's mother was vice president for product development at a large clothing firm. She was busy with work but she also put a high priority on her daughter. Emily never tried to signal her and she did not pick up any warning signs before the fateful night.

During her second week of taking Prozac, Emily's violent obsessions grew steadily more frequent and virulent. Soon they were taking over her mind many times a day. When the obsessions weren't dominating her, they were "lurking in the background." Meanwhile, she continued to take the medication that her doctor had prescribed for her because it was supposed to help.

On the night the compulsion finally overwhelmed her, Emily teetered on the verge of actually getting the knife, and then got ready to do it.

That evening her mother was having a dinner party at the house. Emily went to bed obsessed with the idea of stabbing her mother in the back while she went about enjoying herself and her friends.

People acting under the influence of drugs often have faulty memories for critical moments leading up to horrendous acts. They seldom remember much of what happened to them while spellbound by a drug. Consistent with this, Emily's memory for the next few minutes is blurred.

Emily's mother stepped into her daughter's bedroom to say good night. Emily was sitting on the bed. Her mother asked, "How was your day today?"

In a flat, matter-of-fact voice, Emily replied, "I want to kill you with a knife."

"It was one of those heart-stopping moments," her mother told me. "It was clear she meant it: an out-of-the-blue statement with no hint of joking. She was telling me she wanted to kill me."

Because Emily had declared her feelings, and because her mother took them seriously, her mother is alive today, and Emily did not become a murderer.

Emily's mother quickly gathered her wits and realized that something must have happened to her daughter. "It was not who she was, this gentle soul. Yes, it was horrifying but I knew that something had to be wrong. This was not a child in whom homicidal tendencies had been building for years. Emily was always gentle and loving with people and animals. And especially she wouldn't want to murder me. We had a wonderful relationship. I knew there had to be some other reason for what was happening to her. So it was shocking but also I knew we just had to figure out what was going on with her."

When I expressed surprise at Emily's mother's calm and loving response in the wake of such a shocking pronouncement from her daughter, she explained: "While I took very seriously what Emily said, I just knew it wasn't Emily. And it wasn't like a stranger was at my throat with a knife. It was my child I had known all these years. And she was showing this totally one-hundred-eighty-degree behavior from who she really was. I knew it must be something affecting her."

Emily's mother never sensed the buildup of violence in her daughter. She explained to me, "Emily was always a very self-sufficient child. Not a high-maintenance kid. She was a joy and always had been. She always had a tendency to being more introverted than her older brother, so if she was quiet, it wasn't that unusual." And also, it was summertime when Emily was much more on her own.

Again, like most cases of spellbinding by drugs, Emily's behavior was so out of character that her mother immediately recognized that this wasn't the real Emily. Fortunately, Emily's mother had the confidence in her daughter and in their relationship to search for another explanation—for something outside of her daughter and outside of their relationship. The drug was the only new factor in her daughter's life.

Mrs. Ashton offered to go to an emergency room that night with Emily but her daughter felt so relieved after confessing, she reassured her mother that they could wait until the morning. In some of our cases, a brief relaxation of vigilance will become a chance for disaster, but not this time. In the morning, the family doctor who had prescribed the Prozac gave them a referral to a psychiatrist. That day, Emily and her mother went together to the new doctor. Ten minutes into the session they were discussing the possibility that Emily was having a reaction to Prozac, and the medication was stopped.

LASTING PSYCHOLOGICAL EFFECTS

OVER A FEW PROZAC-FREE DAYS, Emily's compulsion dissipated but its demoralizing effects proved far more difficult to escape. "It definitely left a lot of self-doubts," she told me. She underwent twice-a-week psychotherapy for six months but the guilt never fully left her mind for very long over the next few years. She couldn't forgive herself for harboring those awful thoughts.

A cloud of confusion and guilt about herself settled over Emily and did not fully lift for several years. Emily's grades fell at school and she didn't regain her academic footing until a few years later in junior college. The effort to contain this dreadful secret within herself kept her at a distance from her friends: "I didn't feel as comfortable with my girlfriends anymore." She explained to me that she had to "resocialize myself" over the next few years. "I knew that I wasn't feeling normal about myself after that." Even today—a decade and a half later—she suffers from a lingering emotional aftermath.

Emily became leery of taking medications and somewhat more cautious about doctors. With her mother and her therapist's encouragement, she turned to alternative approaches and imposed self-discipline on her diet, removing all acidic foods, including her beloved pizza. Gradually, she recovered from the chronic nausea without the underlying disorder being diagnosed.

I first heard of Emily's story from her mother at a social gathering. It's the only case in this book that didn't come through my psychiatric practice or medical legal work, and the only one in which the background medical records were no longer available. I phoned Emily to ask permission to speak with her and she later told me that anxieties from the past had been stirred up after she agreed to let me interview her. When we finally talked, she learned from me that her experience was surprisingly and shockingly common—that many people on antidepressants developed murderous and suicidal compulsions. That helped to relieve Emily of some of the lingering guilt and anxiety about the dreadful impulse that had nearly turned her into a murderer and had nearly killed or maimed her mother those years ago.

Even though Emily never acted on her violent impulse, her young life was irreversibly stained by the experience. Imagine how much worse it would have been if she had been unable to confide in her mother or if her mother hadn't been so able to respond in a loving manner. Consider what might have happened if the psychiatrist had rejected the idea that Prozac can drive people into compulsive violence and mistakenly diagnosed her with bipolar disorder or a manic episode. Like many other people who have been misdiagnosed in this fashion, Emily would have learned to view herself as "mentally ill" and potentially violent—and in need of continued medication for the rest of her life. Even worse, imagine if her psychiatrist had continued or increased Emily's medication, driving her further into a state of murderous medication madness with the result being that she killed her mother. Consider the aftermath of how her murderous action would have overwhelmed and even destroyed the lives of the survivors, including her stepfather and her brother.

WHAT IF EMILY HAD ACTED?

AFTER PEOPLE COMMIT horrendous acts that are totally out of character, everything changes in their lives, including how they and other people view their character. As if struck by moral lightning, in a flash the spirit and the flesh are seared and damaged, branding victims of medication madness with their own guilt and the doubts of others. Every self-doubt and every nasty thought that ever crept into their minds, and every mildly aggressive action they ever took, now become amplified in retrospect to verify a flawed character.

Bewilderment and other fearful and negative emotions can creep into every crevice of the person's mental life, changing not only how she views herself now and into the far future, but also how she reinterprets her past. After a drug-induced impulsive act, the perpetrator's mental life becomes newly submerged in guilt, in shame, in anxiety, and in fear.

If Emily had assaulted her mother, it would have been difficult to succeed in court by using a Prozac defense on her behalf. As Eli Lilly, the manufacturer of Prozac, has done with me and other medical experts, in order to protect their drug, the pharmaceutical company might have helped the prosecution mount an assault on Emily and on my testimony. Drug-company and state investigators would quite possibly have ransacked Emily's past life, looking for something minor, like a scuffle with another girl when she was ten, that could be amplified into something momentous. Relatively commonplace and harmless acts of childhood aggression would become enlarged in a retrospective magnifying glass as the prosecution and Eli Lilly tried to show that the drug had nothing to do with the crime—that the perpetrator had a character predestined to violence.

A FORTUNATE EXCEPTION TO ROUTINE PSYCHIATRIC PRACTICE

EMILY ASHTON is now thirty-two years old and the mother of a seven-year-old daughter. These events took place a relatively long time ago in 1991. Yet, of all the cases in this book, Emily's is probably the only one in which a psychiatrist acknowledged the potential role of the medication and prevented a tragedy by stopping it.

Many contemporary psychiatrists would have reassured Emily and her mother, and encouraged Emily to stay on Prozac, explaining that it takes six to ten weeks for antidepressants to have their beneficial effect, and that Emily simply needed to stay on the drug a little longer. Many would have doubled the dose and perhaps thrown a tranquilizer or some other drug into the medicinal stew.

The early 1990s were in some ways a period of enlightenment in regard to the dangers of antidepressant drugs to brain, mind, and behavior. Shortly after Prozac was released on the market, a flurry of clinical reports warned about compulsive suicidality induced by it. Innumerable press reports came out linking Prozac to violence. Hundreds of lawsuits were being brought against Eli Lilly and Company, the manufacturer of Prozac, and I would become the one medical and scientific expert responsible for doing the background scientific research for all of the combined cases.

Today the published cases are fewer and further between. Indeed, my 1994 book *Talking Back to Prozac,* written with my wife Ginger, garnered far more attention than would similar publications today. Why? In these intervening dozen years, as later chapters will document, the drug companies and their advocates marshaled their resources and successfully manipulated the legal system, the media, and health professionals with a barrage of propaganda calculated to dismiss any concerns about antidepressant-induced violence against self and others.

Although clinical experience and research about antidepressant-induced madness mounted, so did the pro-drug propaganda campaign, and health professionals grew less aware of the dangers of antidepressants in 2000 than they had been in 1990. As we'll see, the pro-drug propaganda campaign continues unabated.

CHESTNUT IS DROWNING

EVERY TIME I THINK OF JENNIFER HOPE, I grow sad, and this story initially felt too difficult to write. Unlike most of the stories in this book where the drug-induced violence occurs in situations with little or no provocation, Jennie's story is more complicated by her difficult childhood and by her justified anger at the bully in her sights when she pulled the trigger.

Jennie was born and raised in the rural Deep South and, consistent with their community values, her mother and father raised their children with strict discipline and corporal punishment. They were good people who struggled with their circumstances and their own personal difficulties, but they tried hard, never gave up on Jennie, and would later second-guess themselves about being too tough and at times untrusting of their vulnerable daughter.

Jennie's father, who had been a corrections officer many years earlier, owned a little snub-nosed .22 caliber revolver. By the time Jennie was twelve, the revolver had been sequestered for a decade or more in the shoebox in the bedroom closet and Jennie's parents had forgotten about its existence. The family also owned rifles that were kept loaded in the house.

There were a few traumatic events in Jennie's early life. Her home burned down when she was three, causing considerable anxiety at the time. When she was about seven, her younger brother developed a pituitary tumor that almost caused his death. The tumor and the subsequent radiation treatment partially blinded him.

An "easy child," Jennie wasn't a squeaky wheel and her brother's illness preoccupied the parents at her expense. Jennie was a courteous child, performed well in school, dressed neatly, and took good care of herself. She had fun and especially loved her horse, Chestnut, who was kept on her grandmother's farm.

One day when Jennie was twelve, she was having as good a time as a child could have. It was summer and she was at Grandma's, playing with her younger cousin. They decided to take Jennie's much-loved horse Chestnut down to the creek where all three would cool off together in the water.

To make sure Chestnut did not wander off while she took a dip in the cool creek with her cousin, Jennie tied her horse to a tree, leaving the animal enough rope to graze in the fresh vegetation by the water's edge.

The two girls were having a wonderful time playing in the water hole when something went desperately wrong. Chestnut lost her footing and slid down the slope into the deep pool. The rope around the horse's neck tightened as she fell into the water, pulling her over onto her side. Chestnut was thrashing about on her side in the water as her head began to sink beneath the surface. The rope became so taut that that the desperate child could not loosen it.

Jennie sent her cousin running back to the farmhouse for help. Then Jennie slid deep into the water and struggled with all her might to keep Chestnut's huge head above the surface. When help arrived, an exhausted Jennie was still fighting to lift Chestnut's head above the water, but her horse was dead.

Any adult would praise Jennie for her heroic effort but Jennie could only condemn herself. She was never again the same. She lapsed into guilt, grief, and then unremitting depression. Her mother poignantly remembers how her daughter gave up her love for horses and took all the horse pictures down from her bedroom walls. Jennie gradually withdrew from her parents, lost interest in her studies and sports, turned to more rebellious music, and began to spend time with more troubled peers.

Jennie's mother and father grew frantic and like many parents they tried to get tougher with their daughter. Both confirm that they inflicted harsh physical punishment on Jennie, something they feel genuinely remorseful about.

Almost two years after the drowning of her horse, Jennie overdosed with ten ibuprofen and was rushed to an emergency room. In the ER, laconic Jennie murmured that she was "a big disappointment" to her parents, explaining she felt badly about doing poorly in school.

A urine sample taken in the emergency room revealed the presence of cocaine and barbiturates in Jennie's urine. Jennie vehemently denied any drug use, swearing she would never do anything like that and that she would never lie to her parents about it. Although Jennie's parents were not the type to challenge authority, they asked the ER to send out the urine sample for further testing.

That was the last Jennie's parents heard from the emergency room. They were reluctant to press for the toxicology results and assumed that the drug tests for cocaine and barbiturates had been confirmed.

Jennie felt betrayed by her parents; her parents felt lied to by their daughter. Later, Jennie's grief-stricken mother told me that this mutual distrust put another wedge between them.

Three months later, Jennie's pediatrician mentioned offhandedly to her parents that he had been sent a copy of the follow-up urine test. The more reliable second test turned out to be negative. Jennie had been telling the truth about not using drugs. The emergency room had received the corrected urine test results within days of Jennie's treatment but somehow failed to pass them on to Jennie and her family. From examining Jennie's medical records, I have been able to confirm the negative urine test and the ER's failure to inform the parents about it.

Jennie's parents were, of course, relieved to find out that their daughter had been telling the truth all along, but it was too late to heal Jennie's wounded feelings and sense of betrayal. Mom explained to me, "Jennie had lost trust in us. My husband and I both felt it was a big turning point. She ran away after the false accusation and we were never again as close." With honesty and insight, Mom confessed, "We had decided the problem was drugs, so her problems weren't our fault."

When Jennie was first seen at the emergency room, she was immediately referred to an outpatient psychiatric clinic for evaluation, and her family took her that very day. The intake evaluation found Jennie to be very depressed with "poor concentration, fatigue, anhedonia [loss of pleasure in life], sadness, tearfulness, and poor academic performance." She was thirteen years old.

In yet another medical betrayal, the clinic took three months before finding an appointment time for Jennie with a therapist. Then the master's-level psychologist quickly referred Jennie to a psychiatrist for medication. The therapist saw Jennie a few more times but never sought to include either of the parents in the treatment process.

When dealing with a thirteen- or fourteen-year-old, especially one who is depressed and suicidal, I always involve the parents very closely in the therapy to help them to improve their family life, including their relationship with their child. If grandparents are actively involved in the child's life, I invite them into the office for sessions as well. If there are problems at school, I talk with her teachers, too. Especially if the child is in her early teens or younger, I may spend much more time helping the parents help their child than in seeing the child herself.

No family consultations or therapy were offered by the clinic. Instead, Prozac would become the method of treatment. As is often the case nowadays, especially with children, Jennie would have been better off if she had never been referred to mental-health professionals for help.

On the first and only visit with the psychiatrist, the doctor confirmed that

Jennie was severely depressed. Although his record does not mention Chestnut's tragic drowning and Jennie's overwhelming guilt about losing her horse, the psychiatrist dates the onset of her depression to roughly the time of the horse's death.

The psychiatrist started Jennie on Prozac 10 mg, to be increased to Prozac 20 mg after seven days if the smaller dose proved ineffective. He did not schedule a return appointment until six weeks, leaving it entirely up to the parents to monitor Jennie for side effects and to determine if the dose should be increased after one week. As in all the other cases I've described, Jennie and her parents were not warned that Prozac could stimulate or worsen her behavior, and when it happened, they never guessed it was a drug reaction.

During Jennie's nine days on Prozac, her mother saw her become "confused, and extremely groggy, so she would fall asleep in a sitting position." Her mother also reported symptoms of an incipient manic-reaction. At times Jennie was "hyper and anxious." She was "nervous, jittery, talking a lot, madly cleaning house from one place to the other." Shortly before the incident, she was "silly, giggly, laughing, talking nonstop, doing stuff all day long."

These maniclike behaviors were completely out of character for Jennie who was usually more sullen and withdrawn, and who certainly never wanted to do housework. As we will see documented in our cases and in the scientific literature, any SSRI antidepressant can turn a paralyzing depression into an activated, agitated depression, or into mania—very dangerous mental states that can drive the depressed child or adult into taking impulsive, drastic actions.

Jennie was the victim of so many tragic circumstances and betrayals, I thought that even without a Prozac defense a jury would show the girl sympathy and realize that she needed help rather than incarceration. There was even an element of self-defense in what she eventually did.

Jennie reported that she was being subjected to abuse from a neighborhood boy—a six-foot three-inch 200-pounder who liked to hoist Jennie up and throw her around. Jennie was only five feet four inches tall and weighed 110 pounds. According to Jennie, this giant of a teenager would wrap his arms around her from behind, groping her, and tossing her over his shoulder. On one occasion, she reluctantly told me, he grabbed her breasts and "stomach" and humped her as if having sex. She felt humiliated and terrified.

Although Jennie was never able to express to me or to anyone else why she did what she did, my discussions with her eventually led to how much the boy had "taken advantage" of her. She didn't seem to be trying to sell me on the idea that she had defended herself against abuse; she seemed instead to be reciting in suppressed monotones one more sad detail of her life, never expecting anyone to listen or to care.

Jennie's mother corroborates that when the boy would come to the house asking for Jennie, her daughter would hide and ask her mother to send him away. As far as I know, this abuse was not investigated or confirmed by the police or other authorities.

After taking Prozac 10 mg for six days, Jennie ran away. She eventually was found by friends and relatives, and returned home. At that point, she had been off her Prozac for two or three days. Never attributing Jennie's worsening behavior to the drug, Mom instead concluded that the initial 10 mg dose wasn't working. She did what the doctor had instructed her to do; she began the 20 mg dose. Like so many cases in this book, a dose change occurred in proximity to the perpetration, this time a doubling of the dose on the morning of the incident.

Some time earlier Jennie had happened upon her father's .22 revolver stashed away in the shoebox. She had never fired a gun but that afternoon she decided, apparently on the spur of the moment, to shoot the boy who had been tormenting her. She phoned him and invited him over to her house. He arrived along with two other boys whom they both knew.

In my forensic work, I have often been shocked by the attitudes of district attorneys toward the actions of disturbed children. Often they seem as eager to come down hard on these kids as they would on child abusers, and sometimes more so. Often, these district attorneys seem bent on building up their reputations for toughness on crime at the expense of the beleaguered children. I was told that this DA was a woman determined to build an image for being tough on "teenage crime."

In the trial, the district attorney placed emphasis on the fact that Jennie called the boy on the phone with the intent of killing him. The DA would argue that this proved premeditation and intent, the attributes of first-degree attempted murder. But there's no evidence that Jennie had thought through what she was doing. She acted impulsively in front of witnesses. She made no preparations to escape.

When the alleged bully arrived at her house, Jennie came out the door and stood there briefly before she aimed the gun point-blank at him. The boy refused to back off. Jennie and one of the witnesses report that he lunged toward her. Jennie pulled the trigger.

One of the two boys who witnessed the event reported that "she was wearing a coat and it was a real hot day. For some reason her eyes were all funny-looking, like reddish and glossy." The other boy described Jennie as displaying "basically like a weird laugh. Her face got real red and she had this evil look," he reported, and "she was still calm. It was scary because she was being so calm about it."

Jennie pulled the trigger. What happened next would be a miracle—if it hadn't turned out so badly for Jennie in the long run. The gun jammed. It didn't go off. No one was physically injured. The boys fled. Jennie was found standing in the front yard with the gun and a cordless phone, calling 911 to tell the sheriff that she had just tried to shoot someone. She readily gave up the weapon.

Fourteen-year-old Jennie Hope was charged with first-degree attempted murder. The DA refused to plea bargain. By the time I entered the case, the child had already spent nine months in jail with no prospect of immediate release. To protect Jennie against the adult prisoners, she was kept in isolation without the minimal solace of visual contact with other people. She was allowed to see her family once a week for two hours with no physical contact. Phone-call contacts were only occasional. Without being convicted of anything, she was being subjected to cruel and unusual punishment, especially for a child.

Jennie was so depressed and withdrawn, it was hard for her to communicate with me about what she'd been through or why she had acted in the way she did, except for her distress at the actions of the boy she had tried to shoot. She couldn't recall much about how she felt shortly before the attempted shooting.

I put great effort into evaluating Jennie's case and into writing a report that hopefully would soften the DA's heart toward the child. Unlike many other relatively uncomplicated cases, in Jennie's case I did not view the drug as the sole contributing factor. I made clear that Jennie had always been a good child who showed no inclinations to rebelliousness or violence. Then I recounted the story of how her beloved horse Chestnut had died in her arms, leading to depression and social isolation, and eventually to the suicide attempt that brought her into psychiatric treatment. I described the failure of the emergency room to report that in fact Jennie's tests confirmed her story that she hadn't taken any illegal drugs, resulting in a sense of mutual betrayal between Jennie and her parents. Although I do not like giving an opinion that "mental illness"—rather than drug intoxication—has caused destructive actions, I made an exception for Jennie. In concluding my report, I wrote:

I believe within a reasonable degree of medical certainty that—due to a combination of mental disorder (Major Depression) and involuntary intoxication with Prozac—Jennie Hope was unable to form the intent to commit a crime when she pulled the trigger. This fourteen-year-old girl was unable to control her impulses, to conform them to her understanding of right and wrong, or to understand their consequences. In addition to the mental disorder and the psychiatric-drug intoxication, her behavior was also adversely influenced by inadequate medical care, by a history of family abuse, specifically excessive physical punishment and conflict, and by severe emotional, physical, and sexual abuse at the hands of the boy she tried to shoot.

Notice my use of the phrase "reasonable degree of medical certainty." The law recognizes that the profession of medicine rarely achieves absolute certainty about anything. As I described earlier, what's usually required of an expert is a "reasonable degree" of conviction. Despite the ponderous words, the meaning is simple: As an expert, I need to conclude that it is *more likely than not* that my observations are correct—anything more than a fifty-fifty toss of the dice is sufficient. In all of the cases in this book where I wrote a report or testified, I was more certain than that about the drugs playing a role in the individual's behavior.

I was saddened and outraged that Jennie remained incarcerated. After reading my report, the district attorney would surely reduce the charges against her and set her free under supervision. A first-degree attempted murder charge and potentially an even lengthier jail sentence not only seemed incredibly unjust, it made no practical sense. What could possibly be gained from locking up the child for years on end? It would most likely turn her into a hardened, embittered adult. Jennie needed understanding and help, not a degrading and dangerous continued stretch in jail.

My report did nothing to dent the DA's determination to treat Jennie like an adult who had perpetrated a heinous crime. The DA refused to compromise and we had to go to trial. The state portrayed Jennie as a cunning psychopath who was too dangerous to be set free. The humiliations she had endured from the bully at whom she fired the gun became a double-edged sword. It made her actions more understandable but in doing so it gave her a motivation. In the presence of a clear-cut motivation, it can be harder to argue that a prescription drug or other factors played a role.

The jury did not entirely go along with the district attorney but it did not entirely go along with Jennie's lawyer or my testimony, either. The jurors refused to exonerate Jennie with a verdict of not guilty by reason of insanity, or involuntary intoxication with Prozac. They did, however, reject the DA's charge of first-degree attempted murder and instead found her guilty of a lesser charge, second-degree attempted murder, indicating that she lacked willfulness, deliberateness, or premeditation. Given the uncompromising, aggressive prosecution of the case by the district attorney, Jennie's attorney felt that it was not such a bad outcome. Jennie would probably spend only a few more years in jail.

Jennie's parents were heartbroken for her. I was enormously saddened and wonder to this day how I failed to communicate her story to the jury. Of course, I wasn't the only person responsible for presenting the case. She had an able defense attorney and a family who also tried to explain to the jury what happened. But I felt that I had the most responsibility and had failed her. In my defense, in 1998, my views surely seemed much more "radical" to the jurors than they would today.

Having achieved a criminal conviction, the state then showed some leniency toward Jennie, and she did not have to go back to jail. Instead, she was placed in a supervised residential treatment program for four years until the age of eighteen and then unconditionally released. Jennie could have been kept under supervision until age twenty-one but she did well enough to be released three years early. According to her attorney, Leo A. Thomas, Jennie has been in no further trouble with the law.

How many Jennies might have been saved if the FDA had not delayed until 2004–2005 before formally naming the litany of disastrous mental adverse effects caused by antidepressants, including aggression and hostility? Suppose Jennie's parents had been given the booklet that the FDA now requires doctors to hand to the parents of children who are prescribed antidepressants? As previously noted, the booklet warns parents to look out for the development of the following bulleted items *after* the start of antidepressant treatment:[1]

- Feeling very agitated or restless
- New or worse irritability
- Acting aggressive, being angry, or violent
- Acting on dangerous impulses
- An extreme increase in activity and talking
- Other unusual changes in behavior

How many Jennies might have been saved if the FDA had not procrastinated for decades before admitting that antidepressants have not been proven to help children? Not only would Jennie's defense have been easier to mount, her doctor might have decided against giving her an antidepressant like Prozac. Without the medication, Jennie most probably would not have attempted to fire the gun at the boy.

Chapter 5

Doctors Driven Mad by Medication

BEING SOPHISTICATED, educated, and informed does not fully protect against medication madness. My psychiatric and medical expert practice has included dozens of doctors, scientists, lawyers, professors, and other educated, sophisticated men and women who have succumbed to the adverse mental and emotional effects of prescribed medications. This chapter examines the case of two doctors, one who was driven into a manic state by antidepressants and the other by stimulants.

THE NATURE OF MANIA

INDIVIDUALS SUFFERING FROM medication-induced mania are always profoundly spellbound. They have no idea that the drug is causing them problems, they typically feel better than ever, and they commonly take humiliating, dangerous, and even violent actions that would otherwise have appalled them. Drug-induced mania is the ultimate expression of medication spellbinding and medication madness.

Mania can arise spontaneously or it can be caused by a variety of potentially stimulating substances, such as all of the antidepressants, all of the stimulants, and the tranquilizer Xanax. When mania arises spontaneously in individuals, it is diagnosed as a manic episode, or, if the individual also experiences period of depression, it is diagnosed as bipolar (manic-depressive) disorder. However, when the symptoms are caused by a medication such as an antidepressant, the correct diagnosis is substance-induced mood disorder rather than manic episode or bipolar disorder. This distinction is very important because drug-induced episodes often abate once the drug is removed and because they are not likely to recur without re-exposure to the offending agent.

Mania is an out-of-control or disinhibited state in which the individual loses his or her customary restraint and judgment, and carries out acts that would ordinarily make the individual feel guilty, ashamed, frightened, or even horrified. It can manifest itself as an elevated or euphoric mood, as an expansive or grandiose mood, or as a heightened state of irritability with the potential for violence. Mania can "crash" into depression and suicidality. The following section summarizes the 2000 edition of American Psychiatric Association's *Diagnostic and Statistical Manual of Mental Disorders (DSM-IV-TR)*.[1]

Criteria for a Manic Episode from the *DSM-IV-TR* (2000)

A mood that is abnormally and persistently *elevated, expansive,* or *irritable* with several of the following symptoms:

1. Inflated self-esteem or grandiosity
2. Decreased need for sleep
3. More talkative than usual or pressure to keep talking
4. Flight of ideas or subjective experience that thoughts are racing
5. Distractibility
6. Increase in goal-directed activity
7. Excessive involvement in pleasurable activities that have a high potential for painful consequences

Maniclike episodes, whether caused by drugs or arising spontaneously, can lead to antisocial or criminal actions. In the *DSM–IV-TR,* aggression is specifically mentioned as a feature of manic behavior.[2] It is noted that "antisocial behaviors may accompany the Manic Episode," "ethical concerns may be disregarded even by those who are typically very conscientious," "the person may become hostile and physically threatening to others" and "physically assaultive," and "the mood may shift rapidly to anger or depression."

Compulsive planning and intense goal-directed behavior are features of mania. As described in the *DSM-IV-TR,* "The increase in goal-directed activity often involves excessive planning of, and excessive participation in, multiple activities (e.g., sexual, occupational, political, religious)." Often, the individuals become "intrusive, domineering, and demanding." They suffer from "expansiveness, unwarranted optimism, grandiosity, and poor judgment." Also according to the *DSM-IV-TR,* individuals who are manic "may engage in activities that have a disorganized or bizarre quality (e.g., distributing candy, money, or advice to passing strangers)." The "disorganized or bizarre" qualities are typical of many of our cases. Overall, the actions taken are often self-defeating, bizarre, and irrational.

The *DSM-IV-TR* sums up the seriousness of the dangers associated with a manic episode:

> The impairment resulting from the disturbance must be severe enough to cause marked impairment in functioning or require hospitalization to protect the individual from poor judgment (e.g., financial losses, illegal activities, loss of employment, assaultive behavior).

In other words, maniclike reactions can ruin lives.

The same brief section in the *DSM-IV-TR* on two occasions states that antidepressants can cause maniclike episodes, declaring, "Symptoms like those seen in a Manic Episode may be due to the direct effects of antidepressant medications" and "Symptoms like those seen in a Manic Episode may also be precipitated by antidepressant treatment such as medication."[3] The theme that antidepressants can cause mania, as well as other mood disorders, is repeated throughout the official diagnostic manual.[4]

This section of the *DSM-IV-TR* also repeats the caveat that treatment-induced maniclike episodes should be diagnosed as substance-induced mood disorder, rather than as a manic episode or bipolar disorder.[5] Nonetheless, psychiatrists and other healthcare providers almost never diagnose a patient as suffering from antidepressant-induced mania, instead choosing to diagnose the patient with a primary psychiatric disorder such as bipolar disorder or manic episode. In my clinical and forensic experience, I have rarely seen a doctor diagnose a patient as suffering from drug-induced manic symptoms. In none of the legal cases in this book did the prescribing physician ever acknowledge that his or her prescription caused the manic outburst. I cannot recall in recent years seeing a single patient who had been properly diagnosed with a substance-induced mood disorder even when it was an obvious case. In almost every case, the doctor attributed the drug-induced symptoms to the patient's "mental illness."

What causes such professional blindness toward the adverse effects of psychiatric drugs? In many instances there is probably nothing more at work than the human tendency to deny responsibility for causing harm. However, the prevalence of professional denial of adverse drug reactions ultimately results from the iron grip of the psychopharmaceutical complex on medicine and psychiatry.

HIGH RATES OF ANTIDEPRESSANT MADNESS IN ADULTS[6]

IN 1996, Robert Howland from the University of Pittsburgh reviewed the medical records of 184 patients who had been treated at a university clinic and hospital with SSRI antidepressants including Prozac, Paxil, and Zoloft.[7] He found eleven patients (6 percent) in whom mania was clearly associated with starting the drugs. The reactions were "generally quite severe" and eight of the eleven patients became psychotic, including four who were so agitated that they had to be put into seclusion.

In 1997, researchers carried out a prospective study—they followed ongoing treatment cases to observe their reactions to antidepressants.[8] Of two hundred inpatients treated with Luvox (fluvoxamine), fourteen developed hypomania, which is mania of lesser intensity. Three additional patients developed psychosis with *aggression*. The overall rate of these disturbances in response to Luvox was 8.5 percent.

In 2001, Adrian Preda and a group of researchers from the Yale Department of Psychiatry studied the medical records of 533 consecutive psychiatric patients who had been admitted to the Yale–New Haven Hospital over a fourteen-month period. They found that 8 percent of the admissions could be attributed to mania or psychosis caused by antidepressants. For more than a quarter of these patients it was their first manic episode, confirming that these drug-induced reactions commonly occur in individuals with no prior history of mania. The newer SSRIs were the most frequent culprits but older antidepressants were also involved in causing mania and psychosis. Two of the patients heard voices (hallucinations) commanding them to kill themselves.

Physicians too often mistakenly believe that antidepressants can only cause mania in especially vulnerable people who have already displayed manic tendencies or have some hidden vulnerability to do so. As these and many other studies[9] confirm, that is simply untrue.

HIGH RATES OF ANTIDEPRESSANT MADNESS IN CHILDREN

COMPARED TO ADULTS, children are at even greater risk of developing mania and other behavioral abnormalities when exposed to antidepressants. In

1997, a highly promoted controlled clinical trial conducted by a team led by Graham Emslie from the University of Texas in Dallas found that Prozac caused a 6 percent rate of mania in depressed children and youngsters age seven to seventeen.[10] This is six times the rate found in adult clinical trials. The reactions were severe enough to cause the children to drop out of the clinical study. By contrast, none of the depressed youngsters given placebo in the same study developed mania.

The finding that Prozac caused mania in 6 percent of children—once again, six times the rate in adults—in a brief, controlled clinical trial should have raised a red-flag warning. It should have been highlighted in the introduction, abstract, discussion, and summary of the article. Instead, the pro-drug authors led by Emslie buried the data deep in the report in a brief sentence explaining why some children dropped out of the study. Meanwhile, they pronounced the drug "safe" in their conclusion. Eli Lilly sponsored the study.

Keep in mind that this rate of 6 percent for Prozac-induced mania in children occurred in a carefully supervised, short-term, controlled clinical trial using highly selected patients. Similarly, the high rates of antidepressant-induced mania in adults occurred in scientific studies and clinical rates. The actual rates for adverse drug reactions like mania will be much higher in real-life clinical practice.[11]

In clinical trials, exposure to the drug lasts about one month, while in actual practice it can last for many months and years. The vastly increased number of days of exposure increases the risk of toxicity and serious adverse reactions. In clinical trials, children or adults are excluded from the study if they have preexisting mania, psychosis, or suicidality, while in actual practice the drugs are often given to these very disturbed individuals, again increasing the risk of severe abnormal reactions. In clinical trials, only one drug is administered to the patient, while in actual clinical practice multiple drugs are commonly given simultaneously. In clinical trials, the patients typically are evaluated once a week, often with the help of checklists and tests, while in actual practice the patients are seen irregularly, often with long periods of time between visits, and rarely with any kind of thorough evaluation. In clinical trials, the doctors are often experienced in detecting adverse reactions, and they are working from a protocol that actually tells them what to look for, while in actual practice most physicians have little awareness of adverse drug reactions and have little time or inclination to evaluate them.

Not only will adverse reactions happen more frequently under everyday treatment conditions, they will become much more severe before anyone realizes what's happening. Thus, when 6 percent of children develop manic symptoms in a clinical trial, as a rough estimate double or triple that number are likely to develop these same symptoms in real-life, everyday clinical practice.

THE RISK OF GIVING ANTIDEPRESSANTS TO ESPECIALLY VULNERABLE PATIENTS

ALTHOUGH THE NEWER antidepressants very frequently cause mania in people with no history of mania, they are even more likely to do so in people who have a prior history of displaying maniclike symptoms. Giving the newer antidepressants to "bipolar patients"—that is, people with a prior history of mixed depressive and manic symptoms—is one of the most common and dangerous mistakes made in modern psychiatry. When patients have had past manic episodes, their risk of developing another one while taking antidepressants becomes astronomical.

In 1998, Harold Boerlin and a team of researchers at UCLA published a study of seventy-nine "bipolar patients" who were given routine treatment with antidepressants in a university clinic. A staggering 28 percent of patients developed drug-induced mood elevations, including 10 percent whose reactions were considered "severely disruptive." When more than a quarter of a specific group of patients develop abnormal mental reactions to a drug, it's time to reexamine whether it should be given to them, ever. Another report in 2001, found similar results when observing patients diagnosed with bipolar disorder who were treated with antidepressants—mostly SSRIs—for at least six weeks.[12] They found that 24 percent switched from depression to hypomania or mania. Consistent with many cases in this book, they observed that all of the switches from depression to mania started shortly after the antidepressant treatment began. This is an incredible risk—more than one-quarter of patients with a history of mania suffered a maniclike episode when placed on an SSRI.

Increasing numbers of scientific studies confirm that patients with a prior history of mania are dangerously susceptible to drug-induced mania. In 2003, a group of experienced researchers and clinicians warned, "The risk of antidepressant-induced mood-cycling is high," and "There are significant risks of mania and long-term worsening of bipolar illness with antidepressants."[13] Nor was the risk compensated for by the benefit of suicide prevention: "Antidepressants have not been shown to definitively prevent completed suicides and reduce mortality." Too often, doctors feel compelled to give antidepressants because the patient is suicidal, but, antidepressants don't *prevent* suicide, they *cause* an increased rate of suicidality in depressed patients of all ages.

A 2003 report found, "Antidepressant induced manias have been reported with all major antidepressant classes in a subgroup of about 20%–40% of bipolar patients."[14] The authors concluded, "About one-quarter to one-third of bipolar patients may be inherently susceptible to antidepressant-induced mania."

Of course, these are enormous risks that no informed patient would want to take—and that no ethical doctor should inflict—yet patients with a past history of manic symptoms are commonly given these drugs. I frequently see new patients who have been diagnosed bipolar and then treated with antidepressants, often with disastrous results.

What can we conclude from these studies? In plain English, if you've had a maniclike episode in the past or if you've been diagnosed bipolar, the antidepressants are very likely to push you into a manic episode. The odds are at least one in four (25 percent) that this mental catastrophe will befall you. If you haven't had a manic episode in the past and you're given an antidepressant, the odds nonetheless approach one in ten (6 to 10 percent) that you'll become manic as a result of taking the drugs. In a rational world, this data would lead to pulling newer antidepressants off the market—including drugs like Prozac, Paxil, Zoloft, and Celexa—but not when the government drug-monitoring agency is in reality a drug-promoting agency.

ASSAULTING HIS COLLEAGUE WITH A TACK HAMMER

FRANK KARMACK, MD, had a successful psychiatric practice. He was an active man who mastered and enjoyed many skills from flying and sailing to investing. Then, a number of unfortunate events caused stress in his business and family life, as well as his practice. He ended up in litigation against a female colleague, and she in turn sued Frank's son, who was involved in the business.

Frank started himself on Prozac in the hope of relieving tension and of raising his spirits. When he didn't seem to feel any better, he sought treatment from a fellow psychiatrist. That led to the prescription of other antidepressants while he further deteriorated.

For the first time in his life, Frank attempted suicide while taking Paxil and was hospitalized. This occurred many years before May 2006, when the manufacturer of Paxil at last admitted that its drug increases the rate of suicidal behavior in depressed patients across the age spectrum. The hospital psychiatrist placed Frank on another similar antidepressant, Luvox—the same medication Eric Harris was taking when he assaulted Columbine High School in Colorado. I was a medical expert in two legal cases surrounding Eric Harris and can verify that he was taking increasing doses of Luvox during the year of his mental deterioration into violent madness and that on autopsy he had a "therapeutic level" (that is, an effective level) of the drug in his system.[15]

The label for Luvox as found in the *Physicians' Desk Reference* indicates that 4 percent of children in controlled clinical trials became manic while taking the drug for obsessive-compulsive disorder. Furthermore, although the drug helped children eight to eleven years old, it did not have any effectiveness for children twelve to seventeen years old.[16] Nonetheless, the FDA compliantly approved the drug for all ages of children ages eight to seventeen for the treatment of obsessive-compulsive disorder. Like Eric, Frank Karmack deteriorated on Luvox until he "cracked" and became violent.

Two months prior to the assault, Frank's psychiatrist recorded that Frank was suffering from disturbed sleep, racing thoughts, increased irritability, and emotional instability (called lability). Although these are well-known manic-like adverse effects of antidepressants, the psychiatrist did not recognize that Luvox might be causing Frank to switch from feeling depressed to feeling manic.

One month prior to the assault, Frank's psychiatrist increased the dose of Luvox from 100 mg to 150 mg per day. Meanwhile, Frank grew increasingly outraged at his female colleague with whom he and his son were in conflict. Dressed in only the most meager disguise—fatigues with a hat pulled down over his face—Frank lay in wait for her in the bushes outside her office. When she came out alone, he leaped on her and began smacking her in the head with a small tack hammer. The weapon was not heavy enough to stun her and so she recognized him immediately, but Frank persisted in striking her as if he could somehow get away with it.

Still imagining that the woman would not recognize him, Frank forced her to agree to sign a document exonerating his son in their conflict. When she fulfilled his demand, he stopped beating her and fled, covered with blood.

Frank's attack on his colleague was brutal. He inflicted multiple wounds on her body with the lightweight hammer. Starting early in the 1990s, I noticed that Prozac was causing especially violent acts of aggression and suicide. In 1994, researchers from Johns Hopkins reviewed all the deaths recorded by the Maryland medical examiner over a four-and-a-half-year period to locate cases of suicide where either Prozac or an older antidepressant had been detected in the blood.[17] They found that patients who committed suicide on Prozac were almost three times more likely to use violent means such as shooting, stabbing, suffocation, strangulation, drowning, falling, or jumping in front of a moving vehicle.

If Frank had been in his right mind, he never would have expected the violent assault to have its desired effect—that the victim wouldn't recognize him or figure out that he was the one who wanted to force her to exonerate his son. He would have realized that, of course, she would not honor such a brutally coerced contract and instead that he would be charged with a heinous assault.

Believing that he had now protected his son by forcing his colleague to sign the agreement, Frank tried to complete his plan by killing himself. Instead of using readily available pills (he was a medical doctor) or a gun (he owned pistols), Frank had contrived to disable the catalytic converter on his car so that he could kill himself with carbon monoxide poisoning. Typical of manic planning—elaborate, grandiose, and futile—Frank had bought special tools and obtained detailed instructions on the project. After trying to deactivate the catalytic converter, he climbed into his car and turned on the gas, hoping to poison himself. It didn't work—his car's catalytic converter was not sufficiently impaired—and he survived. After his capture by the police, an elevated carbon monoxide level in Frank's blood confirmed that he had attempted and failed to poison himself with automobile exhaust.

Neither Dr. Frank Karmack nor anyone else involved in his criminal case understood that he was spellbound by an antidepressant and thereby severely disturbed at the time of the assault. No one seemed to realize that Frank remained out of his mind during his defense preparation and trial. The madness induced by medications can long outlast the last dose—people can remain unstable for months afterward—but in Frank's case he continued to take prescribed antidepressants while incarcerated. Before, during, and after the trial he was in the spellbinding thrall of antidepressant mania.

Frank was a psychiatrist with experience as a medical consultant in the courtroom but he did not perceive that anything was the matter with him or his irrational, drug-induced way of thinking and behaving. He was so sure he was normal that he refused to plead insanity. Although he had the psychiatric knowledge to do so, he was too honest to fake an insanity plea!

Instead, Frank convinced himself that he hadn't committed the crime and insisted on testifying on his own behalf. He argued to the jury that his victim, who knew him personally and professionally, had misidentified him, and that he had actually come upon a stranger assaulting her. Frank explained that he had wrestled with the real perpetrator and become covered with the victim's blood. He was a hero but he fled because he thought people might mistake him for the culprit.

Frank's defense was nearly as bizarre as his doomed assault on his colleague. Instead of gaining potential sympathy from the jurors as a person consumed by drug-induced mania at the time of the assault, he offended them by making up a preposterous series of explanations.

Given how disturbed Frank was while taking Luvox at the time of his trial, how was he able to convince his attorney to allow him to testify on his own behalf? People in maniclike states can be very convincing, especially to observers unsophisticated about identifying psychiatric disorders. Even in the throes of a drug-induced manic state, Frank remained a highly intelligent and charismatic doctor.

But if Frank was so emotionally disturbed, how was he able to plan such an elaborate story in his own defense? As described earlier in the chapter, people undergoing maniclike reactions often make and implement elaborate plans. Frank's effort on the witness stand was typically manic in its irrationality and grandiosity in claiming to be the hero rather than the villain.

Dr. Frank Karmack's life and medical career were left in a shambles and he was sentenced to several years in prison. As he gradually recovered in prison from antidepressant toxicity, he began to suspect that the drugs had played a role in his deterioration. Every FDA-approved label for antidepressants mentions the risk of causing mania, and the official *DSM-IV-TR* repeatedly mentions that antidepressants cause manic symptoms. As a result, any psychiatrist should have some awareness of the problem, but while spellbound on the antidepressant, it never dawned on Frank that he was intoxicated. This blunting of self-awareness is a central feature of medication spellbinding.

I was consulted in Frank's case long after his trial when he was considering an appeal based on newly available scientific evidence that I had been evaluating and generating. As I sat interviewing him in a corner of the prison recreation hall, I was struck by what a sober and intelligent man he was, and also by the respect with which the prison staff treated him. Frank had been tapered off the stimulating antidepressants for some time but was still taking Serzone,[18] a more sedating antidepressant less frequently implicated in medication madness.

When I interviewed Frank in jail, there was nothing whatsoever strange or dysfunctional about him. I could have been having lunch at a conference with a respected colleague who was professionally interested in hearing what I had to share with him.

Because Frank had already served much of his sentence, he felt he had little to gain from seeking a new trial. He was most interested in having me shed light on how he could have committed such horrendous acts. Like nearly all survivors of drug-induced mania and psychosis, Frank had been plagued by questions and doubts about himself, especially about how he could have attacked someone so violently. I was able to show him how his behavior fit the classic pattern of antidepressant-induced maniclike behavior. I brought along scientific reports describing in detail how antidepressants drive people into states of madness.[19] It was sad and yet gratifying to take him through the scientific literature to illustrate how commonly antidepressants like Prozac, Zoloft, Luvox, Paxil, and Effexor cause manic symptoms.

No longer feeling suicidal or violent, Dr. Frank Karmack is grateful to be alive. He told me, "I think life's a gift. As difficult as prison is, life is still a gift." In a way that's foreign to real perpetrators, Frank expressed appreciation for the humane and kind treatment he received in jail. If only he had received better treatment from his colleagues in psychiatry—if only his antidepressant-induced suicide attempt, followed by his antidepressant-induced mania, had been recognized and the drugs stopped—he wouldn't have perpetrated violence and his colleague wouldn't have been so brutally attacked.

A DOCTOR COLLECTS CONSTRUCTION MACHINERY

DR. VERNON KIRKLANDER had developed anxiety during his surgical residency in 1996, and began taking 2 mg of the tranquilizer Klonopin each day. His anxiety improved and he stayed on the drug for many years without any noticeable side effects while he went on to become a successful practicing surgeon.

After moving to the country to enjoy more outdoor activity, in 2001, he began self-medicating for allergies complicated by mild asthma. He took two over-the-counter drugs that turned out to be very dangerous for him. One of the medications, pseudoephedrine, is a stimulant that can cause maniclike behavior. Dr. Kirklander took several times the recommended dose. (Although these drug reactions appear to be uncommon, I have personally evaluated two cases of psychosis induced by this common cold medication.)

The other nonprescription medication was a steroid preparation (androstenedione/androstenediol mixture). On March 11, 2005, the FDA issued a warning to manufacturers to stop distributing products containing androstenedione because of its steroidal effects. Like prescribed steroids, the mixture was causing aggression and extreme mood swings. Unfortunately, the removal of the preparation from drugstore shelves took place too late for Vernon. In an effort to control his worsened allergies, he also gave himself a long-acting shot of the steroid dexamethasone, greatly adding to the steroid load in his system, and, thus, to the increasing risk of mania and other adverse psychiatric reactions.

Vernon was also undergoing two serious stresses. Some of his investments had gone bad, and his wife and child were temporarily separated from him. Fortunately, his busy surgical practice continued to do well and was grossing over three hundred thousand dollars per year.

While taking the drug combination of a stimulant, steroids, and Klonopin, Dr. Vernon Kirklander committed his first act of irrational thievery. At the time he was trying to make up his business losses by renovating an office building and he decided he needed an extra air compressor. Although Vernon had no need for it—he and his partner already had a working compressor—he took a bulky 150-pound machine from the hospital where he practiced surgery. He carried it down a flight of stairs, past video cameras he'd seen day after day, and placed the heavy object in his car.

Almost immediately Vernon grasped that he had done something really stupid and he started to return the machine. This time it became apparent to him that surveillance cameras would observe him. So he hid the compressor behind a Dumpster at his office.

As it turns out, hospital surveillance cameras had already recorded him carrying off the compressor, but the photos were too blurred to make a definitive identification. Nonetheless, Vernon confessed the theft to the hospital administrator. No punitive action was taken other than to order him to seek psychiatric treatment.

For reasons that seem mysterious, the psychiatrist decided that Dr. Kirklander had attention-deficit hyperactivity disorder (ADHD) and furthermore that the ADHD had caused him to commit the theft. Vernon would later explain to me that both the psychiatrist and his psychologist colleague had diagnosed themselves with ADHD, so perhaps it was a fad label in the office. No evidence of Vernon's supposed ADHD was put into the medical records and there's no reason to associate the diagnosis with criminal behavior.[20]

If Vernon's psychiatrist had taken an adequate medical history, he would have found out that his patient was taking very large doses of a mild stimulant, additional doses of a dangerous over-the-counter steroid mixture, and a single long-acting injection of a potent prescription steroid. He could have determined that his patient had undergone a maniclike disinhibition and that he should avoid stimulants and steroids in the future.

Instead, as treatment for his mistaken diagnosis of ADHD, Vernon's doctor put him on Adderall, a mixture of old-fashioned amphetamines. Thus, he subjected his patient to increased overstimulation. Soon the dose was raised to 60 mg per day, about double the usual maximum amount. The man who had become manic on large doses of a very mild stimulant, pseudoephedrine, was now being prescribed very large doses of an exceptionally strong stimulant, amphetamine. Meanwhile, Vernon remained on the Klonopin he'd been taking for years.

A few months after prescribing the Adderall, Vernon's psychiatrist decided to cut the dose in half to 30 mg—the usual maximum. Simultaneously, he started Vernon on Strattera 80 mg per day, the ADHD treatment that's been advertised by Eli Lilly as "nonstimulant." While taking Adderall and Strattera, two highly stimulating drugs, Vernon became manic and perpetrated perhaps the most senseless and outrageous series of robberies I've ever evaluated as a forensic medical expert.

In retrospect, Vernon Kirklander's out-of-control behavior in his early forties seems like a caricature of young male fantasies. Men like to acquire and to play with big toys and so manic disinhibition often expresses itself through buying unneeded expensive cars. Vernon's case surpassed the ordinary.

One evening, Vernon rode his eighteen-speed bicycle fifteen miles to a construction site where he had a good time driving a piece of machinery around the various obstacles. When he was finished playing, the forty-plus-year-old doctor decided he was too tired to ride his bike back home. So, he left his valuable (and potentially identifiable) racing bike behind and drove home in a fuel tanker truck. He parked the tanker in his driveway, went to bed, and fell asleep.

Vernon's wife awoke in the night to the unsettling mystery of the tanker truck in the family driveway. When she asked Vernon about it, her husband seemed confused and had no good explanation. In my medical-legal report for Vernon's case, I wrote:

> I asked Vernon's wife about her recollection of the event involving the tanker truck in the driveway. She remembered getting up that night around 1 to 2 AM and seeing the truck in the driveway. It was the type used to deliver fuel to homes. He was acting confused, asking where he had left his car keys. When she asked him about the tanker truck, he gave no explanation.

In retrospect, she thinks she may have partially shocked him back into reality when she confronted him, because he began repeating, "Oh, I gotta take it back." She told me, "He was all over the place and I couldn't have a conversation with him." When she got up in the morning, the truck was gone.

Vernon drove the truck some distance away from his home and left it for the police to find and to return to its rightful owners. It was the kind of stupid prank that might have been committed by two or three extremely drunk high school seniors celebrating graduation, not by a responsible surgeon who hadn't had a drop to drink.

On another occasion, Vernon returned a backhoe to a friend and borrowed a bucket truck from him. Called a cherry picker, it was the kind used by telephone linemen. He then drove the bucket truck through town and onto a construction site. At the site, he stole a large trailer with a backhoe sitting on it, and proceeded to use the bucket truck to pull the trailer and backhoe through town. It was something out of a comedy—the respected surgeon known to many citizens of his small town using a borrowed cherry picker to pull a stolen trailer and a backhoe through the village in broad daylight.

Vernon drove the odd conglomeration of vehicles to his friend's farm where he parked the stolen backhoe and trailer in his barn. The next day, Vernon's friend had no idea where the machinery had come from and called the police who took it away.

What could have motivated Vernon to steal large construction machinery in broad daylight and under such ridiculous circumstances? Neither Vernon nor I could come up with an explanation. He had unlimited access to his friend's backhoe. Why add to his friend's collection of machinery by anonymously depositing a second backhoe on a trailer in his friend's barn?

Under the influence of rising doses of Strattera, Vernon eventually collected and kept for himself two backhoes, two tractors, three industrial trailers, and a pile of lumber. He stored everything in open view near the roadside around his home in the country, never using or trying to sell any of it.

The end of Vernon's thievery came when he tried to use his luxury Lexus sedan to pull a huge piece of construction machinery, a backhoe on a triple-axle trailer. It was Sunday and the site he stole from was a block away from the police station in the center of town. Towing the twenty-five-ton load was too challenging a task for his sporty car, and the trailer and its cargo toppled over on the highway, bashing into his vehicle, and tying up traffic.

Vernon tried to drive his car away from the scene but had to stop to fix a flat tire. A policeman responding to the accident spotted Vernon's battered automobile alongside the road, and put two and two together.

The police obtained a warrant to search the doctor's premises but they might as well as stood out front of his house and looked around, because all the stolen machinery—tractors, backhoes, and trailers—were parked out in the open, much of it visible from the road.

In our interviews, Dr. Kirklander could neither recall nor explain what had been going through his mind at the moment of the thefts, but he thought they might have begun with wanting to fix a broken waterline from his house to his barn—a job requiring hand shovels and sweat, not machinery. Since he knew where the break was—water was bubbling up—it would have been a quick, inexpensive fix. Meanwhile, he never completed the simple waterline repair. Furthermore, Vernon's explanation doesn't fit with how it all actually began—using the tanker truck to ride home after playing with machinery at the construction site.

In reality, no psychological explanation can account for his behavior because he was driven by medication madness with profound spellbinding and maniclike symptoms. Throughout his escapades Vernon never applied his medical knowledge to himself. He never grasped that he was toxic on a huge dose of stimulant drugs, literally being driven mad by them.

During the two months time in which he committed the many thefts of building materials and machinery—none of which he ever sold or used—Vernon became a living demonstration of every category of symptoms listed for mania in the *Diagnostic and Statistical Manual of Mental Disorders,* including grandiosity (grand thefts, to say the least), decreased need for sleep, talkativeness, racing thoughts, distractibility, feverish goal-directed behaviors, and excessive pleasure-seeking activities such as playing with and absconding with huge pieces of construction machinery.

After Vernon was arrested and released on his own recognizance, his psychiatrist perceived that Vernon was displaying maniclike symptoms but did not attribute them to the supposedly nonstimulant Strattera. The recommended maximum Strattera dose was 100 mg per day but the doctor was prescribing him 120 mg. In addition to keeping Vernon on his Klonopin, the doctor now added two more drugs—the antipsychotic Risperdal and the mood stabilizer Lamictal, both in small doses—in an effort to calm his patient's manic symptoms. The other drug effects could not contain the overstimulation caused by the Strattera, and Vernon progressed deeper into mania.

Vernon readily confessed to all the crimes he could remember and did his best to provide details. Then came the day for Vernon to go to the police station to voluntarily sign a formal confession admitting to his various acts of larceny. As the hour approached for his appointment with the police, Vernon panicked. Had he stolen other smaller items that would be found in his house? The police had no plans to push the case any further, but Vernon was still spellbound by his prescribed medication, including Strattera 120 mg per day, and was in a state of tumultuous confusion and fear.

Despite the fact that Vernon had confessed to everything he could remember, he grew afraid the police would find something more. The trouble was, his memory was completely shot for the period of the thefts. So he ransacked his home, dumping odds and ends into his pickup truck. If he couldn't recall where the item had come from, it went into the truck bed. Then, he drove the load of miscellaneous stuff to a local quarry to dispose of it. His bumbling efforts ended in his truck getting stuck in the midwinter mud and slush, and he had to call his wife to pick him up. In his rush to get to his confession, he left the truck behind. But he was late for his confession anyway.

Later, Vernon went back to salvage his truck. This time the owner of the property spotted him and called the police for littering. The local police officer arrived and, not surprisingly, he knew Dr. Vernon Kirklander. He wasn't fooled for a minute when the doctor gave a false name. Besides, as Vernon started to depart, the policeman called him by his real name, and Vernon answered to it. Even if Vernon hadn't been so easy to trap, he was carrying his wallet with all his identification. As a result, two misdemeanors—trespassing and "falsification"—were added to his six felonies.

Was Vernon's effort to hide his identity an indication of conscious conniving—and the capacity to control his thoughts and behavior? No. The anecdote demonstrates that he was so bamboozled by drugs that he'd say almost anything when frightened, however stupid or self-defeating.

As for the possible stolen goods that Vernon had dumped at the quarry, with one exception they turned out to be stuff that he and his wife had owned for years. The police found only one item that didn't seem to rightfully belong to Vernon and his wife. It was a 300-pound motorized scaffold—the sort of thing used for repairing or painting tall buildings. Vernon has no idea when, where, or why he had obtained it, or even how he got it onto his truck.

There was more to come. Four months later in the spring—still taking Strattera 120 mg as well as the other medications—Vernon was allowed to retake possession of his impounded car. He knew his self-control was still shaky, and he was nervous about going to the police facility to pick up his car. So he brought his office nurse along with him to monitor and to reassure him.

When Vernon got to the impoundment area he was told that it was closing time and that he would have to come back in the morning. Meanwhile, Vernon knew that his Lexus still had a flat tire from his doomed attempt to pull twenty-five tons of construction machinery down a highway.

Instead of waiting to pick up the car in the morning, Vernon became impatient and decided to get the tire fixed ahead of time. After dark, now on his own, Vernon returned, easily sneaked onto the impoundment area, removed his flat tire, and rolled it away to get it fixed at Wal-Mart—and in the process was easily spotted by someone at the church next door.

At the time, Vernon thought that he was doing nothing wrong—he was merely eager to fix his flat tire so he could pick up his car in the morning—and so he readily and innocently confessed when the police came around to his office later in the evening. As a result, on top of his six felonies Vernon now had a third misdemeanor charge for trespassing.

Dr. Vernon Kirklander could have been sent to jail for much of the remainder of his life; but he was given only eighteen months by the judge who raised serious concerns about the doctor's sanity and urged him to seek help. Specifically, the judge told the doctor:

> I find at this point in your healing process you've not addressed the problem with your compulsion adequately, you've not addressed the problem of this apparent feeling of omnipotence that you have in conducting these actions in a very blatant open manner. I think that they are problems that can be addressed with proper psychological treatment, psychiatric treatment, but I don't think that you have seriously embarked on that treatment.

The judge's use of the terms *compulsion* and *omnipotence* is remarkable. Compulsivity and omnipotence are typical signs of mania. If the judge could recognize them, we are left to wonder how Vernon's treating psychiatrist missed them. Given that Vernon had been taking Adderall and then Strattera, drugs known to cause mania, the conclusion should have been obvious—but it was missed by Vernon's treating psychiatrist who persisted with prescribing Strattera throughout the entire legal process, keeping Vernon in a medication spellbound manic state.

In a lenient mood toward Vernon, the judge released him after three months, the minimum period of incarceration. In explaining why he was setting him free, the judge told Dr. Kirklander, "I don't believe your offenses were economic in nature. I think there are other forces that drove you and you need to sort all that out."

It was, of course, very fortunate that Vernon was required to spend only three months in jail. But in the process, he lost his medical license.

Vernon would not get a chance to sort out the pieces until he got to my office for a consultation many months later. Despite the judge's concerns about Vernon's mental state, Vernon was too medication spellbound to think that the drugs were harming him in any way. At the time of the sentencing hearing, he was taking the same array of medications as when he perpetrated the last few offenses, including Strattera 120 mg per day, as well as small doses of an antipsychotic drug, a mood stabilizer, and the Klonopin he'd been taking for seven years. The offending agents were undoubtedly the initial combination of Adderall and Strattera, followed by the prolonged exposure to very large doses of Strattera.

Spellbound throughout the legal process, Vernon never made a defense of insanity or involuntary intoxication. He never referred to the medication. He was remorseful, confused, humiliated, and contrite. In a document the court asked him to write, Vernon explained, "In summary, though I take responsibility for what I have done, I now, more than ever, understand the thinness of human frailty and the dangers of a broken spirit that is left in isolation." His spoken statements to the judge at the sentencing hearing again make no mention of medications—he was still taking all of them. He told the judge that he accepted responsibility for what he had done and he expressed remorse. In fact, if ever a man had a right to claim diminished capacity, it was Dr. Vernon Kirklander.

Vernon's medications were continued in jail until, without telling anyone, he decided on his own to stop them. For fear of being forced to take them, he at first he didn't tell the jail personnel. During the withdrawal, he later reported to me, he became overtly psychotic. He was sure he was back in college rather than in jail, and that his cellmate was his college roommate. He was shaky, physically rigid at times, and felt pain throughout his body. But he managed to keep it all to himself, undoubtedly saving himself from a broadside of overwhelming antipsychotic medications.

After stopping all the drugs, and seeing the dramatic improvement in himself, Vernon began to suspect that his behavior had been driven by a massive adverse drug reaction. As a first attempt to figure out what happened, he took himself to one of the nation's leading medical centers for two weeks of inpatient evaluation. Psychological testing most remarkably found nothing wrong with him. In my career, I've seen only a few people escape being diagnosed with something on routine psychological testing. This rare occurrence was further confirmation that his behavior had been caused by something outside himself—in this case, the drugs.

The psychiatrist in charge of the case had trouble making up his mind what was going on with Vernon. To his credit, he recognized that Vernon had undergone a psychotic manic reaction to stimulant drugs. But as so often happens the psychiatrist initially decided that his patient probably suffered from a personality disorder, as well as kleptomania that was unmasked or exacerbated by the drugs. There was simply no evidence for any of this speculation. Indeed, it's wholly improper to diagnose someone with a personality disorder or with kleptomania—or with almost any routine psychiatric problem—when the patient is being driven by a drug-induced psychosis. The medication madness has such an overriding impact that there is no way to ascertain what other kinds of problems might, or might not, be going on. In addition, there was no evidence of a personality disorder or kleptomania before he became manic on the drugs.

Dr. Kirklander came to me a couple of months after his hospital evaluation and almost a year after his sentencing. By now he had become convinced that his craziness had been drug-induced and he had already outlined some graphs linking his abnormal behavior to changes in his medication regimen. He wanted me to help him to better understand what had happened and, if possible, to help him restore his medical license. After spending six hours with him that day, I concluded that he was mania free and entirely normal.

After I wrote my report in which I corrected the mistaken diagnosis of an underlying personality disorder and kleptomania, the doctor at the esteemed clinic rethought his original impressions. He verified my diagnosis, stating in a revised affidavit and letter to the medical board, "In summary, the patient suffered a medication-induced psychosis of severe degree, which was undiagnosed and mistreated at the time, resulting in a worsening of his condition, his personality, and his behavior." He withdrew his previous erroneous diagnoses and affirmed that Dr. Kirklander had been a "normal, law-abiding citizen" prior to the medication reaction. He attributed all of the doctor's criminal behavior to the drug-induced mania and he did not believe that Dr. Kirklander would repeat any of his criminal behavior now that he was medication free.

The medical board hired another consultant, a state hospital psychiatrist who concluded that the drugs had done nothing to influence Dr. Kirklander's behavior.

In early December 2006, the other two doctors testified in person at a hearing of the medical board, and I testified by telephone. I thought the hearing officer had been fair and I hoped that Dr. Kirklander's medical license would be restored. Instead, despite my testimony and that of another expert who confirmed that Dr. Kirklander was intoxicated with psychiatric medications at the time of his bizarre actions, the hearing officer recommended no leniency toward Dr. Kirklander and the board upheld the permanent revocation of his license. Dr. Kirklander's attorney, John R. Irwin, MD, himself a physician as well as a lawyer, explained to me that the state medical board prided itself in being among the toughest in the nation and he held out hope that Dr. Kirklander might in the future be allowed to practice in another state. As exemplified by the medical board's decision, physicians in general remain unwilling to face the hazards posed by psychiatric drugs, even when the effects are grossly apparent and scientifically documented as in this case.

One year after the hearing, Dr. Kirklander continues to do well with no recurrence of his medication-induced mania. Dr. Vernon Kirklander, the former surgeon who collected and played with construction machinery, now works for a friend in the construction industry as a handyman.

KNOWN EFFECTS OF ALL STIMULANTS

VERNON KIRKLANDER was not taking any antidepressants but he was taking a tranquilizer, Klonopin. Unlike Xanax, Klonopin is not especially known to cause extreme maniclike reactions and was not my primary suspect in this case. Also, Vernon had been taking the Klonopin for seven years since finishing his residency training without displaying any markedly abnormal behavior.

Vernon was taking a classic stimulant, amphetamine, when his mania first developed. Stimulants cause adverse reactions very similar to those sometimes caused by the newer antidepressants, including insomnia, nervousness, anxiety, agitation, excessive energy, ultimately mania, and sometimes psychosis. Mania is the extreme of overstimulation. As the American Psychiatric Association's *Diagnostic and Statistical Manual of Mental Disorders* specifically states, "stimulants" can induce "maniclike mood disturbances."[21] The manual further observes:

> Amphetamine Intoxication generally begins with a "high" feeling, followed by the development of symptoms such as euphoria with enhanced vigor, gregariousness, hyperactivity, restlessness, hypervigilance, interpersonal sensitivity, talkativeness, anxiety, tension, alertness, grandiosity, stereotypical and repetitive behavior, anger, fighting, and impaired judgment.[22]

Vernon was taking amphetamines under the trade name Adderall, specifically Adderall XR, the long-acting form.[23] The FDA-approved label for Adderall XR[24] warns: "Psychotic episodes at recommended doses, overstimulation, restlessness, dizziness, insomnia, euphoria . . ." Under "Overdose," the label also notes, "Individual patient responses to amphetamines varies widely. Toxic symptoms may occur idiosyncratically at low doses."[25] Dr. Kirklander was receiving doses as high as 60 mg per day—twice the recommended dose—when he developed his initial manic symptoms before being switched to a combination of Adderall and Strattera, and then to Strattera without Adderall.

Unlike antidepressants, which most often cause serious adverse effects early in treatment and during dose changes, chronic or long-term exposure to stimulants makes abnormal mental reactions even more likely and more severe, and long-term use becomes complicated by addiction.

STRATTERA: THE NONSTIMULANT STIMULANT

DR. VERNON KIRKLANDER WAS EXPOSED to Strattera throughout the period that he committed his series of colossally dumb thefts as well as his later misdemeanors. At no time during his criminal activity or his sentencing was he free of Strattera. Why would a doctor give a stimulating drug like Strattera to a patient who was displaying manic symptoms? In order to avoid the stigma attached to stimulants, the drug manufacturer Eli Lilly promotes Strattera as the "nonstimulant" drug for ADHD. To this day the company's Web site www.strattera.com/index.jsp proclaims on its home page, "Strattera, the first nonstimulant medication that's FDA-approved to treat ADHD in children, adolescents, and adults."

It's a clever but potentially misleading promotional campaign. From producing insomnia and irritability to mania, Strattera is as stimulating as the classic stimulants such as amphetamine. In fact, the 2007 *Physicians' Desk Reference* categorizes Strattera as a central nervous system stimulant.[26] However, unlike the classic stimulants, Strattera has not been shown to cause dependence (addiction) and the Drug Enforcement Administration (DEA) does not consider it a drug of abuse.[27]

For a drug that was supposed to be safer for America's children than other treatments for ADHD—for a drug that was supposed to rise above the stigma attached to stimulants—Strattera developed a surprising first. It became the first stimulant required by the FDA to sport a black-box warning about the increased risk of *suicidality*. As published for the first time in the 2007 *Physicians' Desk Reference,* the label begins with a bold WARNING followed by the black box containing the following information:

> **Suicidal ideation in Child and Adolescents—STRATTERA (atomoxetine) increased the risk of suicidal ideation in short-term studies in children or adolescents with Attention-Deficit Hyperactivity Disorder (ADHD). Anyone considering the use of STRATTERA in a child or adolescent must balance this risk with the clinical needs. Patients who are started on therapy should be monitored closely for suicidality (suicidal thinking and behavior), clinical worsening, or unusual changes in behavior.[28]**

In these short-term, controlled clinical trials (six to eighteen weeks long), the rate for suicidality in the ADHD children taking Strattera was relatively small (0.4 percent), but the rate among the same or similar children given placebo was zero. Most important, notice the warning about "clinical worsening," an apt description for what happened to Dr. Vernon Kirklander.

Later in the FDA-approved label for Strattera, there is another WARNINGS section separate from the black box.[29] It repeats the warning about suicidality and adds:

> The following symptoms have been reported with STRATTERA: anxiety, agitation, panic attacks, insomnia, irritability, hostility, aggressiveness, impulsivity, akathisia (psychomotor restlessness), hypomania, and mania.

The label states that these symptoms may be precursors to suicidality.

Each and every one of the symptoms in that list from anxiety to mania can result from overstimulation of the brain and mind. That in itself is reason enough to fault Eli Lilly when it claims that the drug is a "nonstimulant."

The array of symptoms listed in the label should by now sound very familiar. It is exactly the same list—*word for word*—that the FDA put into its warnings for antidepressants in 2005: "anxiety, agitation, panic attacks, insomnia, irritability, hostility, aggressiveness, impulsivity, akathisia (psychomotor restlessness), hypomania, and mania." This confirms the point that I first began making in 1991 in *Toxic Psychiatry* and that I have repeated in multiple books and scientific articles—that the antidepressants and stimulants produce a similar pattern of overstimulation that is linked to both aggression and suicide, as well as mania.

The FDA was so concerned about the risks associated with Strattera that it also required the following warning in bold text starting with the 2007 label:

All pediatric patients being treated with STRATTERA should be monitored closely for suicidality, clinical worsening, and unusual changes in behavior, especially during the initial few months of a course of drug therapy, or at times of dose changes. Such monitoring would generally include at least weekly face-to-face contact with patients or their family members or caregivers during the first 4 weeks of treatment . . .

Like the new warnings for antidepressants, the label emphasizes the risk of serious psychiatric reactions early in treatment and during dose changes. Vernon worsened dramatically soon after he was begun on Strattera.

The new FDA label also required a warning against giving Strattera to patients with a prior manic tendency because of the increased likelihood of causing a new manic episode. The label for Adderall XR issued the same warning. Dr. Kirklander was already in a manic state induced by Adderall when he was placed on Strattera.

CONFIRMATION OF STRATTERA'S DEVASTATING IMPACT

OCCASIONAL SINGLE CASE REPORTS have been published about Strattera causing mania, mostly in children because they are much more likely to be prescribed the drug for the treatment of ADHD. Then in 2004, a larger study was published including a review of the literature and an examination of a group of 153 children treated with Strattera.[30] The researchers found a wide array of adverse psychiatric events with potentially serious consequences, including manic and violent tendencies: "We have observed extreme irritability, aggression, mania, or hypomania induction in 51 cases (33 percent)."[31] One-third of the children suffered serious psychiatric symptoms! A significant portion of them became very disturbed:

Ten patients developed symptoms severe enough to be considered mania, and three of those were hospitalized . . . whereas three others were incarcerated in juvenile detention centers.[32]

Strattera is a potent cause of medication madness.

If even trained physicians fall prey to severe psychiatric adverse drug reactions without realizing what has happened to them, imagine how impossible it would be for children to grasp that their emotionally disturbed and destructive behaviors were not their own fault but the fault of the drugs and the doctors who prescribed them so cavalierly.

FROM RARE TO COMMONPLACE

DECADES AGO when I was an intern and resident in psychiatry (1962 to 1966), we rarely saw or diagnosed manic-depressive (bipolar) disorder. When a patient was admitted to a hospital in a manic state, the poor soul would be trotted out for a staff review at grand rounds in front of the assembled hospital physicians. I can still vividly recall the few cases of mania that I saw and treated those forty or more years ago.

Today, bipolar disorder is so commonplace that most psychiatrists are treating many patients with that diagnosis in their practice at any one time. What has changed? Partly, doctors are making the diagnosis much more loosely. I am seeing children diagnosed with bipolar disorder because they have temper tantrums or seem excessively irritable, when in reality their parents have not learned how to discipline them properly. Especially in regard to children, drug advocates have openly campaigned to increase the rate of diagnosing bipolar disorder in order to unleash powerful, adult medications on children.[33]

This deluge of children diagnosed with bipolar disorder is quite extraordinary. I never saw a single case of childhood bipolar disorder during my psychiatric training and none that I can recall from the early years of my practice through the late 1980s, but nowadays I see many cases each year. A 2007 study in the *Archives of General Psychiatry* estimated the annual number of office-based visits for a diagnosis of bipolar disorder in children and youth between the periods 1994 to 1995 and 2002 to 2003.[34] The researchers found a fortyfold increase in children being diagnosed and treated for bipolar disorder. Ninety percent of these children were being treated with medication. More than 47 percent were being treated with antipsychotic drugs, none of which were approved for children. Thirty-four percent were being treated with antidepressants, which can cause or exacerbate maniclike episodes, and 36 percent were being treated with stimulants, which also increase the risk of mania.

However, the bipolar diagnostic fad does not account for the frequency with which full-blown, obvious cases are actually being seen in both inpatient and outpatient practice, even among children. The diagnostic fad cannot explain the greatly increased admission rate to mental hospitals for documented manic-depressive mood swings.

THE COVER-UP

WHAT'S THE CAUSE OF THE INCREASED RATES of severe cases of mania? Antidepressant medications, and to a lesser extent stimulants and tranquilizers, especially Xanax, are causing the upsurge of manic episodes. In almost all the adult cases that I have evaluated in the last decade, and in *every* child and teenage case I have seen in my office, the manic symptoms had begun after starting antidepressants and, more occasionally, stimulants or Xanax.

In the cases in this book, none of the children and their parents, and none of the adults who were driven into mania by prescription drugs, was told by the treating doctors that he or she had a medication-induced disorder. When occasionally the drug was implicated in any way, it was portrayed as a benign agent that happened to "unmask" a preexisting, underlying bipolar disorder—a theory based not on science but on the physician's impulse to avoid blame for the disaster.

The two men mentioned earlier in this chapter, and many others in stories to come, fit nicely into the official *DSM* criteria for a diagnosis of manic episode with one big exception—their reactions were drug-induced. According to the official diagnostic manual, when a drug causes a maniclike episode, it is improper to make a diagnosis of manic episode or bipolar disorder. As emphasized earlier, when a drug is the suspected cause of maniclike symptoms, the proper diagnosis is substance-induced mood disorder.

Unfortunately, this commonsense and officially approved diagnostic standard is largely ignored in the practice of psychiatry. In almost every case I have evaluated, and perhaps every case in this book, the substance-induced mood disorder has been mistakenly diagnosed as bipolar disorder, laying the blame on the patient's "mental illness" rather than on the doctor's prescription. Like the proverbial elephant in the living room, the drug's obvious role in producing the mania will go unmentioned in the medical record.

It is very prejudicial to the patient to be labeled with bipolar disorder rather than with a substance-induced mood disorder. A diagnosis of bipolar disorder stigmatizes the victim for life as suffering from a serious and potentially recurrent "mental illness" or "psychiatric disorder." Without any scientific basis, the diagnosis is used to push lifetime medication, and in criminal cases, it becomes a justification for lengthy incarcerations in institutions for the criminally insane. The bipolar diagnosis makes it more difficult or impossible to get health insurance or long-term care insurance.

In contrast, a proper diagnosis of substance-induced mood disorder identifies an acute neurological disorder that typically goes away after the medication is discontinued. Instead of lifetime medication, the proper diagnosis discourages further use of the offending drug. *None of the dozens of individuals described in this book went on to repeat their criminal or dangerous behaviors after they were removed from the drugs.*

Chapter 6

Killing Loved Ones to Save the World

THOSE WHO KILL their family members often attribute their actions to commands from God or orders from internal voices. Sometimes, they believe they are saving the souls of their loved ones or even the world itself. Can prescribed medications cause this kind of extreme madness?

ONE OF THE NICEST PEOPLE

MELVIN WORTHY is one of the kindest, nicest people I have ever met and yet he committed one of the most horrendous acts I've ever encountered. Unlike most of the stories in this book that draw on my legal cases, Melvin sought me out for psychiatric treatment after he'd been tried and eventually released, so I've had the opportunity to confirm my good impression of him over the years as he healed his life.

Melvin was in his late thirties at the time of the catastrophe. He had been a contractor renovating homes for a number of years before deciding to return to college to become a teacher. He had finished three years of college toward his degree and was beginning to student teach. He was happily married at the time and was in love with his wife. He had no history whatsoever of being emotionally disturbed or aggressive. He never had fights as a schoolboy and never abused his wife.

Always a shy person who didn't like to exert control over other people, Melvin was nervous and worried about his ability as a student teacher with high school students. His family doctor prescribed Zoloft to help him manage his worrying. It was Melvin's first exposure to psychiatric drugs. He was told to start with a sample package of 25 mg per day. After seven days, he was supposed to incrementally increase the dose to 100 mg. He never got past the seven days of 25 mgs per day.

On his second day on Zoloft, Melvin decided to take a walk through a cemetery near the school where he was teaching. He happened upon a bench with his initials carved into it and concluded that it must be a message from God that he was going to hell. When he heard a motorcycle outside his home that night, he knew it was the devil coming to get him. All of this came over him out of the blue. The ideas were entirely alien to him and to his nature.

Melvin began to search for explanations for what was happening to him. In his medication spellbound, psychotic state he decided that Earth was made up of two species—the more intelligent ones who were out to kill the less intelligent ones. He began to think that his wife represented the more intelligent species and that she was colluding with his family to murder him.

That night he barred the door to the house with a chair and in the morning he feared that his wife's coconspirators were hiding in the woods around their home, waiting to shoot him in the head when he left the house.

By day three on Zoloft 25 mg, Melvin began to see aliens hiding in normal bodies all around him. They were already taking over the world. In a frenzied state of terror, he realized that the alien leader had already taken over his wife's body. When she drove them to dinner at a restaurant that night, he kept the car door unlocked in case he had to jump out to escape with his life. In the restaurant, he made sure he could quickly grab the car keys in case he had to run for his life to the car in the parking lot. His mind was racing fast as he decided she had poisoned his coffee.

In desperation Melvin insisted on leaving the restaurant with his wife to walk around downtown where he hoped to feel safer among crowds of people. There, they bumped into a couple, their neighbors, and he became convinced they, too, were in on the murderous conspiracy against him. He found himself backing against the walls of buildings to keep an eye on everyone.

When it started to rain, his wife offered to give the neighbors a ride home with the two women sitting in the back. Now, Melvin visualized his wife getting ready to attack him from the backseat.

Throughout this period of several days, Melvin Worthy often felt terrorized but at other times he was "high" and giddy with excitement. The night before he went berserk, Melvin was sitting in bed looking at his wife while she slept. She seemed to have the hard shell of an insect beneath her skin. He could see the new underlying structure showing through the skin of her face. He got up and checked himself in the bathroom mirror. He, too, was changing. He was becoming bigger, more hairy and stronger, as if he would "come thundering out of himself as someone who had the power to kill her."

Psychotic breakdowns, whether spontaneous or drug-induced, often have a nightmarish quality. Like awakening from a nightmare, the vividness of psychotic episodes usually diminishes over time and eventually fade from memory. I have reviewed prior hospital records with patients who could recall almost nothing about their thoughts, feelings, or behavior during the time that they were overcome with terrifying hallucinations or delusions. For unknown reasons, Melvin had a more detailed recollection of these horrifying experiences. However, when it came to the actual perpetration of violence, he had the more typical spotty amnesia for what took place. Like almost all the people I have interviewed a few months or more after a drug-induced mental breakdown, he had reconstructed the events from a combination of his unreliable memory and what he learned from others, and he felt ashamed and guilty about what he had done.

The night before the assault on his wife, Melvin couldn't sleep and he got up to drive around by himself for a while. He described "being alone in the world, looking down on a more intelligent species wiping out those of us with lesser intelligence. It was all very clear as if I had it all figured out. My wife was actually the leader of her species. I was going to be the leader of our species."

It was becoming a hopeless situation. Melvin Worthy saw his wife killing him and thought, "When she has killed me, the people near me will spontaneously die off. It was like I was the queen bee for our species."

On day seven of Zoloft, while driving down a highway with his wife sitting beside him in the passenger seat, Melvin became certain that he had to kill the alien inside her to save himself and the world. With delusional thoughts racing wildly through his mind, he drove his car full speed into a head-on collision with a road barrier.

Melvin has a vague memory of reaching over at the instant of the crash to unsnap his wife's safety belt. She was thrown from the car. He staggered out, found her lying on the ground, and began to bang her head against the concrete and then to choke her.

He told me, "As I'm choking her, I remember looking in her eyes and realizing that this was my wife and I'm doing something very bad and that this was wrong."

Melvin's memories are very spotty for the next few hours but he remembered picking up his wife and carrying her three blocks toward a hospital. Along the way, he decided instead to throw them both over the side of a bridge but a high wire fence impeded him. When his wife called out his name, the sound of her voice began to bring him back to his senses.

Melvin was almost run over while flagging down a car for help. The driver was so frightened by Melvin's appearance that he called for help on his cell phone and then sped off.

Melvin doesn't recall when help arrived. In the police reports at the emergency room, he is described as realizing that he had made a terrible mistake, that there is "something wrong with animals like me." He attempted to hang himself but was stopped, and was then committed to a mental hospital.

Within hours of being at the hospital, doctors wanted to start medicating Melvin. At first, they tried to make him continue on Zoloft—the drug that had made him psychotic after the first day or two of exposure. When Melvin refused, they forced him to take Effexor, a close cousin that causes similar problems to the SSRI antidepressants like Zoloft. It made him worse. Finally one of the physicians noted in the record that Melvin was "exquisitely SSRI sensitive." Eventually they subdued him with antipsychotic and mood-stabilizing drugs, and then added yet another risky, stimulating antidepressant, Wellbutrin.

PSYCHIATRY'S COMPULSION TO DO "MORE OF THE SAME"

MUCH LIKE MELVIN WORTHY, patients are often continued on the medications that have driven them over the edge. Sometimes it seems as if the doctors become defiant. Confronted with the possibility that their medications have caused a disaster, they go into denial and compulsively continue or increase the dose of the same or similar drugs. From a more charitable viewpoint, they fail to appreciate that adverse psychiatric-drug reactions often occur after only one or two doses, and instead they decide the drugs haven't had "enough time to work." The result is the same, as they continue prescribing the drug and even increase the dose.

Before continuing with Melvin Worthy's story, a detour into a once venerable private mental hospital may prove enlightening as well as disillusioning. I'll call the young man Uri Updike. To this day, I think of him with regret.

Several years ago I was asked to give grand rounds for the psychiatrists and staff at Chestnut Lodge, a famous private hospital in Rockville, Maryland, immortalized in the novel, *I Never Promised You a Rose Garden*. Once a bastion of drug-free intensive psychotherapy, and the home base to great names in the field like Harry Stack Sullivan and Frieda Fromm-Reichman, the Lodge had already betrayed its traditions and become a typical drug-oriented psychiatric facility. Having already shown its belly, it would shortly expire and close its doors in 2001.

When I arrived to give my presentation at Chestnut Lodge, some of the old-timers still worked at the facility. Their presence lent a sadly nostalgic air to the meeting. I hoped to rekindle some of their spirit, their flagging therapeutic zeal, and their broken confidence. In my own private practice of psychiatry conducted since 1968, I have always worked with the most disturbed patients without resorting to psychiatric drugs. Most of my extensive hands-on experience with psychiatric drugs comes from taking patients off their medications, often after years of exposure to multiple drugs.

To provide discussion material for the grand rounds, I was given Uri Updike's lengthy case record to read and to comment on to the hospital staff. Uri was a young man in his twenties who was proving to be, in the euphemistic language of biological psychiatry, "treatment resistant."

The voluminous records were nonetheless incomplete so I made a special request to obtain Uri's earliest medical and psychiatric records. Uri had been hospitalized for several years since having a psychotic schizophrenic-like breakdown at age nineteen. I was able to track his story back to his first hospitalization and first psychiatric encounter at a well-respected acute treatment hospital in Washington, D.C. When he entered the hospital, he was feeling anxious and depressed in reaction to obvious environmental conflicts and stresses in his life. The medical record acknowledges the psychological causes for his problems.

On the ward, Uri was given an older antidepressant, Elavil (amitriptyline), and soon afterward he became psychotic. The doctors treated Uri as if his psychosis had inexplicably materialized on the wards and he was continued on the offending drug, Elavil.

For the next five or six years, Uri was never removed from psychiatric medications. He was never given a drug holiday to see if he could recover from drug toxicity. He in turn never stopped showing signs of the psychosis that had first overcome him shortly after starting the antidepressant.

I was shocked when I evaluated the Uri Updike's current condition at Chestnut Lodge and found he was taking a variety of antipsychotic and mood-stabilizing agents, including Elavil—the drug that had originally driven him crazy all those years ago. It's as if he'd lost his mind taking LSD and then his doctors had continued him on the hallucinogenic drug for the next half-dozen years.

Of course, I was eager to tell the Chestnut Lodge staff my revelations about the boy Uri, now grown into a young man. I had discovered why Uri originally became psychotic years ago, and I may have discovered how to help him recover at last—by removing him from the original offending antidepressant, followed by gradually removing him from all his medications.

With a couple of exceptions, the hospital staff responded to my evaluation of Uri with a mixture of coolness and hostility. Despite my most earnest efforts during my presentation, the hospital doctors did not agree to change anything about how they were medicating him.

Seeing their reluctance to face the strong probability that Uri was a long-term victim of psychiatric mistreatment, I offered to act as an ongoing consultant in his case or to treat him myself in my private practice. He could remain at the Lodge and come back and forth to see me in my office, as many other Chestnut Lodge patients did with their private doctors. My offer fell on deaf ears.

Uri himself was so demoralized by the years of drugging and incarceration, he was incapable of making decisions. My hands were tied, unless I wanted to take a very radical step by trying to contact his family on my own. I might have found the name and address of his parents in the record but such an action would have raised complicated ethical and legal issues, and I decided not to take the step. As I write this, I remain uncomfortable with my decision not to interfere more drastically during that brief window of time when I might have obtained sufficient information to contact his family.

LIKE ABUSERS IN THE FAMILY

THERE IS SOMETHING in human nature that rebels against being found wrong. When parents are caught abusing their children, or when husbands are caught abusing their wives, often their first tendency is to escalate the abuse. It's as if they are saying defiantly, "I'll show you that you can't stop me!" For this reason, it's important to take strong action against abusers rather than to rely on simply warning them.

I cannot exaggerate how reflexively my colleagues reject any suggestion that their drugs could be making their patients worse, let alone crazy. Consider this additional example. I was giving a seminar to the staff of a local Bethesda, Maryland, hospital—the kind of presentation that has the lofty designation of grand rounds. I was presenting on the subject of antidepressant-induced suicide and violence. It was the mid-1990s when the controversy was becoming well known but no other psychiatrists in the country were willing to speak openly about it.

In the discussion period following my lecture, a psychiatrist stood up and described how one of his patients, a government official with no history of violence, started an altercation at a gas station and hammered an innocent victim with a tire iron. The doctor had prescribed his patient Prozac a few days before the incident. After hearing my presentation, the doctor was obviously shocked to consider for the first time that his prescription might have transformed his patient into a madman.

After he sat down, another psychiatrist stood up. The new speaker puffed up with indignation as he dismissed my warnings as nonsense concocted to gain undeserved publicity. In response to the doctor who thought that Prozac might have driven his patient to violence, he defiantly declared, "The Prozac didn't have time to work. I would have doubled the dose."

None of the assembled physicians contradicted him. Probably none of them knew that adverse drug effects, including loss of emotional control and impulsivity, often occur after the first one, two, or three doses of a drug. Although I would soon be writing about this phenomenon, which would eventually be incorporated into the labels of antidepressants, the drug companies had thus far kept secret that serious adverse psychiatric reactions commonly occur after only one, two, or three doses. Or, perhaps no one wanted to break the conspiracy of silence that has ruled the profession for at least a hundred years since we first denied the abuses perpetrated in state mental hospitals and more recently with drugs, electroshock, and lobotomy.

MISSING THE CORRECT DIAGNOSIS

TO RETURN TO MELVIN WORTHY'S story of psychosis and violence inflicted on his wife while he was taking Zoloft, psychiatrists employed by the state usually act on behalf of the state, that is, on behalf of the prosecution. They are loathe to "let criminals off" by finding them not guilty by reason of insanity, especially if the state is determined to prosecute them. In Melvin's case, however, even the state psychiatrists and then the state prosecutor determined that Melvin was "not criminally responsible," and the judge found him not guilty by reason of insanity. The role of drugs in causing the disorder was never raised in his legal defense. To find him not guilty, it was sufficient that he was ruled insane at the time he committed the violence, regardless of the cause of the insanity.

However, the role of the drug was relevant to his future treatment plan. If his doctors had more forthrightly recognized the cause of Melvin's psychosis, hopefully they would not have treated him with the cocktail of psychiatric drugs, including antidepressants, which made it harder for him to recover.

The hospital doctors diagnosed Melvin with bipolar disorder, severe, with psychotic features. This was incorrect. When a person suffers from a maniclike episode induced by an antidepressant, as I've mentioned several times, the correct diagnosis is substance-induced mood disorder with manic features. Melvin became another example of how psychiatrists almost never honor this clearly defined distinction that's available for all to see in the American Psychiatric Association's *Diagnostic and Statistical Manual of Mental Disorders* (1994 and 2000).

After spending three months in a facility for the criminally insane, Melvin Worthy was committed under court order and transferred from the state facility to a very highly respected and expensive private psychiatric hospital where he spent the next year. Unfortunately, he was treated with the same dumb reflexes that characterize too much of contemporary psychiatric treatment. He was loaded up on drugs, including the antipsychotic agent Zyprexa, the mood stabilizer Depakote, and the extremely stimulating antidepressant Wellbutrin. This cocktail of toxic agents impeded Melvin's recovery. Ironically, he'd been driven crazy by only a few days exposure to low doses of an antidepressant but the doctors wanted to keep him on a raft of drugs, including more antidepressants, for the rest of his life.

Eventually Melvin recovered sufficiently to be released and went to work for a relative. He remained court-mandated to receive psychiatric treatment and also remained heavily medicated. If I hadn't been invited into his treatment, he would probably still be numbed by drugs and unable to recover.

FINDING HIS WAY TO ME

MELVIN WORTHY'S psychotherapist—not his prescribing psychiatrist— decided that Melvin would probably be better off without so many drugs fatiguing him and clouding his brain. Although the psychotherapist was not medically trained, she suspected that the drugs might be reinforcing Melvin's interminable depression, apathy, and lack of energy. The therapist was familiar with my work, so she referred Melvin to me.

Melvin was eager to find help in tapering off his medications, and after evaluating him, I consulted with his current psychiatrist. My colleague thought it was worth a try to reduce Melvin's medication, but he did not want the responsibility and was happy to pass on that seemingly risky task to me. His cooperative attitude toward my efforts was crucial because Melvin was still under the control of the courts and as Melvin's current physician he could easily have interfered with a transfer of medical responsibility to me.

Like most heavily drugged patients, Melvin had little idea how much his current medications were stupefying him and crushing his spontaneity. He suffered from a subtle and potentially devastating kind of spellbinding, the flattening of emotions and will seen in patients taking potent antipsychotic drugs like Risperdal, Zyprexa, and Geodon, as well as mood stabilizers like lithium and Depakote. They often become "snowed under" without realizing how subdued they have become. His therapist told me that Melvin was obviously slowed down, but the same toxic effects that crushed Melvin's mental processes also made it difficult for him to perceive his drug-induced deficits.

I also talked on the phone with, and later met, Melvin's mother who graphically described the medication transformation. Melvin had been a high-energy, bright, and communicative person before being put on the drugs.

Melvin was suffering from psychomotor retardation, a generalized suppression of mental life and physical movement caused by antipsychotic drugs like Zyprexa. The experience feels like a mental and physical straitjacket, or as one patient told me, "like cement in the brain." Part of the mental suppression results from a chemical lobotomy caused when the drugs block neuronal pathways to the highest mental centers in the front of the brain. A similar blockade of neuronal pathways, this time deeper in the brain, produces symptoms that are identical to Parkinson's disease with its flattened facial expression, rigid muscles, stooped gait, and tremor. These neuronal pathways to the frontal lobes and also deeper in the brain depend on a neurotransmitter called dopamine and almost all "antipsychotic" drugs are potent dopamine blockers.[1] In the extreme, patients taking antipsychotic drugs like Haldol, Zyprexa, Abilify, and Risperdal become robotic-looking and even zombielike. A list of these drugs can be found in appendix A.

Other than understandable sadness and remorse, compounded by the psychomotor retardation, Melvin seemed normal. Specifically, he had no signs of psychosis and no paranoid, suicidal, or aggressive tendencies. His former psychiatrist, his therapist, and his mother confirmed the absence of any signs of mental disturbance.

Melvin and I decided together that Zyprexa was causing him the most difficulty and so we began by weaning him off the antipsychotic. Over the next several months, with the permission of the court monitor and supportive help from his therapist, I removed Melvin one by one from all of his medications. As I've found with most patients, his well-being improved as his brain recovered from the drug-induced biochemical imbalances in his brain. He was more able to benefit from his regular therapy sessions and from his more occasional consultations with me.

Gradually, Melvin's confidence and sense of competence returned. He regained his energy, was able to work more effectively, and began to enjoy life again. He became bonded as a contractor and resumed renovating homes and selling them. He still loved his wife, and felt deeply saddened about injuring her and about her subsequently divorcing him, but he understood how she felt. He was remorseful and felt no resentment about her decision.

Melvin Worthy eventually found another woman to love—an intelligent and wise health professional—and a few years ago he brought her to visit me for a couple's session. Melvin wanted to make sure his fiancée fully understood the implications of marrying him. They did get married and have done well together for several years, and I was happy to help him obtain his unconditional release from court supervision.

Not long ago I had another visit from Melvin and his new wife in my Ithaca office, and they both confirmed that he is continuing to do well.

WOMEN KILLING THEIR CHILDREN

MURDER OF SPOUSES, parents, and even children is not uncommon in our world and most of the time it's not related to a psychiatric drug. But sometimes it is, as in my case of a mother who murdered her child. Mrs. Sally Grimm shot and killed her ten-year-old son and nearly killed her sixteen-year-old daughter by beating her with a baseball bat. Sally was thirty-seven years old at the time of the assaults, a married woman with a high school education. In addition to raising her children, she was an active churchgoer. On a trip to her hometown, I interviewed her ministers and friends, who described her as quiet and not very communicative but showed no obvious signs of "craziness."

At the time she attacked her children, Sally had been suffering from depression for six years following the death of her father from lung cancer. After two difficult years, she had sought psychiatry treatment and been given a variety of drugs, none of which seemed to help much. She was briefly hospitalized and was described as being mildly euphoric or hypomanic, probably due to the Luvox she was taking.

The case was very complicated but basically came down to several switches and a drastic increase in her medication shortly before the assault.

Sally had last seen her psychiatrist three weeks prior to the assault when he stopped Lexapro 20 mg and immediately began her on Zoloft 200 mg, a hefty dose for a small woman. To add to the potential for toxicity, she was already taking another antidepressant, Remeron 30 mg. Plus, she was also being prescribed a high dose of Klonopin, a total of 6 mg per day. It was a polypharmacy prescription for medication madness.

In the three weeks leading up the assault, Sally called her doctor several times to complain about worsening anxiety and depression. The doctor responded by making large adjustments in her medication, at first reducing and then increasing her Zoloft, and then reducing it again, while he increased her Remeron. The last phone call and medication change took place the night before her tragic outburst of violence.

The vicious attacks were entirely unprovoked. Sally cannot recall the events but our reconstruction indicates that she probably shot her son twice while he was sleeping on a couch. After that, she awakened her sleeping daughter Celia with blows to her head from a baseball bat. When Celia tried to flee, her mother caught up with her in the kitchen and resumed beating her. It's unclear what happened next but the brutalized, terrified girl managed to hide in an empty bathtub where she nearly bled to death.

Sally's reaction was similar to that of Melvin Worthy who was also taking Zoloft for a short time when he hallucinated his wife as an alien and tried to kill her. Sally's daughter heard her mumbling about God while assaulting her. At one point during her rampage, Sally explained to me, she saw her daughter as a menacing ghostlike figure stalking her.

When Mr. Grimm returned home after work an hour or two after the murder and mayhem, he confronted carnage. The kitchen was splattered with blood and his son lay dead on the floor in the living room. Then, he found his wife in bed trying to asphyxiate herself with a plastic shopping bag. After taking the bag off her head, Mr. Grimm heard his daughter calling faintly from the bathroom.

While Mr. Grimm phoned for help and attended to his badly injured daughter, his wife fled from the house. She sped off in her car, eventually parking it in a secluded area near town. There she napped and awoke to find herself in an alien world peopled by strange-looking little figures living amid quaint old-fashioned cottages. She tried ineffectually to kill herself by scratching her skin with whatever was available in the car, including the pop-up tops of beer cans. Still suffering from medication madness the following morning, Sally drove pell-mell through the middle of town in rush hour in the direction of a busy shopping center while a hot pursuit took place behind her.

Sally was defended by two very able, hard-working North Carolina attorneys, Robert Campbell and Lisa Dubbs. Together we retraced her route by car in rush hour and it became apparent she had been heading into a bottleneck of traffic in the heaviest shopping area. If she had wanted to escape capture she could have taken one of several routes that turned off the road leading away from town. Why was she driving like a madwoman into town? She explained that she was heading to the drugstore in the mall to obtain over-the-counter medicines to commit suicide.

A local sheriff spotted Sally's car and gave chase. At high speed she jumped the median, drove wildly on the wrong side of a busy main thoroughfare, and smashed into an oncoming car, fortunately without seriously injuring anyone.

Police officers almost never report information that will support or encourage an insanity defense. Instead, they are likely to write down questions and answers that confirm the perpetrator's rational state of mind. Also, they rarely allow themselves to be interviewed by medical experts hired by defendants. But the sheriff was kind enough to tell me that Sally's driving was the wildest car chase of his entire career.

When the sheriff reached Sally in her car, he found her sitting upright, apparently uninjured, but stupefied and unresponsive. In the emergency room, she showed no signs of head injury but she was so delirious she couldn't identify herself.

When I saw her several months later in a maximum-security facility for the criminally insane, she was the most depressed person I had ever interviewed. It was difficult to create any rapport with her or to obtain information from her. She was so distraught and depressed about murdering her son that she did not want her life to be spared. She had absolutely no desire to mount an insanity defense or a defense of involuntary intoxication with Zoloft.

Sally did tell me that her family doctor had given her Zoloft several years earlier and "it made me feel dead—like I didn't have the strength to live." When she then told her psychiatrist, "I don't like Zoloft," she says that he told her, "Zoloft is a really clean drug." He said she would do better on the higher doses.

After she was on Zoloft, Sally began to suffer extreme irritability. When I told her that I knew she had turned off the air-conditioning and the furnace in her home, she explained, "Sounds drove me nuts." She felt "really anxious," "numbness in my legs and arms," "sometimes tingling," "sometimes like drunk," and "unstable going up and down basement stairs like drunk."

Finally, she told me that she didn't want an insanity defense, that she wanted to be electrocuted, and that she wouldn't tell me anything more.

I left the facility, feeling profoundly sad. It didn't get any better on the following day when I met with Sally's daughter, Celia, and her husband to learn their viewpoint on what had happened. Mr. Grimm believed that his wife had been driven insane by the psychiatric drugs and that realization somewhat enhanced his effort to find forgiveness for her within himself. It wasn't easy for him. For their daughter, Celia, it was impossible. She had lost her brother and been beaten nearly to death by her mother. She vividly described the terror that overwhelmed her on being awakened by her mother smashing her with a baseball bat.

When I explained that her mother had been made psychotic by the drugs, the youngster understandably refused to express any sympathy. Instead, she displayed her facial and shoulder scars to me. I left that interview feeling more saddened than when I left her mother in the locked facility for the criminally insane. Medication madness cuts a wide, deep swathe of misery through the lives of family and friends.

Court-appointed attorneys Robert Campbell and Lisa Dubbs worked hard on the case and pushed their experts as well. In addition to my devoting hours to reviewing the case and educating the attorneys about psychiatric drugs, they had me spend two very long and emotionally exhausting days visiting the site of the tragic events and conducting face-to-face interviews with Sally's family, her friends, and her ministers. However, it turned out that my testimony about involuntary drug intoxication wasn't needed and I didn't have to testify. Sally Grimm was so grossly mentally deranged that there was no need to argue before the jury that it had been caused by an adverse drug reaction. Her attorneys rightly decided that she was so obviously insane under the law that more subtle arguments to the jury about the role of medication in causing her condition were unnecessary and potentially controversial and confusing.

I've already said this was a complex case. I had some reluctance to testify because of an incident in Sally's life several years earlier in which she had shot someone who was threatening her and her mother. That case was ruled self-defense by the police and no charges were brought. In her trial for murdering her son, the judge ruled that the earlier incident was inadmissible and it was never brought up in front of the jury during the trial. For that reason, I will not give further details in this book, but in the interest of accuracy I want to mention there was this complicating factor in her past history. Nonetheless, Sally had never been psychotic before the weekend that her Zoloft was doubled and I was convinced that the Zoloft, in combination with the other drugs, had made her psychotic at the time she attacked her children.

Chapter 7

Drug-Induced "Happy Faces"

NOT ALL SEVERE adverse psychiatric reactions to medications result in physical violence and not all are experienced with grim purposefulness. Instead, the manic individual may feel convinced of the harmlessness of his behavior and even enjoy its outrageousness. He feels as if he's finally cut loose in order to have a good time. In more extreme drug-induced maniclike episodes, the individual feels high or euphoric, has wildly unrealistic expectations about what he can accomplish, feels invulnerable to consequences, and persists at some outrageously irrational behavior until he is doomed by it—all the time thinking he's having a good time and operating at the peak of his powers.

This chapter tells three stories of drug-induced manic reactions from my practice as a medical expert.

ACTING STUPIDLY—AGAIN AND AGAIN

I DON'T KNOW how many of us yearn to be famous bank robbers or cat burglars, but most people probably never go beyond filching a few extra sugar packets to take home from a fast-food restaurant. In regard to medication madness, I'm sure it mostly gets expressed in the same small ways when it comes to thieving. An individual becomes disinhibited on antidepressants, stimulants, or tranquilizers, and crosses a line they usually would respect. I've had several consultations about women who have shoplifted items of small value under the influence of drugs. I've often heard from people how their driving became more reckless while taking the newer antidepressants. Again, we're talking about a continuum. The more flamboyant drug-induced felonies described in this book are the extreme tip of an iceberg of much larger numbers of smaller crimes and misdemeanors committed under the influence of psychiatric drugs.

Some kids seem to lack ambition. Adam Madison was bright enough, his teachers and parents agreed, but he never settled down to work in school. He did well on aptitude tests and his college boards, and his grades were good enough to get him into a respected college; but no one thought he was working to his potential. His father, Abraham, was patient with his son, maybe to a fault. When you're a successful businessman you want your boy to have the best things that you can give him. But maybe school wouldn't end up mattering that much. His son could always join the family business.

Abraham and his wife, Sarah, contented themselves with realizing that Adam was a good kid. He had friends, never got into fights, and didn't abuse drugs. He'd been in trouble only once in his life while working as a grocery-store cashier at college. He was caught letting some of his friends get through the checkout without paying for everything. It was more like a college prank than a crime.

Adam continued to seem at loose ends about working toward a future. He began drinking too heavily at school and eventually told his parents that he wanted to take a break from college. Fortunately, money was no problem for the family and as long as Adam found some kind of job he could live at home and be given as much pocket money as he needed. His parents also hoped he would figure himself out and they suggested he see a psychiatrist, especially for his drinking.

Adam was placed on Paxil by the psychiatrist's nurse practitioner and soon began to deteriorate into an agitated depression—a combination of anxiety mixed with depression and suicidality. As I've seen in numerous cases, the overstimulation caused by antidepressants can drive people to escalate their alcohol intake in a self-medicating effort to calm down. However, these individuals do not realize that they are suffering from drug-induced overstimulation, and are not consciously aware of using alcohol to sedate feelings of overstimulation.

After Adam started Paxil in April, his mental condition and behavior deteriorated. A little more than a month later, Adam's parents noticed he was drinking more and having trouble sleeping. One day they found him at home crying and curled up on the floor, babbling about wanting to die, and they took him to an emergency room. The ER record reported that Adam had drunk seven to eight beers, and was "belligerent," and was yelling, "I'm insane."

He was also described as "incoherent" at times and making sexually inappropriate comments to the staff. I wrote in my report to the court:

> Unfortunately, the emergency room doctors did not recognize Adam's condition as most probably related to the combination of Paxil and alcohol. This degree of incoherent, inappropriate, out-of-character behavior in a young man is more typical of a Paxil-induced manic state than of alcohol intoxication. Adam had never before become out-of-control while drinking. His blood level, while over the legal limit for intoxication, was not very high for an individual who was accustomed to drinking heavily. Most important, Paxil had been started within the past six weeks, suggesting a close association to his abnormal behavior.

At the time, Adam had been taking a relatively small dose of Paxil 10 mg for less than two months. Two weeks after the emergency room visit and a few days after the Paxil dose was doubled to 20 mg, Adam began a robbery spree, holding up eight local gas stations in eleven days. Once again, his case fits the familiar scenario of a recent escalation in dosage.

There is no evidence that Adam was drunk during any of the robberies. Instead he was described as very calm and seemingly rational with no evidence of slurred speech or impaired gait. He reported to me and to the police that he did not drink at these times and the police found no evidence of alcohol intoxication.

During each of the many gas-station robberies Adam drove his family car—the same vehicle that he and his family had driven to several of the same local stations on innumerable occasions over the years to purchase gas and snacks. Some of the robberies were perpetrated in broad daylight and most were at busy sites with employees and customers present.

Adam wore no disguise whatsoever. At one point, a gas station attendant looked at him with dismay and pointed to the video camera that was recording Adam's every facial expression. Adam paid no attention to the common-sense warning. On another occasion, he parked his car so close that people were able to run after him as he drove off.

For a weapon, Adam carried a blue-handled kitchen knife taken from a set in his home. He would brandish the little weapon in front of groups of mechanics, some of them with large hammers, wrenches, and other potential weapons within easy reach. Adam was tall but slender, and not at all intimidating. Perhaps it was Adam's almost innocent appearance that restrained the men. Perhaps his sheer audacity caught people off guard. None of the men decided to subdue or to shoot him, and no one was physically injured.

Seven out of eight of the targeted gas stations were near Adam's home. He and his family regularly patronized most of them. As the one exception, Adam robbed a gas station near his girlfriend's house. There a surveillance camera captured his image and Adam's photograph was put on the local television. A member of his girlfriend's family easily identified him as the young man on the TV screen.

After the eight robberies, Adam pleaded guilty and received a six-year jail sentence. When he was released on bond for a short period of time prior to serving his sentence, no one imagined that he would use the brief window of opportunity to repeat yet another identical gas station robbery.

In his medication-spellbound state, Adam had no flexibility in his choices and actions, and so he repeated the same type of robbery for a ninth time. Again, he strode into a local gas station in broad daylight. Again, the establishment was so near to his home that he and his family frequently visited it. Again, he wore no disguise. Again, he drove the same family car and used an identical blue-handled knife from the same set in his mother's kitchen. He was easily apprehended after a brief police chase.

There was no evidence that Adam was trying to get money in order to leave town to flee his jail sentence; he had not taken any of the cash that lay around the house. Nor had he taken any clothes or other articles that would indicate an intention to flee. Besides, his gas tank was nearly empty.

Having been recently convicted and sentenced to six years for the identical bizarre offense, Adam now faced spending much of the rest of his life behind bars. At this point, even the judge began to scratch his head. What could be the matter with this kid? Adam was too medication spellbound to attribute any of his behavior to the Paxil. Fortunately, his family began to search the Internet for an explanation and they discovered my work and the controversy surrounding Prozac-like antidepressants such as Paxil.

Adam was not mentally disturbed—not before he began taking Paxil. Adam was not retarded; he was bright. Adam came from an affluent family and had no desperate need for money. Although he drank too much on occasion, alcohol played no apparent role in his irrational actions and he was never drunk during any of the nine robberies. On a few occasions he bought cocaine after the robberies, but that was a new behavior for him and most probably part of the ongoing maniclike reaction.

The robberies weren't motivated by the desire for street drugs. Adam had plenty of money lying around his home that he could have used to buy illegal drugs. The insane quality of the robberies wasn't driven by cocaine because he wasn't high at the time—he never took any illegal drugs before or during the time he perpetrated the robberies. Plus, cocaine addicts are usually far more cunning and hostile.

As in almost every case I've evaluated, Adam's memory was jumbled up and spotty for the robberies, and it was very difficult to reconstruct each of them. I spent hours reconstructing events from the police records and interviews with family and friends. Without knowing anything about Adam's subjective state of mind, the bizarre behavior pattern would indicate that he was mentally disturbed. However, lack of any prior history of criminal behavior or mental disturbances; the presence of symptoms of drug overstimulation such as emotional instability, increased agitation and irritability, insomnia, weight loss, and paranoid fears; the utter irrationality of the acts; the recent increase in his dose of Paxil—everything confirmed for me that this was a case of medication madness.

As in all the cases in this book, Adam and his family had not been warned by the prescribing doctor, nurse, or physician's assistant that the drug could cause abnormal behavior. His parents became suspicious of the drug only after Adam committed the ninth similar robbery while on bond after having committed the initial eight holdups.

Fortunately, his criminal attorney, Steven Wilutis, supported my intervention into the case, and as a result of my report, Adam was given a much lighter sentence than he might otherwise have endured. Instead of spending most of his life in jail for multiple armed robberies, including one committed after he had already been sentenced, he will be released in a few years.

A FIVE-AND-ONE-HALF-YEAR MANIC REACTION

MOST OF THE DRUG-INDUCED manic episodes in this book were relatively brief in duration. They were so abrupt in onset and severe that the individual was unable to stay out of trouble with the law for more than a few weeks. Many were incarcerated in jails or mental hospitals. However, an unrecognized maniclike episode can go on for a considerable period of time, even for years, as the catastrophe for family, friends, and coworkers slowly builds to a crescendo.

To Henry Rodgers's wife, Annette, life seemed financially secure. If anything, she and her husband had been living the high life for the past few years. An old friend of Henry's had decided it was time to repay him for all the work he had put into his friend's business years earlier, so Henry was regularly depositing extra checks and spending lavishly on Annette and their son, and on their home. In addition, he was doing well as an accountant with executive-level responsibilities at a large nonprofit in the health industry. The only stress in their lives was Henry's growing irritability and insensitivity. He bragged much too much about his newfound wealth, spent too much on foolish things, and seemed to have lost much of his genuine feeling for his family.

Everything changed overnight. Henry came home from work to announce that he was in trouble, not serious trouble from his viewpoint, but trouble enough. He'd been caught embezzling funds at work.

"How much?" his dismayed and shaken wife wanted to know.

Well, he really couldn't be sure, but it was a lot.

Without contacting a lawyer, Henry had quickly confessed to embezzling from the organization and voluntarily spent the afternoon helping the independent auditor pick his way through the innumerable forged checks. Appreciating the impending catastrophe, Annette decided to find an attorney.

An Unblemished Past

Henry Rodgers had lived a remarkably normal and responsible life, never abusing drugs or alcohol, never having any trouble with the law. As a high school teenager he was an Eagle scout and began a lifelong habit of working hard to earn money. He finished college and later received a master's degree in finance. He was married with a son whom he adored, and had recently accepted the position as an accountant at the nonprofit.

The same week that he started his new job, Henry was prescribed a psychiatric drug for the first time in his life. It was Paxil. It came about in an unexpected fashion. Henry had gone to his family doctor to ask if anything could be done about his problem with premature ejaculation. The medical doctor referred him to a social worker for counseling and after the first visit the social worker called the doctor with a novel idea. Paxil might help Henry's sexual problem.

Paxil commonly causes sexual dysfunction . . . so why prescribe it for sexual dysfunction? The imaginative social worker thought that Paxil's side effects might benefit Henry by slowing down his sexual response. She was not alone in making this unsound recommendation but it was unusual, and hardly in the professional arena of a social worker.

For the next five and one-half years, Henry dutifully took 20 mg of Paxil every day. He stopped seeing the social worker because he didn't feel she was helping. Meanwhile, his family doctor saw him only once a year for his annual physical exams, so medication monitoring was minimal and psychological monitoring was nonexistent.

When I asked him, Henry thought in retrospect that the Paxil had somewhat improved his premature ejaculation but his wife told me that little or no benefit had been achieved. Patients taking drugs are often the least reliable when it comes to assessing improvement.

Like most patients undergoing serious abnormal mental reactions to antidepressants, Henry Rodgers was so spellbound that he had no idea that he was being adversely affected. As happens especially often when the drug reaction is maniclike in quality, he thought he was doing better than ever. He had proof, too: He was bursting with energy and drive, and doing incredibly well at work where he had even taken over two or three additional jobs as their occupants left the nonprofit.

Although the first signs of mania appeared soon after starting Paxil in the form of his enormous energy bursts at work, Henry's criminal activities did not begin until a year after starting Paxil, when he began to embezzle money from the nonprofit association by writing checks to himself in amounts under ten thousand dollars. By the time he was caught, he had deposited over one million dollars in his joint checking account.

Henry carried out his embezzlement in an absurdly transparent fashion by recording all the checks in the online bank account he had created for the company. After teaching his staff how to access the new accounting system, it quickly became obvious to everyone that he'd been writing innumerable checks to himself.

He made no attempt to hide the checks, instead depositing every one into his readily identifiable joint family account at his bank. At the same time he bragged to friends and family in an offensive maniclike fashion about how rich he had become.

Henry boasted about his newfound wealth to the outside independent auditor who would eventually confront him about his embezzlement. No one in possession of his rational faculties would risk alerting the man most responsible for eventually discovering and proving his embezzlement. Henry was completely medication spellbound.

With increasing intensity over the five-and-a-half-year period of time on Paxil, Henry displayed multiple symptoms of mania, including excessive energy, insomnia, agitation, irritability, aggressiveness, social insensitivity, emotional instability, grandiosity, entitlement, the pursuit of bizarre and doomed plans, and a sense of godlike invulnerability. He was so unstable that two family members wondered if this normally levelheaded man was using cocaine. Although he was not using cocaine, he was taking a prescribed medication that often has cocainelike effects, causing overstimulation and mania.

In the days after he was caught, the consequences of his crimes began to dawn on Henry, and he precipitously dropped from a state of mania into a state of severe depression, culminating in a failed attempt to hang himself. He then tried to overdose on his Paxil, was found by his wife with rope burn marks on his neck, and then was hospitalized. Although Henry had ample reasons to feel that his life was floundering, Paxil probably also contributed to his switch from mania into suicidal depression.

I was called into Henry Rodgers's case as a medical expert within a very short time after his arrest. When I first saw him, he had been off Paxil for several weeks but continued to suffer from severe depression mixed with manic symptoms, such as racing thoughts and irritability.

During my initial evaluation I also met in my office with his wife, brother, mother, and father. Afterward, I brought everyone together again to warn Henry and his family about his continuing vulnerability and the need for more frequent psychotherapy with the therapist he was seeing in another city. When I saw him for his second evaluation with me about two months later, he had been hospitalized again and placed on several potent psychiatric medications. One doctor had wanted to put him on another SSRI antidepressant but Henry had regained his senses sufficiently to refuse.

Like the other stories of medication madness in this chapter, Henry Rodgers's case reflects the "happy face of mania." His activities fit the description of a manic episode in American Psychiatric Association's 2000 diagnostic manual: "Ethical concerns may be disregarded even by those who are typically very conscientious (e.g., a stockbroker inappropriately buys and sells stock without the clients' knowledge or permission; a scientist incorporates the findings of others)."[1] Again, as noted in chapter 6, the diagnostic authority also states unequivocally, "Symptoms like those seen in a Manic Episode may also be precipitated by *antidepressant treatment* such as medication . . ."[2]

Again, typical of individuals in a manic state, Henry was transformed from a responsible and caring person to a self-centered, arrogant, irritable, and controlling man who constantly offended family and friends. At the same time, he was transformed from a frugal financial expert into a spendthrift who spent extravagantly on himself, his home, and his family.

Unfortunately, as in almost every case I've ever seen, Henry Rodgers's physicians were unwilling to document anything in the medical record that impugned the treatment rendered by a colleague. So, Henry was falsely diagnosed with bipolar disorder, even though the history in the same medical chart traced the onset of his problem to taking Paxil.

However, Henry's criminal attorney, James E. Long, was able to grasp the value of what I was saying about involuntary intoxication. In my report on Henry Rodgers's behalf, I wrote:

> Due to the involuntary intoxication caused by Paxil, Mr. Rodgers was incapable of forming the intent necessary for the commission of the crimes associated with embezzlement. His medication-induced disability was a mental disease or defect that caused him to lack the substantial capacity to know or appreciate the nature and consequences of his actions from 2001 through May 2006. He was also unable to control his impulses and unable to conform his behavior to the law. Although somewhat improved, he was still impaired in this regard when I evaluated him in my office on July 31, 2006. When I evaluated him again on October 3, 2006, he was considerably improved.

In order to conform to the letter of the law, I had to describe Henry's disorder as a "mental disease or defect," when in reality he was suffering from something much more specific and concrete: a drug-induced brain dysfunction.

Henry became painfully aware of the damage he has done to others and in a most remarkable fashion he sold most of what he owned, including his home, in order to make as much restitution as possible. He has a very supportive family: His parents and his wife's parents combined their resources and mortgaged their properties in order to pay his bail, and along with other family members they helped to pay his legal and medical costs.

I recommended to the court that Henry Rodgers be allowed to remain in society. He was already suffering punishment in the form of a catastrophically severe medication reaction, public humiliation, depression and suicidality, psychiatric hospitalization, the loss of his professional status and income, financial collapse, and the suffering of his entire family.

Henry was able to negotiate a plea bargain that resulted in a sentence of three to ten years with the possibility of parole after two years. Ordinarily, embezzling one million dollars would have led to a sentence of eight to twenty-five years. According to Henry and his attorney, my report influenced the prosecution and especially the judge in regard to the lighter sentence.

Four months before Henry's sentencing hearing, a news story in the *St. Petersburg Times* described a remarkably similar Florida case in which a company executive embezzled 1.8 million dollars over a two-year period while taking Paxil.[3] He cut 179 checks to himself and to his creditors. After pleading guilty to a felony, the U.S. Attorney's office recommended that he spend forty-one to fifty-one months behind bars; but U.S. District Court Judge James Moody, Jr. gave him only twelve months of home confinement and five years of probation. The judge agreed that Paxil was partially responsible for the embezzler's manic behavior.

There is no way to begin to estimate the number, but undoubtedly there are many unrecognized cases involving embezzlement, fraud, and other white-collar crimes perpetrated by individuals driven into manic states by psychiatric drugs.

THE ENTERTAINING HOME INVADER

MOST OF THE DRUG-INDUCED psychiatric disturbances in this book seem to materialize out of nothing. There's no indication in the person's background to account for a "nervous breakdown," "going crazy," or "losing it," other than the drug reaction itself. By contrast, Earl Cobbler was certainly going through a tough time when he became the jolly robber, but most of his problems became severe after he was placed on psychiatric medication. There was nothing in his background to suggest a potential for these bizarre criminal antics.

Earl had received a bachelor's degree in real estate and urban development and went on to become a real estate specialist at one of the nation's largest stock brokerage firms. From there he went to work as an official in a federal agency handling complex real estate matters. He then became a consultant to several nonprofit organizations concerned with community development and became a successful professional. He had no criminal record and his business activities and community projects were untarnished by scandal.

For many years, Earl had suffered from occasional attacks of anxiety. When he experienced an especially terrifying episode of panic attack, his general practitioner prescribed the tranquilizer Ativan. Probably in an effort to control his anxiety, Earl increased his alcohol intake. Ativan may also have exacerbated his drinking. Not only does the tranquilizer have similar effects to alcohol, it can become a gateway drug to abusing alcohol. Alcoholics are often cross-addicted to tranquilizers like Ativan, Xanax, and Klonopin.

Earl's personal projects and business continued to do well, but his anxiety and his drinking became increasingly worse. He sought help from a psychiatrist who prescribed a variety of medications, including several different antidepressants in succession. Although Earl was too medication spellbound to make the connection at the time, his judgment deteriorated while taking the drugs. He began to make very bad decisions in his real estate deals, landing him deeply in debt and alienating him from his business partners. His wife also separated from him. One might suspect that these stresses could have pushed him toward desperate solutions, but not only was he much too intelligent and emotionally stable to have sought the solutions that he did, literally no one in his right mind would have so cavalierly thrown his life away. That behavior began only after he was begun on Prozac.

Earl's former wife described his deterioration after he started taking Prozac: "It caused him to be extremely delusional. When he started the drug, it was—he had a definite behavior change . . . he was kind of in a dream world about everything, about business, about what was going on in our life, and that was not normal for him." She explained, "He could not think straight. He couldn't control what was coming out of his mouth and I'd have to say, 'I can't understand you, what are you saying?' "[4]

Earl lost so much weight and looked so haggard while on Prozac that his ex-wife worried about his having cancer. She was sure he was "not in his right mind" when he committed the outlandish crimes.

None of the medications made Earl's anxiety go away. When Prozac caused a side effect, Earl stopped using it but later resumed. At the same time, he was being prescribed Xanax during the day and Klonopin at night to help him sleep. Xanax is so short-acting that it wears off during the day, frequently causing rebound anxiety and insomnia, with a worsening of the individual's overall condition.

PROZAC AND XANAX IN A DEADLY COCKTAIL

SOMETIMES TRANQUILIZERS can ameliorate the symptoms of activation (stimulation) caused by antidepressants, including anxiety and insomnia. Unfortunately, the two don't always balance out, and sometimes the combination makes things worse. Tranquilizers have alcohol-like disinhibiting effects and they can be very spellbinding, leading to abuse and addiction. Xanax can cause mania. For some people, mixing antidepressants and tranquilizers exaggerates the disinhibiting, spellbinding effects of both drugs, and results in catastrophic episodes of loss of control.[5]

Xanax belongs chemically to the group of drugs called benzodiazepines—including Valium, Klonopin, and Ativan—that are commonly used to control anxiety and to treat insomnia. They are often called "benzos." A more complete list of tranquilizers, sleeping pills, and other drugs that share similar characteristics will be found in appendix A.

As I document later in the book, all benzodiazepines can cause "paradoxi-cal effects" such as disinhibition or loss of self-control, sometimes leading to violence. They can also cause depression. All of them produce tolerance, abuse, and dependence, commonly known as addiction.

Among the benzos, Xanax is especially likely to cause stimulation, includ-ing agitation, anxiety, disinhibition, loss of control, and ultimately mania. Its po-tential range of effects is surprisingly similar to the stimulating antidepressants and the stimulants themselves—although it more often produces a quieting and sedating effect.

The brain and mind, when healthy, provide the individual with a seemingly unlimited potential for thinking, feeling, and acting, often in unanticipated and creative ways. However, when damaged, the brain and mind possess a much more limited variety of ways of reacting, and, therefore, many intoxicating substances cause similar adverse psychiatric effects. As a result, drugs as dissim-ilar as antidepressants, stimulants, and benzodiazepine tranquilizers can produce similar adverse psychiatric effects from depression and suicide, to mania and violence.

Earl was also taking Antabuse, which discourages impulsive drinking by causing nausea and other symptoms when alcohol is consumed. As a result, Earl had stopped drinking for several years before his life unraveled and alco-hol would play no role in what unfolded. Soon after Earl's psychiatrist doubled his dose of Prozac to 40 mg, Earl's life completely fell apart. He was forty-six years old at the time.

As an added complication to his drug treatment, Earl began to take an over-the-counter cold medication containing ephedrine. Although it is a rela-tively mild stimulant compared to Ritalin or Dexedrine and Adderall, ephedrine nonetheless shares some of the risks, including anxiety, insomnia, and, in rare cases, mania. Although ephedrine was at the time a nonprescription medication, the FDA would later remove from the market any nonprescription (OTC) preparations and supplements containing the drug due to stimulating adverse effects on the cardiovascular system.

Meanwhile, Earl had been reduced to working as a telemarketer for real estate investments and he used the over-the-counter stimulant to stay awake and focused while on the phone. The ephedrine most likely added to the over-stimulation of his brain and mind that the Prozac was already causing. Earl, of course, had no idea that his prescribed medications could turn him into a crazy person. The nonprescription compound with ephedrine in it seemed so harm-less that he never mentioned to his doctor that he was taking it.

To this day, Earl cannot explain what was going through his mind when everything started to spin out of control. He broke into a home and stole a gun. He tried to wave down two young women who were horseback riding in a park but they sped away unharmed. These initial events remain very vague to him. About one month later, he went across the street to his neighbor's house, used a key that their families had previously exchanged, and stole a credit card. The first name on the card was Phyllis but Earl took it into a jewelry store and bought a six-thousand-dollar Rolex watch with it.

First, he signed the credit slip with his real name. When the clerk raised a question about it, Earl took back the slip and signed it with the name on the card, Phyllis Gorman. When questioned again, he explained that Phyllis was a family name and that people called him Phil.

It seems incredible that the clerk would fall for such a story, but people in the early stages of a maniclike reaction can be very engaging. Sheer bluster must have gotten Earl through this improbable bit of lying. Using Phyllis's credit card yet again, he purchased a laptop computer and a handheld personal organizer.

There was, of course, no hope whatsoever that Earl could get away for long with using his neighbor's credit card to buy big-ticket items. He was doomed to get caught, but in his drug-spellbound state he felt invincible.

Having carried out the credit-card thefts, Earl went to his psychiatrist for his first session in two months and received renewals of his prescriptions. According to the doctor's note, Earl told him, "Lots is great," and that he had received five job offers. Gross exaggerations are common signs of incipient mania. Earl also told his psychiatrist that he was late for the session because his car had been broken into. None of this was true but his psychiatrist failed to pick up on the seemingly manic tone.

"It was like I was in two different worlds," Earl told me when I conducted my first telephone interview with him from jail.

Twelve days after the credit-card thefts, Earl was driving from his parents' home to work when he passed by a motel. At an earlier time as a real estate consultant, Earl had evaluated this building on behalf of a chef who wanted to turn it into a restaurant. The deal had never materialized and instead a new owner had turned the site into a motel with little cabins. As he drove by it on this day, Earl resented the new motel whose cabins were "tacky" and an "eyesore."

Earl decided that he ought to rob some of the people who were staying at the motel; that way he would get even with the proprietor for ruining the ambience that had once surrounded the original building. It seemed like a really good idea at the time. No hesitations or fears clouded his determination. He told me, "I just pulled off the road and thought, 'This will be an interesting scene to enact.' " It was as if he was an actor in an artificial drama rather than being in real life.

Although he cannot recall why, Earl had a Halloween mask in his car. It might have been a present for his son for the upcoming holiday. It could have been part of a planned disguise, but it's not clear that he had formulated any plan in advance.

Earl took the stolen gun, put on the mask, and crept up to the window of one of the cabins. Two people were naked in bed and making love. He didn't want to "inconvenience" or disturb them at such an intimate moment, so he moved on to the next cabin, knocked on the door, and announced that he had brought a bottle of complimentary Champagne from the management.

When the vacationing young couple saw Earl with his mask and gun, they got "excited," as Earl perceived it at the time. He tried to reassure them by saying "I'm good at this," and that no harm would come to them.

After collecting a purse and wallet from the couple, instead of fleeing the scene, Earl stood around for a while chatting amiably with his victims, trying to calm them before departing. In the process he came to realize—apparently to his surprise—that his theft might ruin their vacation. "You're here to have a good time. What do you need to have a good time?" Earl asked his victims.

The girl replied, "Please just give me back my checkbook and my driver's license. That's all we need." With a checkbook and identification, they could continue with their vacation plans, she explained.

Earl met the woman's request. "I told them that I hope you have a good time. We had a lot of conversation about the cabins. It was very lighthearted in my mind." He added in retrospect, "I'm sure it was very intense as far as they were concerned."

All the while he was pointing a revolver at them.

Two days later, Earl attended Sunday church. He prayed and asked God to give him direction for the upcoming week because he felt he might end up committing another robbery. Earl believed at the time that he got a positive response from God. It went like this: "You're not really hurting anybody, Earl. You're adding a little excitement to their lives." Earl explained to me with embarrassment, "I came out of church knowing it was okay. In retrospect, that blows my mind. I walked out of church thinking that what I'd done was okay."

On Monday, one impulse would cascade into another as Earl took his crime spree to a new level with a dangerous and terrifying home invasion. It began as he was driving by a general store outside of town, when he recalled an incident in the store from several months earlier. While shopping there, he had witnessed the owner behaving in a very rude manner toward his wife, who ran the store with him.

Earl decided to retaliate against the rude husband by robbing his family store. He pulled his car up to the porch in front of the store and got out, never occurring to him that someone coming in or out might later be able to identify it.

Before entering the store, Earl put on a new Halloween mask as his disguise. He had seen neighborhood kids at his dad's home having a great time with a similar mask and had gone to the local Kmart to buy one for his son. The mask was shaped like a white plastic skull. When he squeezed a bulb, fake blood circulated through the mask as if he were bleeding. The kids had loved it and Earl thought it was hilarious.

In addition to his gun, Earl had obtained pepper spray. He remembered thinking it would be "nicer" to pepper spray the people he robbed rather than to shoot them, and he believes he never had any intention to fire the gun under any circumstances.

Possession of the pepper spray and the gun, and perhaps the mask as well, indicates that Earl had been preparing for a robbery, while leaving the specific circumstances up to chance or impulse. As already described, a person can be manic and psychotic—out of touch with reality—and yet be able to make elaborate plans; but the plans are likely to look crazy and futile, and to go drastically awry.

Earl explained to me, "When I walked into the store I said to myself, 'Isn't this wild? This will be another place for another interesting crime.' I thought it was something lighthearted that was somewhat interesting."

Two women were in the store, including the proprietor's wife. Earl made "little jokes" about the robbery and showed off his mask by pumping fake blood through the face. A couple of customers who were wandering about the store thought he was putting on a show. Earl was sure he was doing nothing really wrong. Despite suffering from chronic anxiety on a daily basis, he now felt no fear. Instead he felt exhilarated and even elated.

Earl took a purse from one of the women and when she grabbed it back from him, he let her keep it without a struggle. He scooped money from the cash register. Then he told the two women to go into the back of the store. They refused to budge. "I asked, 'Pretty please,'" he told me, but they still refused to obey his pleadings. Before departing with a small amount of money from the cash register, he instructed them not to follow him out of the store.

As Earl stood momentarily on the porch of the store, he realized the error in parking at the front of the building, and a glimmer of reality dawned on him. "I got the first realization that there was a penalty to this."

As he got into the car and drove off, Earl spotted the two women looking after him from the porch. Feeling little fear of the man they would describe as the Happy Burglar, they had ignored his admonishment not to follow him out the door.

Now Earl realized that the women must have seen everything about his car from the dents on his fenders to the numbers on his license plate. He felt like the "whole world would be looking for me" including the National Guard. He saw himself being surrounded.

Feeling panicky for the first time as a robber, Earl drove his car for a few miles and then turned into an unfamiliar neighborhood. He picked out a house and drove around back, where he parked.

Earl's description of what happened next was more confused than his recollection of earlier events. I have reconstructed the events from interviews with him, depositions of victims, and police reports that include victim interviews.

Earl recalls driving his car behind the house and breaking in through a window. He recalls covering the car with a sheet. He also pulled out the phone lines inside the house—an act he quickly regretted. He wanted to call the store that he had robbed minutes earlier to ask the two women if they had called the police and reported his license plate numbers. In his medication spellbound state, he hoped that they might have found his antics so entertaining that they decided not to report him. But he couldn't phone the store because he had ripped out the phone cords.

Earl tried to collect his wits. "I was sitting in the house, thinking I'd stay there for a while," he explained to me. "I didn't imagine someone coming home."

Then two girls, age ten and twelve, arrived home from school and let themselves into the house.

Earl realized that he had frightened the children and so he did everything he could to reassure them. He convinced himself that they eventually "got pretty close" as they listened to music and talked about their parents.

Earl also wanted their help. He asked the children if they could figure out how to fix the phones to make them usable but they had nothing to offer. Earl confided to me with chagrin and dismay, "I was asking this ten- and twelve-year-old child, 'Do you have any ideas?'"

Uncertain what to do, Earl decided to stay with the girls for a while longer. "The house was a wreck," he remembers. He told the children that they should be ashamed of not helping their mother keep their home neat and clean. He thought, "We'll just clean up the house and the parents will be happy when they get home." Harboring the notion that the parents would be pleased by what he was doing, he put the two preteens to work on bathroom and kitchen detail. After a while, one of the kids declared, "I'm bored," and Earl told them, "Watch TV or whatever you want."

At the time, Earl hoped he was bringing a healthy excitement and "zest" into the lives of the children whose home he had invaded. Later, the family members would say that he didn't seem very threatening and that he talked an unusual amount, a typical sign of someone who is manic.

The police questioned the children about how close Earl might have come to using the gun. Had he cocked it and pointed it at them? The children said he hadn't done anything that seemed very threatening.

Eventually, Earl found out from the children that their mother would be arriving home very soon. Trying to get some help with his precarious situation, he asked the children if they thought their mother would do "anything goofy" when she found him in the house. Would their mother be upset when she came upon him holding her children at gunpoint in their home? The two kids informed him that Mom would be very upset.

Earl wanted to make their mother feel more at ease when she arrived. He learned from the children that she drank wine to relax. So he cleared off a chair in advance for her, poured a glass of wine, and placed it on a nearby table.

When the mother arrived, Earl held her at gunpoint while doing everything he could to reassure her that he wouldn't hurt her or the children. He told her to sit in the chair and then he bound her feet with duct tape. But he neglected to bind her hands and absentmindedly left the scissors on the floor within easy reach.

Earl left the house briefly to hide his car but the mother and children were sufficiently intimidated not to flee while he was gone. Earl returned, obtained the keys to the family's SUV, and drove off.

Before departing, Earl left the children a bullet as a memento of their "exciting" time, feeling certain it would be cool for them to share the bullet in show-and-tell with their friends at school. By accident, he also left his wallet with all his identification on the mantel of the fireplace. In retrospect, Earl had no idea how he managed to leave his wallet in plain view.

After leaving the children and their mother, Earl drove directly to his friend Mary's house and watched TV with her without saying anything about what he'd done. Then he drove to his parents' house where he lived. When he stepped outside on the deck to have a cigarette, he found the police looking over the stolen SUV. They arrested him and took him to jail.

In jail and still taking Prozac and Klonopin, Earl continued to have racing thoughts and compulsive, unrealistic fantasies. He stayed up at night in his cell, plotting his flight to South America, something that seemed entirely plausible at the time—although he had not the faintest idea how he would escape from the prison. Meanwhile, the crimes he had committed didn't seem "bad" even though he was facing a lengthy jail sentence. He felt "ten feet tall and bullet-proof." He felt no remorse while continuing to take the Prozac in jail.

A year later Earl told me, "Even when I got to jail I didn't think I'd had a negative impact on that mother or those kids, and then, [after stopping Prozac] it hit me, and it hit me pretty hard—that I had possibly scarred these people for life." The medication spellbinding was broken and the realization came only after the medications had been withdrawn for many weeks.

As in many of my cases of medication madness, Earl continued to benefit from the loving support of his family who could not believe that he would have committed any of these crimes while in his right mind. His father helped research the case and communicated with the attorney and with me on numerous occasions. He lent his son moral and financial support.

The toll on family members in these cases is enormous. They not only bear witness to the suffering and humiliation of a loved one—a husband or a son they feel was innocent of criminal intentions—they also become drained of their spiritual and financial resources.

As soon as I finished my report, Earl's defense attorney carried it by hand to the local district attorney. The district attorney quickly read it. Probably because Earl's behavior was so inexplicably ludicrous and self-defeating, the DA believed what I wrote about prescription medications causing Earl's mentally disturbed condition. A plea bargain resulted in a relatively short sentence that pleased Earl, his family, and his attorney.

Chapter 8

Not Quite Twelve Years Old

FROM BEGINNING TO END it was almost exactly thirty days.

Nearly twelve years old, Andy Jordan seemed to be having a great summer filled with fun activities. His father told me, "Andy did a lot of things for a short life. He ice-skated, played basketball and baseball, tried waterskiing, even got to drive a car on some private land of family's. He had lots of extended family and was well liked." His mother added, "Andy had a best friend since third or fourth grade. They went places together and with both of our families."

As far as Andy's parents can recall, everything was going fine. Then on an evening in early September not long after the start of school, Andy told his mother that something was bothering him but he couldn't tell her what it was. He said it would make it worse to talk about it. He said it had to do with missing his friend and missing Grandpa. To his mother, other than his expressions of concern, he seemed normal. Since he couldn't talk about it, she suggested that he write her a note.

Mrs. Jordan understood her son's references to his grandpa and his friend. Grandpa—her father—had died four years earlier in 1998 after a long bout with cancer. Andy was eight at the time and had been close to his grandpa.

Almost two years after Grandpa's death, when Andy was ten years old, a friend next door accidentally hanged himself. They were neighbors and played together but as far as Andy's mother could tell they weren't very close buddies. The boy was climbing by himself in a tree swinging from a length of dog chain when he jumped from the tree and became entangled as he leaped. "He was a daredevil. We were always afraid he would get hit by a car," Andy's mother explained to me. "Other than wanting his friend to be back, Andy never seemed that upset." Although it raised red flags for me, Andy's mother feels certain that her son never thought of his friend's death as a suicide.

Soon after his friend died, Andy began to complain occasionally about headaches and chest pain. The first note in his pediatrician's chart in early 2000, described Andy as staying home from school because of those complaints. With a question mark, the doctor suggested a possible explanation: "Reacted to stress of fatal accident to next-door neighbor." Andy's pediatrician never did anything to follow up by talking further with the boy and his family or by recommending counseling.

Childhood problems like these are common and a part of growing up. Children face losses, learn about death, react emotionally, and eventually integrate the new experiences into their maturing experience of life. Children are most helped by the presence of at least one adult who cares enough to spend time with the child during difficult times. Ideally, there's also an extended family—brothers, sisters, parents, grandparents, aunts, and uncles—surrounding the child.

Nowadays, when our children run into difficulties we often turn instead to physicians—family doctors, pediatricians, and, more rarely, psychiatrists—who may have minimal personal interest in or connection to the child, who may know little or nothing about children or families, and who too often handle distressed children clumsily at best. Having little time to spend with each child and typically knowing nothing else to do anyway, they become technologists administering drugs with much less acumen and even less success than an auto mechanic addressing a knocking sound in the motor.

Andy's occasional stomachaches and headaches continued for the remainder of the year and persisted occasionally thereafter. In November 2000, Andy was seen at an emergency room on several occasions for recurrences of his stomach pain. Without any psychological discussion, his pediatrician noted at this time, "He is in the fourth grade at St. James parochial school. He is a good student and good basketball player. He is a very sensitive child, though." Nothing more was said or done.

As an added stress, Mr. Jordan developed pneumonia in July 2001. He was only forty-eight and the infection struck him out of the blue without any apparent underlying cause. After the initial hospitalization, he was discharged home but had to return to the hospital two weeks later for insertion of a chest tube to remove the fluid on his lungs. The routine procedure went awry, the tube missed its mark and cut Mr. Jordan's spleen, causing internal bleeding and a sudden loss of blood pressure.

By chance, Andy and his mother arrived at Dad's hospital room in the middle of the emergency. His mother remembers it vividly. It was "like the typical doctor movie on TV where something goes wrong."

For several terrifying hours, Andy thought his father was going to die. He had already lost his grandfather and friend. As often happens when adults are involved in life-threatening emergencies, no one at the time fully grasped the impact on Andy. Naturally everyone was caught up with his or her own anxiety and then so relieved when Andy's father survived that they never thought about the effect on the boy. The evening of the hospital emergency, Andy had written in his journal, "My dad almost died last night."

So, Andy had been through three tough life experiences: his grandfather's death, his friend's death, and his father's near death. According to his parents, Andy seemed to bounce back each time. With the exception of occasional stomachaches and headaches, Andy acted as if nothing fazed him. He never looked especially anxious or depressed. He dutifully went on with his schoolwork and dove into sports and social activities.

The evening when Andy's mother asked him to write down what was bothering him, she wasn't apprehensive. She imagined he'd been missing his grandpa and his friend but nothing more than that.

The next morning Andy gave his mother a note. He wrote about feeling very sad since the death of his neighbor: "Mom, sometimes when I get really mad and frustrated, I feel like I don't want to live . . . Mom, just call someone that can help me. I am sorry, but I still love you!"

We will never know why the experiences began to prey on Andy's mind in September 2002, but we can imagine the possibilities. It was the beginning of school. Andy's stomachaches and headaches often coincided with going to school. According to Mrs. Jordan, Andy didn't love school and didn't hate it, but he was sometimes uncomfortable in groups. He didn't like crowds and commotion and that may have discouraged him about school. His grades were above average and he enjoyed his friends and sports.

Andy's friend had died during the fall four years earlier and perhaps Andy was reacting to an upcoming anniversary of his death. As best as I could reconstruct, in previous years some of his worst stomachaches had been in the fall.

Andy was not a troubled child. As far as I can tell from the medical records and from his parents, no one saw him as seriously emotionally distressed until that last month of his life—after he'd been given psychiatric drugs. Many children undergo severe losses in childhood but few end up attempting suicide as they approach the age of twelve. Andy in particular was not a gloomy, sad, or withdrawn child. He was outgoing and full of life.

Many children do feel guilty about the death of family members and especially friends. They ask themselves, "Why am I alive? Why should I be the one who's alive?" If they are sensitive and thoughtful like Andy, they go through a time of self-examination, something close to an existential doubt, and they come through it. If they can find one adult to share their feelings with, they more readily come out stronger and more mature. But nowadays, if they voice anything that sounds potentially self-destructive, they are likely to be rushed off to the pediatrician, family doctor, or psychiatrist to be turned into lifelong consumers of psychiatric drugs.

Medicating Andy

Immediately after receiving the note asking for help, Andy Jordan's parents took him for an emergency visit to a clinic where a psychologist began testing him on the first visit. The psychologist quickly became concerned about Andy's level of anxiety and depression. She noted, "Severe anxiety in all areas, probably exaggerated as a plea for help. Recommendations: Go ahead with med trial to address anxiety disorder and panic attacks."

The clinic's psychiatrist was unavailable so the psychologist called Andy's pediatrician to recommend medication. The pediatrician in turn immediately started the boy on Zoloft 25 mg to be automatically increased to 50 mg in one week. It appears as if the nonmedical psychologist initiated the medical treatment and that pediatrician merely took orders but he would soon turn over Andy's treatment to a psychiatrist.

The pediatrician's record indicated he was medicating Andy for "adolescent depression" and "anxiety with secondary somatization." Somatization is the physical manifestation of emotional problems, such as a headache, a stomachache, or a rash. The reference is probably to the stomachaches that the pediatrician had previously evaluated without finding any physical cause.

One week later on September 17, Andy's parents doubled the Zoloft to 50 mg as prearranged. One week after that, Andy's father e-mailed the psychologist, "Everything seemed to be progressing fine with Andy until this morning. The medication does not seem to be helping."

Two to three weeks after starting Zoloft, Andy began to beg not to have to go to school. When being dropped off at school, he would sometimes curl up and refuse to get out of car. At the urging of the clinic, his parents enrolled him in a partial hospitalization program where he spent much of the day in a treatment setting before returning home each night. The partial hospitalization staff identified him as suffering from "anxiety, depression, grief and loss, and suicidal thoughts." As I've so often seen in retrospect, he quickly deteriorated on the Zoloft. This is consistent with FDA's new warnings about children undergoing "clinical worsening" on antidepressants (see chapter 3).

Andy's behavior became increasingly difficult, puzzling, and strange. He sat in the family van and used his cell phone to call his parents in the house asking to go to the airport. He wanted to go on a trip. Doing their best to calm him, his mother took him to the local library to read about travel.

Within a week or two of starting Zoloft, Andy began to look "agitated" and to complain that his head was hurting worse than ever. His mother poignantly recounted how her son would hold his head and say, "Mom, I can't take this anymore." She cried as she told me how she had unwittingly given her son false reassurance, telling him, "You're on the medication and it takes time." She was reassuring him that the medicine was going to help when it was destroying him.

When Harry Henderson in an agitated state drove his car into the policeman to get his gun to kill himself, he wanted to end the pain in his head that was caused by the antidepressant. As a child, Andy was so demoralized by the pain inside his head that he could only throw desperate temper tantrums.

Andy at times lay on floor screaming and kicking, holding his head. Sometimes he rocked back and forth, sometimes he flailed about and screamed, and at others he banged his head in an apparent effort to relieve the pain. All of this was entirely new behavior. "It just wasn't Andy," both his parents explained, but they never guessed that medication could be driving their child mad.

Adding to the confusion, most of the time Andy seemed just fine—his normal self. This kind of waxing and waning is typical of adverse drug effects but it baffles parents and inexperienced doctors alike who don't know what to make of it. Because they assume that an adverse drug reaction would be continuous, they mistakenly end up attributing such extreme and episodic bouts to "mental illness" in the victim.

It never crossed the mind of Mr. or Mrs. Jordan that the medicine could be making their son worse. "When the doctor prescribes medicine you assume it's going to make you better," Dad explained to me. Later, they would be outraged to learn that antidepressants had never been proven to relieve depression in children—that doctors were prescribing them without FDA approval and without scientific justification—a mistaken practice that continues to this day.

Toward the end, Andy confided in his parents that he thought he heard Jesus or God telling him it was time to come. What were they to do about these alarming signs? Their son was already seeing a psychologist, going to partial-day hospitalization, and taking medication. They hardly ever let him out of their sight. Meanwhile, Andy had come apart so quickly, a rapid four-week downhill course that no one could explain, leaving his parents no time to gather their wits.

Why had the nonmedical psychologist at the clinic been directing Andy's medication through the pediatrician? As it turned out, the young psychiatrist who did prescribing duty at the clinic was preparing to take her boards. Although she had not seen Andy, she called the pediatrician to discuss the boy's treatment, and then described their conversation in the clinic record:

> Called [the pediatrician] at request of Andy's dad to discuss his case. Three weeks ago Andy became quite depressed and was refusing to go to school. He wanted to be dead. He was started on Zoloft 25 mg for one week and then 50 mg since then. After one week he became more anxious and more vehemently refused to go to school. He was especially resistant to going to church at school. He will increase the Zoloft to 75 mg.

The note clearly indicated that Andy had gotten worse on the Zoloft, yet the doctor reflexively increased the dose.

After the psychiatrist at the clinic made her sight-unseen decision to increase the dose of Zoloft, responsibility for prescribing Andy's medicine was picked up by the psychiatrist at the partial hospitalization program. He followed through on the recommended increase to Zoloft to 75 mg, citing "anxiety, agitation, and psychosomatic complaints," all of which are more likely to be caused by than to be cured by Zoloft.

Risperdal: Another Potential Medication Catastrophe

At the same time that the day-hospital psychiatrist doubled Andy's Zoloft, he added the antipsychotic drug Risperdal 0.25 mg to the boy's regimen. While there was virtually no hope of anything good coming of treatment with Risperdal, there was considerable risk of developing severe and life-threatening drug-induced disorders. Among other things, Risperdal causes potentially fatal diabetes, pancreatitis, and neuroleptic malignant syndrome. The latter is a potentially lethal reaction similar to a life-threatening viral encephalitis in how it causes fever, global mental disruption, rigidity, coma, collapse, and death.

Risperdal also can cause tardive dyskinesia, a persistent and usually irreversible disorder that causes disfiguring grimaces and tics and potentially disabling abnormal movement of arms, hands, legs, and neck, as well as the muscles of speaking, swallowing, and breathing. In my own clinical and forensic practice, I have seen at least two dozen cases of tardive dyskinesia in children given Risperdal. Some of these stories will appear in later chapters, where tardive dyskinesia will be discussed in more detail.

Despite all this, many doctors prescribed Risperdal for children at a time when the FDA had not given approval to do so. More recently, in late 2006 the FDA approved this dangerous drug for the control of extreme irritability in autistic children, and then for the control of psychosis and bipolar disorder in older children and teens.

On the day after his psychiatrist started him on Risperdal, Andy's parents had to take him to the emergency department of a facility for children because of his increasing depressed feelings. There a brief comment was made in the record, "Sometimes hears voices unrecognizable—commanding at times. Won't say what they say." Despite this ominous report, the facility did not find that he met the criteria for emergency admission.

Most likely, Andy was having an adverse drug reaction to the increased dose of Zoloft, the start of the Risperdal, or both. Consistent with most of the cases in this book, severe adverse psychiatric reactions often take place within a day or two of starting or changing a dose of SSRI antidepressants, or adding other drugs.

It's a pattern I've seen all too frequently in my clinical practice as well as in my legal consultations. A child develops a relatively straightforward problem— grief and sadness over the death of a friend or relative—and then becomes mired down in psychiatric medication treatment, progressively worsening until he's put on mind-crushing, extremely dangerous antipsychotic drugs like Risperdal, Zyprexa, Seroquel, or Abilify.

The following day Andy's therapist contacted the family. The boy had spoken about wanting to join his deceased grandfather and friend but he voiced no plan. The psychologist was worried but foresaw no imminent danger.

Andy's psychiatrist at the clinic, the place where his treatment had begun, finally saw the boy for the first time. This is the doctor who had originally recommended the doubling of Andy's Zoloft before she ever met him. Now she seemed to make a decision—to reduce and then stop Andy's Zoloft.

Since Andy's deterioration began with the taking of antidepressants, he deserved a good long holiday from them. Instead, the psychiatrist started him on another antidepressant, Effexor (venlafaxine) that posed the same mental hazards as Zoloft. Effexor stimulates serotonin in much the same fashion as Zoloft by blocking the removal of serotonin from the synapse between nerve cells, but it adds a few additional potent effects as well. The new FDA-mandated black-box suicide warnings for Effexor are the same as those for Zoloft and the other SSRIs.

The doctor transitioned from Zoloft to Effexor by reducing the Zoloft dose and starting Effexor at the same time, so Andy was being exposed to both drugs at once with unpredictable effects at the time disaster struck.

Andy's parents by now were frantic. As I've seen time and again, in the midst of poisoning a child with medications, doctors begin to shift the blame from themselves to the child's distressed parents. Notes in the record began to show thinly veiled hostility toward the parents. Instead of reexamining their own misguided medical decisions, the doctors began blaming the parents for supposedly overreacting to their son's deteriorating and increasingly desperate condition.

After beginning the switch from Zoloft to Effexor, the clinic psychiatrist at last met with Andy's parents. She then wrote to the boy's pediatrician, "Neither he nor his parents have seen much improvement with Zoloft over the last four weeks. In many ways, he seems to be worse." Her note read, "We discussed treatment options, including increasing his Zoloft dose or trying a different medication." Despite enough bad experience to make me cynical, I still could not believe it: The doctor really wanted to increase the Zoloft! So why did she shift to Effexor? The doctor changed to Effexor only because Andy was getting diarrhea on the Zoloft. Simply put, the onset of dramatic mental deterioration while taking a psychiatric drug was not sufficient reason to stop it, but the onset of diarrhea was.

Mrs. Jordan picked Andy up from the day hospital. Andy enjoyed visiting the dogs at the humane society and so they drove to the shelter. Andy had a pug at home and now for the first time he found another pug at the humane society. The family would consider a second dog but this pug had already been spoken for.

After they arrived home, Andy was planning to have a snack before going to play with a friend. That night the family was supposed to have their picture taken for the church directory. Andy's mother had set out her son's clothes for him. Andy was in the middle of one of his typical busy days and he seemed fine.

It was time to pick up Andy's fifteen-year-old sister at the end of her school day. Knowing that he'd been feeling self-destructive at times, Andy's mother wanted to keep a close eye on him, but she also didn't want her daughter to wait by herself at school. Mr. Jordan was due home any minute. The trip back and forth to school was a matter of minutes. Andy at this moment did not seem at all depressed. He reassured her and smiled cheerily, telling her as she left, "I'll be fine, Mom. You can call to check on me while you're gone."

Mr. Jordan arrived as expected a few minutes later. He had forgotten the key to the garage entrance to the house and went around front to let himself in. Later he would lament that every second might have mattered, but he had no way of knowing that at the time. Andy was probably already dead.

Andy committed suicide on that Friday afternoon in October 2002. At that point in time, he had been taking Zoloft 50 mg for two or three days and Effexor 37.5 mg for the same amount of time. He was also continuing to take Risperdal. A count of his remaining pills after his death confirmed that he had been taking them as directed by his doctors.

Andy had been in the hands of mental health professionals and been taking medication for one month. He was not quite twelve years old.

Andy's method of death was eerily similar to several other victims of medication madness whose cases I have evaluated. He hanged himself on gym equipment in a manner that required him to hold himself aloft while he strangled and lost consciousness.

Staff from the family treatment center wrote a posthumous case summary, stating that "Andy had never made a previous gesture toward suicide or self-harm, and had never identified a plan to harm himself." The note continued that the clinic staff had contacted the partial hospitalization staff and that they, too, had seen "no warning signs." Shortly before his suicide, he had left the unit "in an upbeat mood, talking and joking with peers. He was excited about getting to go on a field trip with his school class today, and was to start half-days at school again next week."

When I called Andy's parents to follow up on his story, the wound was still raw. "Four years sounds like a long time but it really isn't—at least not for us," Andy's mother explained to me. "I don't think I'll ever be able to talk about him without getting upset. Hard, when you see his friends, and they're grown up—and he's not. We know that life's not fair and you just try to deal with it as best you can." Andy's parents have not resumed their previous normal social life. "We're no fun to be around," she explained. "That one person missing has the biggest impact on all of us, me and my husband, and our three other children."

Andy was usually the only one in the family to go to church with Mom every Sunday and now the day of worship inevitably brings renewed sorrow for her. "I've never gotten mad at God. But it's hard to go to church because you're reading about where you're going to go some day [to heaven]—and that's where Andy's already gone." She explained, "It's just an awful, awful, thing, and it just happened yesterday. You miss him so darn much."

Andy's parents cling to reminders of their son's life like his beloved pug. "And we still have him . . . the dog," his mother told me plaintively. They had managed to stay close to Andy's best friend for a time but he gradually drifted away from them.

Mr. and Mrs. Jordan are a long way from recovering from what happened in their family four years ago. As sad as they remain, their biggest concern is for their other children. Andy's older sister with whom he was the closest was fifteen going on sixteen at the time of his suicide. Andy also had a good relationship with his oldest sister who was twenty-one at time and living outside the home. The oldest of their children, a twenty-seven-year-old son, was hit very hard as well. He still breaks down thinking about what happened to his little brother. Everybody's been deeply hurt.

Mr. Jordan confirmed the unrelenting pain of the tragedy: "It is now the same as four years ago. Devastating impact on everyone's life in the family. Everybody's changed forever. This whole thing happened in a month. We did everything we thought we needed to do, and the end result was Andy committing suicide, hanging himself, in the ten minutes between when his mother left and I got home."

Bringing Lawsuits

Andy's parents almost missed the two-year deadline for bringing their suits. The statute of limitations—the time beyond which a lawsuit can no longer be initiated—had almost expired. Then their oldest son read in a newspaper about the 2004 FDA hearings where so many parents had told about tragedies involving their children who took antidepressants. The stories sounded like exactly what happened to Andy.

At that time, almost two years had passed since their son's death, but it had never occurred to Andy's parents that the prescribed medications could have been to blame, and so they had never even tried to look it up on the Internet. Now, with this lead in hand, they discovered a virtual flood of information on the Internet concerning suicides in children caused by antidepressants.

The family's attorney asked me to read the medical records and to give an opinion concerning potential lawsuits against the doctors and the drug companies. With the exception of the pediatrician, I concluded that all of the health practitioners had been negligent in their treatment of Andy. As a result, malpractice suits were brought against the psychologist at the clinic who initiated the medication phone call to the pediatrician, the psychiatrists at the clinic and at the partial hospitalization, and the facilities where Andy was treated. Product-liability suits were brought against the manufacturer of Zoloft (Pfizer) and the manufacturer of Effexor (Wyeth) for negligence in the development and marketing of their drugs, specifically in regard to hiding drug-induced suicidality.

Before the case went very far, all parties involved settled the case with Andy's parents without admitting to any wrong doing. The defendants required the parents to keep secret the settlement amount. However, the attorney described the settlement as "significant" and "generally satisfactory" to the parents. I was gratified when he attributed the settlement to my presence in the case.

The parents remain dismayed that so many professionals were involved in treating Andy and yet not one of them considered that the drugs might be making him worse. Andy's mother puts it simply, "I will never understand how or why it happened." Yet it's a pattern repeated in almost every case of medication madness. Even with the new warnings—and the demonstrated lack of efficacy—leading experts in the field have publicly declared that antidepressants remain an important method of treatment for children. The plain truth is this: Except for a temporary, slight reduction in the numbers of prescriptions for children, it's business as usual in regard to prescribing antidepressants to children and adults. Indeed, the profession is hell bent on reenergizing the push for these useless, toxic agents, touting the antidepressants at every opportunity, claiming that the "benefits trump the risks for kids."[1]

Chapter 9

Sleeping Pill Madness

ON AN AFTERNOON in June 1990, a hotel maid noticed a man wandering around the tenth floor of the glass-and-steel-enclosed tower of the Hyatt Hotel. He was dressed appropriately and looked about the age of many businessmen who came to the hotel but he looked tense, nervous, and was as white as a sheet. Thinking that he seemed harmless, the hotel maid went on with her duties without reporting anything amiss.

Of course, the maid had no way of knowing that the man was intoxicated by the sleeping pill Halcion, one of the most emotionally devastating drugs in the psychiatric armamentarium.

SEDATIVES, HYPNOTICS, AND ANXIOLYTICS

TRANQUILIZERS—technically called "sedatives, hypnotics, and anxiolytics"—are probably the most spellbinding drugs of all. Many of them share a common chemical structure called benzodiazepine, hence the familiar name benzos. These drugs are usually used to treat anxiety or insomnia. Halcion is the shortest-acting with the most biochemical punch and, therefore, the most toxic. It is used exclusively to induce sleep. Xanax is a close second to Halcion in its capacity to cause medication madness. It is mainly prescribed for anxiety but also for sleep. The Upjohn Company manufactures both drugs.

The tranquilizers have an enormous capacity to produce mental and behavioral impairment, even with the first dose, and they often do so without the individual grasping what is happening. Often, the individual feels better than ever. Especially with Xanax, the drug-induced euphoria can progress to outright mania, bringing the medication spellbinding to tragic outcomes.

Xanax, Valium, Klonopin, and Ativan are among the most frequently prescribed benzodiazepines. There is no essential difference between the benzodiazepines that are sold as tranquilizers and those that are sold as sleeping pills, such as Dalmane. The manufacturers have simply chosen to evaluate and to market some of them for treating insomnia. All of the benzodiazepines are controlled substances (narcotics) and are classified in the Drug Enforcement Administration (DEA) Schedule IV to indicate a serious risk of addiction. The nonbenzo sleeping aids Ambien, Lunesta, and Sonata are also classified in Schedule IV (see appendix A) and pose similar risks.

Halcion is a benzodiazepine approved exclusively for the short-term treatment of insomnia. It is so highly potent and short-acting that individuals frequently go into withdrawal within hours of taking it. This short duration of action was touted as a positive attribute for a sleeping medication on the grounds that the individual would awaken in the morning without a "hangover" of persistent sedative effects. Instead, so much of the drug is gone by morning that people can wake up in a state of withdrawal.

HIGH UP AND ON HALCION

ABOUT AN HOUR or two after the maid noticed the ashen stranger wandering around the hotel corridor, one of the hotel staff saw the reflection of a man through a window in the main hotel building. He appeared to be doing something on the tower roof. She called the superintendent's office to see if anyone had permission to be working up there. The answer was "no" and security was contacted.

The front-desk manager quickly reached the roof of the main building where he observed a man sitting on the edge of the tower roof across the way. The individual was described as having glazed eyes, moving slowly, and acting confused.

The manager called out, "Are you a guest here?"

"No," the man replied. Showing no emotion, the man sitting on the edge of the roof explained, "I'm from this area and I wanted to see how it looks from up here."

The security officer arrived and poked his head through the hatch on the tower roof not far from where the man was perched on the edge of the roof and told him, "You'll have to come down from there."

"Okay," the man replied. He stood up and took a few steps toward the security officer.

The security officer felt a shudder of fear when he saw the glazed, robotic look in the man's eye.

The man said to the officer, "Wait just a minute." He returned to the edge of the roof, sat down, turned onto his stomach, eased his body over the edge, held on momentarily, and then pushed off. He fell 120 feet, crashed into a bed of gravel, and was killed. He did not make a sound as he fell.

Afterward, it was discovered that a hatch to the roof in the stairwell of the top floor had been left open to accommodate construction workers.

The deceased was Martin Quick, a fifty-three-year-old salesman of business machines. He was survived by his wife and daughters, age twenty-six and twenty-nine.

Martin's personal effects included a wallet with photographs of his family, business cards, the usual array of identification and credit cards, and fifty-eight dollars in cash. Also in his pockets, the police found a prescription bottle for Halcion 0.25 mg with one pill remaining.

Martin's widow sued the manufacturer of Halcion and the doctor who prescribed it to her husband. In both the product-liability case against the manufacturer and the malpractice case against the doctor, the key issue was our ability to show that Halcion could cause suicide. If we could show the judge that Halcion had the potential to cause suicide, then we would then be allowed to argue that Halcion caused Martin's suicide. We would also have to show that the drug company and/or the doctor had done something negligent that caused Martin to kill himself.

Not a Typical Suicide

In my deposition under oath before the trial I explained why Martin Quick's suicide was so unexpected:

> Martin had never been suicidal before. He did not have any of the major criteria we see in people who commit suicide. He is not hinting. He is not leaving notes. He hasn't previously attempted suicide. There isn't a recent suicide in his life. His economic life has not gone to hell. That is, he hasn't lost his job. He hasn't lost a nearest and dearest loved one. He has not

lost social contacts. He has many. He has family around him. He has not displayed loss of all joyful connections to life. He plays golf. He has fun relationships with people. He is nonalcoholic, doesn't drink at all. He is not a drug addict. He is not elderly. He is not retired. He has literally none of the typical constellation of future suicide [indicators] at that point in time.

Martin was in good health in 1990, when he developed pain in his lower abdomen and went to an emergency room where he was diagnosed with an acute inflammation in his prostate gland. Although he was usually very healthy, this incident may have started him worrying about himself and his mortality but we don't have much information about what he was thinking during this period of time.

Eight days after his ER visit, Martin saw his internist for the first time in a year. The doctor noted that Martin complained of the "recent" onset of insomnia, and that he was "slightly" anxious. He was also experiencing some malaise, weight loss, and decreased appetite. His appetite, however, was now improving. The doctor wondered if his patient might be developing hypothyroidism or if he was experiencing stress secondary to the prostate infection that might have been percolating beneath the surface for some time. He prescribed him 15 tablets of Halcion 0.125 mg for the insomnia even though the problem was described as recent and probably caused by the discomfort from the infection in Martin's prostate.

When the prescription was about to run out, Martin called the doctor to ask for an increased dose. According to the office note, "Patient said he was sleeping better but wanted the next increase in dosage." Without talking with him directly, the doctor prescribed fifteen tablets of Halcion 0.25 mg—double the dose. That was thirteen days before Martin climbed onto the roof of the Hyatt.

Friends and family began to notice changes in Martin during the last week or two of his life. An unusually friendly guy who enjoyed himself with people, Martin gradually became less talkative and somewhat withdrawn. At some point, his wife began to hear a note of suspiciousness, a hint of paranoia, creeping into her husband's conversation. This is not unusual in cases of drug toxicity.

Martin's neighbor described him with affection as "handsome, cheerful, and easy to talk to. I never saw him smoke or drink. He took care of his property, keeping the grass mowed, etc. He would play golf almost every Sunday. He also enjoyed playing racquetball." But the neighbor told me that Martin had changed dramatically during the weeks when he was receiving Halcion. "He lost weight and no longer looked cheerful. In my estimation, he looked depressed. He was just not himself. He looked sick." But Martin never confided anything in his neighbor, leaving her and her husband in shock over his death.

Martin's wife testified in deposition and trial that she called the doctor's office several times to express concerns about her husband's worsening withdrawal and depression. However, there is only one telephone message from her noted in doctor's office notes, recorded twelve days after the dose was doubled. Martin was due in the office for a prescription renewal and a visit in two days but his wife wanted to bring him in with her on an emergency basis. The busy doctor tacked Martin onto the end of his day.

Not long before his appointment that evening with the doctor, Martin went from his place of work to the hotel, and jumped to his death. The one remaining Halcion tablet in the bottle in his pocket indicated that he had been taking the medication faithfully at the rate of one per day. It's a mystery why he was carrying the bottle with him.

Although we cannot ask Martin what he was experiencing, it's safe to say that Halcion had spellbound him. As his mental condition deteriorated, he never suspected the drug, and asked for the dose to be doubled. He took Halcion every night as directed—probably wholly unaware that the drug was driving him to suicide.

Halcion Causing Madness

As we went to trial in 1990, I was out on a limb testifying to an adverse drug effect of suicide, which the FDA had not and would not officially recognize. Although the defense would try to discredit me in trial as a radical for claiming that Halcion could drive anyone that crazy, I felt that I had the scientific literature on my side.

In 1979, C. van der Kroef, a psychiatrist in The Hague, Netherlands, noticed abnormal psychiatric reactions to Halcion in four of the eleven patients he treated with the drug. Here is van der Kroef's vivid description of one of his patients:

> The insomnia improved at once, but psychically she rapidly went downhill. Progressively she became paranoid. Several times she asked me what the hypnotic contained—LSD, perhaps?—for she felt that she was bordering on psychosis. She felt shut off from the world; it was as if she no longer belonged to society. Her friends asked her what was happening to her, so

strangely was she behaving. . . . After two months I, too, began to suspect, particularly in light of experience with an earlier patient, that all this might be a consequence of her taking triazolam [Halcion].

The doctor and his patient agreed to stop the Halcion and to replace it with another kind of sleeping medication. The doctor reported, "Within a day she felt herself again. The people around her noticed the difference and recognized her old self again."

In 1980, commenting on van der Kroef's findings, M. N. G. Dukes stated, "virtually every known drug in this class" has produced "hallucinations, delusions, paranoia, amnesia, delirium, hypomania—almost every conceivable symptoms of psychotic madness . . ."

According to Dukes, all the benzodiazepines prescribed for the control of anxiety are implicated in causing violence:

> More than a dozen papers in the literature speak of irritability, defiance, hostility, aggression, rage, or a progressive development of hates and dislikes in certain patients treated with benzodiazepine tranquilizers; all those products which are widespread have been incriminated at one time or another. The phenomenon has been demonstrated in animal studies and it has even been proved possible to show in human volunteers that these drugs can release pent-up hostility, particularly in highly anxious or action-oriented individuals.

British researchers Charles Medawar and Anita Hardon in 2004 provided a concise history of the cover-up surrounding benzodiazepine madness, concluding, "Of all the benzos, Halcion had the most troubled history of all." Halcion was eventually banned in England, the Netherlands, and other countries—but not in the United States. Few Americans realize that due to the FDA's growing dedication to industry interests, it has in many cases fallen behind other countries in protecting the public.

Halcion Causing Depression and Suicide

Although complicated by his acute prostatitis, Martin was already showing symptoms of depression when he saw his internist. He was having trouble sleeping and suffering from weight loss, loss of appetite, and just plain not feeling well. Setting aside that Xanax and Halcion are especially risky drugs to take, it's been known for a long time that all the benzodiazepines can cause or worsen depression.

In a 1991 handbook on psychiatric drugs intended for doctors, G. Arana and S. Hyman, stated:

> *Depression:* All benzodiazepines have been associated with the emergence or worsening of depression; whether they were causative or only failed to prevent the depression is unknown. When depression occurs during the course of benzodiazepine treatment, it is prudent to discontinue the benzodiazepine.

The American Psychiatric Association's 1990 in-depth task force report on benzodiazepine tranquilizers cited scientific sources to bolster its observation:

> Benzodiazepines have also been reported to cause or to exacerbate symptoms of depression. This, too, is not a frequent side effect, although the depressive symptoms may be potentially serious.[1]

Benzodiazepine expert Heather Ashton observed in 1995 that benzodiazepines could blunt the emotions in general, producing "emotional anesthesia." She reported, "Former long-term benzodiazepine users often bitterly regret their lack of emotional response to family events during the period that they were taking the drugs." Ashton also observed that the drugs could precipitate suicide in already depressed patients.

Great Britain's Committee on Safety of Medicines—that country's drug monitoring agency—recommended in 1988, "Benzodiazepines should not be used alone to treat depression or anxiety associated with depression. *Suicide may be precipitated in such patients.*"

The most interesting evidence for use at the trial had come hot off the griddle—secret FDA documents that had come into my hands.

Data from the Spontaneous Reporting System

The FDA's Spontaneous Reporting System, now called MedWatch, consists of a computerized record of all reports sent to the agency concerning adverse drug effects. Many of the reports come from drug companies as required under FDA regulations and many come spontaneously from other sources. During the early and mid-1990s when these studies were done, almost all spontaneous reports came from practicing physicians and from hospital pharmacists, but nowadays an increasing number also come from consumers who have had bad experiences with drugs.

In an in-house executive summary written for the FDA's Division of Epidemiology and Surveillance (September 19, 1989), agency official Bob Wise compiled and analyzed all reports sent to the agency concerning Halcion and Xanax as causes of hostility including "anger or rage, aggression, and some actual assaults and murders." The paper was meant for FDA eyes only but was somehow obtained by attorneys involved in Halcion litigation and passed on to me. In his unpublished paper, Bob Wise stated:

> More such reports of this type have been received by the FDA for triazolam [Halcion] and alprazolam [Xanax] than for any other drug product regulated by the Agency. Reporting rates, which adjust for differences in the extent of each drug's utilization, reveal much higher ratios of hostility reports to drug sales for both triazolam and alprazolam than for other benzodiazepines with similar indications.
>
> The public health importance of these reactions lies in their severity, with occasionally lethal behavior unleashed, in the context of large population exposures as the popularity of both drugs continues to rise.

The computerized reporting system was sending up flags for an unusually high rate of violence from Halcion and Xanax, including "a reaction in which a fifty-seven-year-old woman fatally shot her mother two hours after taking one-half milligram of triazolam [Halcion]." Wise further explained that the rate of violence on Halcion was even greater than that on Xanax. At the time, Xanax and Halcion together were among the most widely prescribed psychiatric drugs in the world, and Xanax continues to be extensively used.

Wise found 113 reports of suspected Halcion-induced hostility. Xanax was next with 79 reports. No other drugs came close to Halcion and Xanax in regard to reports of drug-induced hostility. Among 318 other medications, the vast majority (75 percent) had only one or two reports each of hostility. The pattern seemed obvious: In comparison to other drugs, Halcion and Xanax were causing a great deal of destructive behavior.

Wise summarized, "This apparently excessive number of rage and similar reports with triazolam and alprazolam, after adjusting the differences in frequency of drug use, provides strong suspicion that a causal relationship may obtain." Wise concluded that these reports cannot "prove the presence of a causal relationship" to the drug, but that they do "imply a substantial public health importance for the potential hostility syndrome."

Wise missed an extremely important aspect of his own data. Not only were Halcion and Xanax first and second in total reports of hostility, Versed was third in order. The total numbers of reports were Halcion (112), Xanax (77), and Versed (46). Another benzo, Valium (34 reports) was fourth.

Versed, like Halcion and Xanax, is a very short-acting, highly potent benzodiazepine. It is used exclusively as an intravenous injection for preoperative sedation and memory impairment. Because Versed is used for anesthesia, it is given to the general population rather than to patients with psychiatric problems. Therefore, its powerful association with psychiatric reactions such as hostility confirmed that the drug, and not the patient, was the source of the problem.[2]

In summary, the database for all drugs in the spontaneous reporting system of the FDA, which includes all prescription drugs in the United States, shows that three short-acting, highly potent benzodiazepines come in first, second, and third for reports of hostility as an adverse drug reaction. Furthermore, the three drugs are typically used under very different clinical conditions: Halcion orally with one daily dose at night for sleep, Xanax orally with several daily doses for daytime anxiety, and Versed intravenously for preoperative purposes, usually on one occasion only. Despite their different uses, dosage schedules, and even routes of administration, they cluster at the very top of the list for producing hostility and aggression. This is convincing and seemingly irrefutable evidence that these kinds of agents can cause violence. Another benzodiazepine, the very long-acting Valium, came in fourth—giving the benzodiazepines an across-the-board victory, finishing in first, second, third, and fourth place.

In contrast, the antidepressant Prozac was a distant sixth with twenty reports of hostility—but the data had been collected through August 1989, and Prozac had only been on the market for eight months. Prozac would soon become the champion of drugs in the FDA's spontaneous reporting system in regard to adverse mental effects including violence and suicide.

Two weeks before Bob Wise completed his report in 1989, Charles Anello, FDA deputy director of the Office of Epidemiology and Biostatistics, wrote a separate in-house agency memo comparing rates of abnormal behavior reports for Halcion to another benzodiazepine, Restoril, that's used as a sleeping aid. The shorter-acting, more potent Halcion racked up far more reports of causing abnormal psychiatric reactions such as "agitation, anxiety, and nervousness," "psychosis, hallucinations, paranoid reaction, and acute brain syndrome," and "hostility and intentional injury." There were nineteen reports of hostility on Halcion and one on Restoril. These striking differences between Halcion and Restoril confirm that even among the dangerous benzodiazepines, Halcion stands at the top, probably due to its higher potency and shorter duration of action, which combine to give extra punch to the drug.

Finally in 1991—too late to warn the doctor who prescribed Halcion to Martin Quick—Diane Wysowski and David Barash from the FDA's Division of Epidemiology and Surveillance published a report in the scientific literature based on some of the agency's previously in-house data.[3] Once again reviewing spontaneous reports to the FDA, the authors compared triazolam and temazepam through 1985, for "confusion, amnesia, bizarre behavior, agitation, and hallucinations." Taking into account differences in prescribing rates, they concluded "rates for triazolam [Halcion] were 22 to 99 times those for temazepam [Restoril], depending upon the reaction." With citations to bolster their conclusions, the FDA authors summarized:

> Factors that confirm a causal association between triazolam and adverse behavioral reactions include corroborating case reports and sleep laboratory studies in the literature, reports of reactions in otherwise normal persons, acute onset and temporal relationship to reactions with initial dose, spontaneous recoveries and return to normalcy with drug discontinuation, and occurrences of positive rechallenge. Also, the high benzodiazepine receptor affinity with triazolam has been postulated as a possible biological mechanism.

In November 1991, the FDA implemented new required labeling for Halcion.[4] Martin Quick had been dead by suicide for a year and a half. The new label emphasizes that triazolam is indicated for short-term use and it adds new warnings about adverse psychiatric effects:

> A variety of abnormal thinking and behavior changes have been reported to occur in association with the use of benzodiazepine hypnotics, including HALCION. Some of these changes may be characterized by decreased inhibition, e.g., aggressiveness and extroversion that seem excessive, similar to that seen with alcohol and other CNS depressants (e.g., sedative/hypnotics). Other kinds of behavioral changes have been reported, for example, bizarre behavior, agitation, hallucinations, depersonalization. In primarily depressed patients, the worsening of depression, including suicidal thinking, has been reported in association with the use of benzodiazepines.

The warning concludes with an observation that psychiatric reactions have been reported in "therapeutic doses," and also that Halcion may cause more amnesia than other benzodiazepines. Despite the improvements in the label, it still fails to communicate the enormously elevated rates of adverse psychiatric reactions on Halcion in comparison to all other drugs monitored by the FDA at that time.

GREAT BRITAIN TAKES STRONG ACTIONS

GREAT BRITAIN TOOK A STRONGER STAND and banned Halcion in 1991. On December 9, 1991, the Committee on Safety of Medicines (CSM) responded to Upjohn's appeal to rescind their decision with a definitive scientific conclusion about the dangers of Halcion. The agency found a clearly established causal relationship between Halcion and adverse psychiatric effects. These adverse effects occurred, in the committee's opinion, far more frequently with Halcion than with other tranquilizers.

Why would Great Britain take a tougher stand against Halcion? The answer lies partly in the greater power of the drug industry and its medical lackeys in America, and, in particular, the lavish spending of Upjohn in the maintenance of its self-avowed partnership with the American Psychiatric Association. In response to my criticism, in a letter published in *The New York Times*,[5] the medical director of the American Psychiatric Association[6] responded with a letter of his own defending the APA's actions in accepting a gift of 1.5 million dollars from Upjohn. He declared that the drug company and the psychiatric association have a "responsible, ethical partnership." Upjohn reconfirmed the "partnership" in a letter of its own to *Clinical Psychiatry News*.[7] Even after the controversy, the American Psychiatric Association continued the theme of "our partners in industry" in a mass mailing to its membership.[8]

THE TRIAL IN MARTIN QUICK'S CASE

THE DRUG COMPANY knew that the FDA was soon going to blow a whistle, however muffled, on Halcion, drawing more attention to its capacity to cause behavioral abnormalities. Perhaps because of foreknowledge of what was to come, and also because of its desire to keep company documents secret, Upjohn settled with Martin Quick's widow without going to trial. The company did so without admitting any fault. The defendant doctor refused to settle and we went to trial.

If we won this case, it would be the first successful malpractice victory based on the premise that Halcion can cause suicide. It would be a courtroom test of the scientific basis for holding this viewpoint. The judge would have to decide if the evidence was scientific and, therefore, admissible in court. If the judge allowed the evidence to be presented, the jury would then have to decide the merits of the testimony and the malpractice case.

Barry Chafetz of the Chicago firm Corboy and Demetrio put together a team of several experts, including another psychiatrist and a pharmacist as well as M. N. G. Dukes, the international authority on drug monitoring.

Dr. Dukes, known as Graham to his friends, testified on the specific issue of Halcion's capacity to cause suicide. Dr. Dukes is a former research manager in the pharmaceutical industry. After that he became medical director for the Netherlands equivalent of our FDA, then head of pharmaceuticals for the World Health Organization (WHO) in Europe, and then a professor of drug policy studies in Norway. I especially admire his enormous expenditure of effort in traveling around the world to help establish drug-monitoring agencies for third-world countries. He also recently retired from the editorships of the largest annual compendium on adverse drug reactions, *Meyler's Side Effects of Drugs,* and the peer-reviewed *International Journal of Risk and Safety in Medicine.* After we got to know each other, Dr. Dukes invited me to be the psychiatric editorial consultant for his international journal. In 2006, I had the honor of presenting him an award at the annual meeting of the International Center for the Study of Psychiatry and Psychology (www.icspp.org).

We had to show, first and foremost, that Halcion *could* cause suicide. In doing this, we had to convince the judge that our scientific evidence had sufficient merit to justify his allowing us to testify about it to the jury. Using material similar to that in this chapter, we passed that hurdle and Dr. Dukes and I were allowed to present our conclusions that Halcion can and does cause suicide.

Then we had to show that Halcion, in fact, *did* cause or contribute to Martin's suicide. This was largely a matter of ruling out other factors, such as family problems, and then showing the temporal relationship between his taking the drug and becoming suicidal. In Martin's case, there were no other complicating factors beyond evidence that he showed signs of depression, probably over his prostate inflammation. Many people become depressed, but relatively few commit suicide. Martin possessed none of the risk factors commonly associated with suicide such as prior suicide threats, alcoholism, drug addiction, chronic and severe pain, a deteriorating illness, job loss, or loss of loved ones.

Finally, we had to show that Martin's internist was negligent in prescribing the drug. His record documented one serious error. Despite warnings put into the drug label several years earlier and despite scientific literature, he gave Halcion to a person who showed signs of depression. He should not have prescribed Halcion under those circumstances. In addition, according to Martin's wife, she had called the doctor's office several times with concerns about her husband's deteriorating condition and had been disregarded. Furthermore, there was no indication in the record or elsewhere that the doctor had given any warnings to Martin about behavioral aberrations caused by Halcion, and he admitted that he did not do so.

In my opinion, had the drug company been more forthcoming about the hazards of the drug, the doctor would have had a better chance of practicing medicine in a safe and effective manner. Nonetheless, a prudent physician did have sufficient warnings about Halcion causing or exacerbating depression to have avoided prescribing it to Martin.

The jury awarded Martin's wife 1.2 million dollars. It was a major victory for the family. It also demonstrated that a judge would allow evidence of Halcion-induced suicide into court and that a jury could be convinced that the drug can and did cause medication madness and even suicide.

SPELLBOUND BY THE NEWER SLEEPING PILLS

APPROVED BY THE FDA in December 1992, Ambien is one of a few relatively new sleeping medications that have been heavily promoted to the profession and the public. Although Ambien has a different chemical structure from the benzodiazepines like Halcion and Xanax, it affects the same neurotransmitter system, GABA, producing very similar effects, including abnormal behaviors and addiction. Too many physicians have been fooled into thinking it is really "different" from the benzos.

The 2007 FDA-approved label for Ambien CR as found in the *Physicians' Desk Reference* contains a WARNINGS section that focuses on potential behavioral abnormalities, while painting a clinical picture of potentially severe spellbinding:

> A variety of abnormal thinking and behavior changes have been reported to occur in association with the use of sedative/hypnotics. Some of these changes may be characterized by decreased inhibition (e.g., aggressiveness and extroversion that seemed out of character), similar to the effects produced by alcohol and other CNS depressants. Visual and auditory hallucinations have been reported as well as behavior changes such as bizarre behavior, agitation, and depersonalization. Amnesia, anxiety and other neuro-psychiatric symptoms may occur unpredictably. In primarily depressed patients, worsening of

depression, including suicidal thinking, has been reported in association with the use of sedative/hypnotics.

The Ambien CR label also describes how patients in brief three-week controlled clinical trials developed hallucinations, disorientation, anxiety, depression, psychomotor retardation (mental and physical slowing), depersonalization, disinhibition, euphoric mood, mood swings, and stress symptoms. Hallucinations occurred in 4 percent of the patients taking Ambien and in none of the patients taking placebo.

The label for Ambien CR also contains a SPECIAL CONCERNS section with separate subheadings for "Memory problems," "Tolerance," "Dependence," and "Withdrawal." Many of the problems are very similar to those associated with the addictive benzodiazepines (see appendix A). A fifth subhead, "Changes in behavior and thinking," offers a series of seven bulleted drug reactions:

- more outgoing or aggressive behavior than normal
- confusion
- strange behavior
- agitation
- hallucinations
- worsening of depression
- suicidal thoughts

Most people taking Ambien have no idea about the existence of these medication madness risks. I'm sure many readers who have been prescribed Ambien, Lunesta, and similar drugs will be surprised by the litany of mental and emotional risks to which they were unwittingly exposed.

On March 14, 2007, the FDA issued a new warning for a broad range of sleep medications, including every one listed in the appendix, but the real culprits are the newer drugs like Ambien and Lunesta that brought these starting phenomena to medical and public attention.[9] The new warning describes the following risk:

Complex sleep-related behaviors which may include sleep-driving, making phone calls, and preparing and eating food (while asleep).

It can be very difficult to wake up sleepwalkers, and on awakening they are often confused and usually have no memory for what they have been doing. Although spontaneous sleepwalking is fairly common among children, it is rare among adults. A drug that causes sleepwalking in adults poses serious risks. Needless to say, unconscious driving, walking, and cooking can be hazardous to oneself and to others. Sleepwalkers have been known to step out of open windows or into busy streets.

Less appreciated is the risk of violence. Sleepwalkers have been known to commit unprovoked violence and in some legal cases sleepwalking has been used as a defense in criminal trials. One textbook recommends against trying to wake sleepwalkers by "grabbing, shaking, or shouting," because "in their confused state, sleepwalkers may think they are being attacked and may react violently to defend themselves."[10] It is safest to gently lead a sleepwalker back to bed.

Guiding a Spellbound Sleepwalker

A friend of mine recently found himself needing to handle a series of sleepwalking episodes with his father who was hospitalized for surgery on his foot. His dad is a strong and mentally stable man in his seventies who had never before sleepwalked. In the hours after the surgery, he got up in a dream state and began running down the hospital corridor. The reaction was probably caused by anesthesia but perhaps by postoperative morphine injections as well. The hospital staff responded by calling two security officers. After a considerable tussle, they pushed his dad back into bed and restrained him. Then the nurses gave him a shot of Haldol to quiet him down.

Based on his familiarity with my work, my friend knew about the hazards of drugs like Haldol. One of the risks is akathisia—the same extreme hyperactive agitation that we've seen in patients taking SSRI antidepressants. In a tragic irony, Haldol, the drug most often given to subdue patients, can also drive them into an anguished hyperactivity. The patient becomes even more agitated and wild, leading to escalating measures to subdue and control him. So my friend asked the doctors not to resort to Haldol again but instead to allow him to spend the night in the hospital room with his father.

My friend's dad got up several times that night in a dream state and started to sleepwalk from the hospital room.

In one of the incidents, my friend asked, "Dad, where are you going?"

Completely asleep and immersed in his dream, his dad explained, "To a book convention."

He replied, "Sorry, Dad, the convention was canceled, so we'll just have to go to bed."

The father complied and got back into bed where he fell into a normal sleep again.

My friend had communicated through his father's dream to guide him back to bed. He was enormously grateful to be there for his dad and to prevent further potentially humiliating and dangerous scuffles, and even more dangerous injections of Haldol.

The story illustrates several important themes: the capacity of drugs to make normal people behave abnormally, the reflexive medical response of using force and giving more drugs as restraints, and the capacity of a caring individual to handle the problem without resorting to restraints or mind-suppressing drugs.

Chapter 10

Tranquilized Into Violence

TRANQUILIZED INTO VIOLENCE? We know by the name, *tranquilizer*, that these drugs are meant to make us calmer—and sometimes they do. At least, they can sufficiently suppress overall brain function to make us feel more relaxed and ultimately sleepy. But can they have the opposite effect of unleashing aggressive and violent emotions?

FROM CIVIL RIGHTS ACTIVIST TO RACIST

BOB BELLO was a successful entrepreneur and a business school professor. Yet he went on a rant against his students in class. It cost him his teaching job and his reputation in the community, and damaged his sense of himself.

Bob had been prescribed Xanax 1 mg twice a day for tension by his general practitioner and within ten days he showed up at an emergency room stating that he was afraid he was going to have a "nervous breakdown." In the emergency room, Bob looked anxious, confused, and emotionally unstable. Although he was not diagnosed as psychotic, he was so out-of-control that he was given the potent antipsychotic drug Haldol (haloperidol) by injection.

The emergency physicians noted Bob's recent exposure to Xanax but failed to consider the drug as a potential culprit. Doctors often hold an unrealistically benign opinion of tranquilizers like Xanax. Medication spellbound, Bob could not figure it out for himself. Because benzodiazepine tranquilizers can cause drunklike intoxication without the telltale slurring or staggering, no one suspected he was under the influence of the drug.

During his ten days on Xanax, Bob's friends and colleagues thought he was having a nervous breakdown. Typical of maniclike medication spellbinding, he was agitated, verbally aggressive, and seemed at times obsessed and fixated on matters of little or no importance. Unable to eat or sleep, he was described as "wired," "all wound up," "freaked-out," "goofy," "speeding," "burning up," and "disintegrating." He thought his office was bugged.

Bob ran out of Xanax and did not obtain any more. Because his exposure was so brief, he did not experience, or at least notice, any withdrawal effects. Xanax mania left Bob and his life in a shambles.

EXTENSIVE SCIENTIFIC LITERATURE

FOR MANY YEARS, the label for Xanax has contained a number of surprising admissions about this drug's destructiveness. Under "Precautions" the FDA-approved label for Xanax warns that it can cause mania:

> Episodes of hypomania and mania have been reported in association with the use of XANAX in patients with depression.

Under "Adverse Reactions," the label states:

> As with all benzodiazepines, *paradoxical reactions* such as *stimulation*, increased muscle spasticity, *sleep disturbances, hallucinations,* and *other adverse behavioral effects* such as *agitation, rage, irritability,* and *aggressive* or *hostile behavior* have been reported rarely.[1]

These adverse drug reactions echo much that's also in the antidepressant labels, except that the Xanax list displays even more graphic language, including "stimulation" and "rage," as well as "hallucinations."

Although drug companies almost always place their drug labels in the *Physicians' Desk Reference* (PDR), which is private and not a governmental publication, they are not legally required to do so. In 2006, the drug company Upjohn dropped the Xanax label from the *PDR,* although it kept selling the drug. In that year, it introduced Xanax XR, the long-acting preparation, and placed it in the *PDR*. In the label for the XR formulation, the precaution about causing hypomania and mania remains verbatim. A new table describes the most common drug-induced symptoms that surfaced during short-term (six to eight weeks long) placebo-controlled clinical trials:

Sedation—45.2 percent

Somnolence—23.0 percent

Memory impairment—15.4 percent

Fatigue—13.9 percent

Depression—12.1 percent

Dysarthria [drunken speech]—10.9 percent

Abnormal coordination—9.4 percent

Mental impairment—7.2 percent

Ataxia [drunken walking]—7.2 percent

Libido decreased—6 percent

Impaired balance—3.2 percent

Disturbances in attention—3.2 percent

Lethargy—1.7 percent

Dyskinesia [abnormal movements]—1.7 percent

Disorientation—1.5 percent

Confusion—1.5 percent

Depressed mood—1.3 percent

Hypersomnia [excessive sleeping]—1.3 percent

Side effects like sedation, somnolence, fatigue, depression, lethargy, depressed mood, and hypersomnia result from global suppression of brain function. Even taking substantial overlap into account, these figures make clear that this drug disables the brain and mind, causing both physical and emotional manifestations of depression. Xanax XR was formulated in the hope that a long-acting preparation would cause fewer acute side effects. Clearly, the result failed to meet the hype.

Also, if we add together the physical side effects that mimic drunkenness—dysarthria, abnormal coordination, ataxia, balanced impaired, and dyskinesia—they occur in 32.4 percent—or roughly one-third—of patients.

Since Xanax is very spellbinding, many patients would not recognize or report their psychiatric and mental side effects, which would then go unrecorded in the clinical trials. Therefore, the numbers of patients who experience these adverse effects must be considerably higher than even these ominous figures suggest.

But the story isn't over. Perhaps the drug company (Upjohn morphed into Pharmacia & Upjohn) realized that the facts in the label would drive physicians away from using Xanax XR. After a mere one year in the *Physicians' Desk Reference,* Pharmacia & Upjohn decided not publish the Xanax XR label in the 2007 edition of the book, something I do not recall ever seeing before in regard to such a brand-new drug. There are no Xanax formulations in the 2007 *PDR.* This will work greatly to the advantage of the company and greatly to the disadvantage of doctors and patients who will no longer have ready access to the FDA-approved label through the easily available *PDR.* Other sources for the complete label, such as the company or FDA Web site, are rarely used by physicians or consumers due to their inconvenience. Lacking ready access to the more threatening information that appears in the newer labels, most physicians will probably continue to prescribe Xanax and Xanax XR too freely based on older misconceptions about its relative safety.

We might also ask how the FDA could approve a drug with so many *admitted* hazards. There's no way to explain it other than the agency's greater devotion to drug companies than to public safety.

Meanwhile, it's been known for decades that benzodiazepines can cause disastrous mental reactions.[2] Writing in the prestigious drug textbook, *The Pharmacological Basis of Therapeutics* (1990), T. W. Rall summarized:

> *Adverse psychological effects:* Benzodiazepines may cause paradoxical effects. . . . Euphoria, restlessness, hallucinations, and hypomanic behavior have been reported to occur during the use of various benzodiazepines. Antianxiety benzodiazepines have been reported to release bizarre uninhibited behavior in some users with low levels of anxiety; hostility and rage may occur in others. Paranoia, depression, and suicidal ideation occasionally also accompany the use of these agents.[3]

THE BRAIN-DISABLING EFFECTS OF TRANQUILIZERS

BENZODIAZEPINES LIKE Halcion and Xanax graphically illustrate how psychiatric drugs produce their sought-after effects by disabling the brain. They disable the brain by ratcheting up GABA,[4] the main neurotransmitter system in the brain that suppresses or dampens down overall brain function. Given that the benzodiazepines are turning down the entire brain, there is no way that they could have a specifically "therapeutic" effect on anxiety, panic, or insomnia. Much like alcohol, which is a drug with very similar effects on the brain and mind, a low dose of benzodiazepine may seem to "take the edge off anxiety;" but it is actually blunting overall mental acuity and function. It is a continuum of effects, so that large doses of a benzodiazepine will cause a deep sleep and eventually coma, and can be used to produce generalized anesthesia for surgery.

Because Halcion, Xanax, and other sedating drugs inhibit or turn down brain function, the brain compensates by raising the level of its activity. That is, the brain fights off sedation by making itself become overstimulated.

The brain's attempt to compensate for the suppressive drug effects will eventually backfire by producing withdrawal reactions. When the benzodiazepine dose level can no longer suppress the overstimulated brain, or when the dose is reduced, withdrawal symptoms break through in the form of overstimulation along a continuum from worsened anxiety, panic, and insomnia to psychosis and seizures.

EVEN ONE OR TWO DOSES

GERRY SHANNON had a prescription for Xanax that she rarely used. It had been given to her by her family doctor to be taken as needed for anxiety and mostly she kept it in reserve. This was a time she needed it. She was recently separated from her second husband and the marriage seemed to be over. Gerry suspected him of having an affair with a neighbor but had no evidence to support her accusations. Now she was going to pick up some of her things from him in his trailer in the country where they used to live together.

The night before driving to see her husband, Gerry took a small dose of Xanax 0.25 mg to help her sleep. After awakening too early in the morning at 6:00 AM, she took a second tablet. Too tense to eat, both doses hit an empty stomach, increasing the immediacy of their impact. Four hours later she arrived earlier than expected and found her husband having breakfast with the neighbor she had suspected of having an affair with him.

As Gerry's husband protested that nothing irregular was going on, the neighbor, Angie, said nothing and hurried from the trailer to avoid trouble. When Gerry's husband followed Angie outside to say good-bye to her, Gerry rummaged through the trailer until she found the powerful .357 revolver that he kept out of sight.

By now Angie was one hundred yards away, heading toward the nearby farmhouse where she lived. Gerry came out of the trailer, saw Angie in the distance, pointed the heavy gun and fired. For an inexperienced shooter firing a high-power pistol, hitting a pie plate at five yards can be a challenge. A distance of one hundred yards might as well be infinity. Gerry sent one shot whistling into a tree near to Angie—and the other into her body. Angie was seriously wounded.

Gerry Shannon was one of my first drug-intoxication cases and retrospectively one of my most difficult. I couldn't point to a buildup of drug intoxication leading to an agitated or manic state. There were no witnesses to her state of mind prior to the shooting except for her husband who barely saw her in the seconds between when she arrived at the trailer and when she fired the shots. Nor was Gerry taking large doses or abusing Xanax. In telling me what happened, Gerry was honest to her own disadvantage in explaining that the two doses of Xanax seemed to have no perceptible effect at all on her.

Fortunately, more than fifteen years ago, there was already an extensive scientific literature implicating the benzodiazepine tranquilizers in suicide and especially in violence. I was able to write a report for the court in which I stated:

> Few negative behavioral effects of drugs are as thoroughly and persistently documented as the association between impulsive, violent behavior and benzodiazepine minor tranquilizers, including Xanax. . . . While Gerry on many occasions in the past had been "made jealous" by her husband, she had never committed any form of violence against him. In a lifetime that endured many past provocations, such as her physically abusive first husband, she had never committed violence or injured anyone.

I attached five scientific reports published over the previous two decades (1971 to 1991) implicating benzodiazepines as a cause of violence.[5]

There was no evidence of any premeditation. Gerry considered herself "good friends" with her husband and rarely grew angry with him. This was true despite his tendency to womanize at times. After Gerry realized that a bullet had hit Angie, she made no further attempt to injure her. Instead she ran to get her truck, drove it across the field to get as near as possible to Angie, and then drove her to the hospital.

Gerry does not fit into any of the criteria of the perpetrator profile (see chapter 1). Gerry blamed no one but herself for her actions and only decided to ask me for an evaluation when others urged her to do so. Although living at a poverty level, she decided not to sue her prescribing family doctor for malpractice because she believed he had no awareness that Xanax could have caused her to lose her inhibitions. She felt that he meant well and didn't wish to "ruin his life" with a malpractice suit. None of these attitudes seemed consistent with the kind of person who relishes or intentionally commits violence.

Gerry had been in jail briefly before being released on bail but now she faced the possibility of spending many years incarcerated for attempted murder. After reading my report, the prosecution and the judge decided that Gerry lacked criminal intent. Her charges were reduced and she did not need to spend any further time behind bars.

Chapter 11

A Courtroom Christmas Story

UNLIKE TV MOVIES about the courtroom, the trials in which I have testified have seldom produced much humor; they are deadly serious and incredibly stressful. This particular case was no exception, except for the storybook ending. The case also illustrates the dangerousness of even mild spellbinding that leads an individual to underestimate the degree to which a drug has made him sleepy.

Once again, I was working with Barry Chafetz from Corboy and Demetrio in Chicago. Attorney Chafetz had tried to reach a reasonable settlement in this case but the defendants who were being sued refused to settle, necessitating a trial. Perhaps the defense attorneys so resented their mammoth loss in the Halcion suicide malpractice trial described in chapter 9 that they were determined to put Mr. Chafetz and me in our respective places.

Gary Glass was fifty-two years old and was otherwise in good health when he developed an array of symptoms—numbness and tingling, dropping things, and short-term memory problems—that raised concerns that he might be suffering from small strokes or some other problem in his brain. He was sent for an MRI. Although the MRI study would turn out negative and the symptoms would disappear, events surrounding the study would nearly destroy him.

On two previous occasions Gary had become anxious when sliding inside the magnetic resonance imaging (MRI) machine. He had obtained considerable relief from one dose of Valium 5 mg taken shortly before his last MRI. For an undetermined reason, the new neurologist told Gary that he had an even better drug to give him for his anxiety. He prescribed Ativan (lorazepam) at a dose of 4 mg.

Ativan is roughly five times stronger than Valium by weight, so that taking 4 mg of Ativan is equivalent to taking 20 mg of Valium—a much larger dose than Gary was used to. A single dose this large is likely to impair reflexes and coordination, and to induce sleep, especially in someone who is unaccustomed to it.

Not knowing that it was an excessive dose, Gary dutifully took his 4 mg of Ativan after arriving at the MRI facility. He was scheduled to undergo the MRI in about twenty minutes, leaving plenty of time for the drug to take effect on an empty stomach.

Descriptions by the MRI staff would indicate that the dose had an intoxicating effect on Gary. An incident report written afterward observed:

> Before he went to change [his clothes] the patient asked for a cup of water to take some medication. After his MRI the patient appeared unsteady on his feet. He was told by the tech to wait in the waiting room for his films. He asked for a cup of coffee and this was given to him. The patient subsequently asked if his MRI films could be sent UPS and how long this would take. The patient apparently decided to have his film sent UPS and left without waiting for his film. I did not see the patient leave.

Another incident report again described the patient taking medication before the MRI and its aftermath:

> After the exam the patient appeared very groggy and somewhat uncoordinated. At some point he told me he had taken two 2 mg tablets of "something like Valium." I asked the patient if he had someone to drive him home. He stated that if he felt unable to drive, he had someone he could call.

A third incident report confirmed, "When the scan was complete he seemed groggy and unsteady."

The MRI log kept by the technician stated that Gary repeatedly fell into a restless sleep: "Patient reminded repeatedly to stay awake and not move." The MRI radiology report confirmed that Gary had been moving during the procedure, blurring some of the pictures.

Gary left the MRI facility, began to drive home, felt sleepy, and then crashed his car into a tree. He survived but sustained painful injuries. Fortunately, no one else was harmed.

Gary's case illustrates drug spellbinding, albeit in a more limited form than shown in our other stories. Much like someone who has had too many drinks of alcohol, the Ativan mildly intoxicated Gary while simultaneously undermining his judgment about his condition.

In his deposition, the prescribing neurologist contradicted himself, at first saying that 4 mg of Ativan was a "very strong" dose but that he had warned the patient about it. Later in the same deposition, he said it was a "relatively low" dose. The doctor admitted that the drug effects would begin a short time after taking the drug and that the sedation would last for a few hours. Meanwhile, the doctor's medical record gave no indication of anything he might have said to the patient warning him about the strength of the dose or the risk of driving under its influence. Regardless of what the doctor said, the facts spoke for themselves. The neurologist had prescribed five times the effective dose of Valium that Gary had used in the past—a sufficiently large dose to impair function and to induce sleep.

The malpractice case against the neurologist and the MRI clinic should have been settled for a modest amount of money—perhaps forty thousand dollars—but the defendants refused and forced us to go to trial.

The defense attorney cross-examined me in a most degrading manner, attempting to characterize me as a money-grubbing hired gun who would ruin the career of a fine colleague for mere money. It led to a charming conclusion. To understand the charm of that conclusion, you need to know that the trial was held in late December, shortly before Christmas.

The judge in the case was very elderly. He displayed a very sweet manner toward the jury, regularly asking them how they were holding up, if they could hear everything being said from the witness stand, if they needed bathroom breaks, and so on. He fussed over them much like a grandfather with his grandchildren. At the same time, he was hard of hearing, and tended to speak loudly, adding to the paternalistic effect. He was also visibly aggravated with the attorneys on both sides of the case, especially the defendant's attorney when he was so roughly cross-examining me. The judge warned him not to make faces at me when I answered questions, not to slur his voice in derision toward me, and to comport himself more respectfully. I found this gratifying because judges sometimes fail to prevent lawyers from badgering expert witnesses.

Throughout the withering cross-examination, I tried to comport myself with dignity, calm, and even good humor. It wasn't easy and I wasn't sure if I was succeeding. As I often do when under attack in public, I thought about my wife Ginger, and I reminded myself that I'm a decent person doing worthwhile work. I might have silently prayed for help in doing my best under this attack.

Due to enormous preparation and to whatever communication skills I've been granted, I usually hold my own during these courtroom cross-examination contests, even though they are loaded in favor of the cross-examiner. Nonetheless, I always feel the need for reassurance when it's over.

The cross-examination did not end until late in the afternoon, when it was time to end the trial for the day. As I stepped off the witness stand, the judge rapped his gavel and recessed the trial until the following morning. Meanwhile, my testimony was finished and I could return home, as I was eager to do, especially since it was so near Christmas.

After getting off the witness stand, I walked across the front of the courtroom to say good-bye to attorney Chafetz at the plaintiff's table. As I got there, a commotion broke out behind me from the direction of the judge's bench. I turned to see three or four members of the jury rushing up to the judge.

The jurors were pointing at me. In my career, I had never seen anything like it.

"Who does he remind you of?" the several jurors in unison asked their elderly judge.

"What? What?" the judge asked loudly, trying to hear from high up on the bench.

"Who does he remind you of?" they asked the judge again as they pointed toward me, this time with big grins on their faces.

Having trouble hearing or making sense out of what they were asking, the judge shook his head uncertainly.

Finally, one of the jurors pointed at me again and blurted out loudly, "He's like Clarence the Angel in the movie *It's a Wonderful Life*." The jurors were comparing me to the kind and gentle, if somewhat bemused, unsophisticated and rotund angel who saves Jimmy Stewart's life in America's favorite Christmas movie.

I tried to think of something to say back but attorney Chafetz wisely restrained me from interfering with this perfect courtroom moment.

Clearly the attack on me had utterly failed. I had not only kept my composure but communicated a degree of spirituality to them. If the defendants had been sensible, they would have settled the case on the spot, but they insisted on taking the trial to the bitter end. In a lawsuit that could have been settled for forty thousand dollars, the jury awarded Gary Glass eight hundred and forty thousand dollars.

Chapter 12

A Vicious Addiction

SPELLBINDING OFTEN OCCURS RAPIDLY in an overwhelming fashion, often within the first few doses of a psychoactive drug. However, especially in regard to tranquilizers and sleeping pills, spellbinding can occur gradually, creeping up on the individual over time. Eventually the individual becomes completely disabled without having any idea what has happened. Over a period of months the unwitting victim of medication spellbinding can become desperately drug dependent, easily manipulated, emotionally unstable, depressed, and suicidal.

THE MAN WHO COULDN'T TELL A LIE

SPELLBOUND BY PRESCRIBED XANAX, Sam Rudolf was so impaired in his judgment that he voluntarily subjected himself to a government deposition at a time when he was too befuddled to adequately testify or defend himself. It took almost five years of prescribed Xanax to put him into that vulnerable state and he would remain on Xanax through his tragic courtroom trial for a total of six and one-half years.

From looking back at his medical and work records, and from interviews with people who knew him, Sam's life seemed to have been going well before he sought psychiatric help. As a young man, he and his dad started a small company that made precision machinery, and the company thrived. When his dad retired, Sam took over managing the company. He kept innumerable phone numbers in his head and calculated razor-thin dimensions for cutting tools without resorting to a calculator.

In addition to thriving at work, Sam was a devoted father and husband, and had few bad habits. He gambled occasionally but rarely lost substantial amounts. His annual income was well into six figures. As a result of hard work and providing a needed service, he was gradually becoming wealthy.

At the age of thirty-nine, Sam developed a physical disorder that remained undiagnosed for many months. It would turn out to be cystitis—inflammation of the bladder—an uncommon disorder in men that was easily cured with appropriate antibiotics. His internist mistakenly thought the disorder might be psychological and referred him to a psychiatrist. Sam had no particular history of anxiety, but he felt considerably distressed after being told the abdominal pain was all in his head.

The psychiatrist started him on Prozac and then followed up several months later by adding Xanax. Because SSRI antidepressants frequently cause agitation, anxiety, and insomnia, doctors often end up adding a sedative or tranquilizing agent to calm the patient down. Usually these doctors mistakenly attribute the overstimulation to "mental illness" and incorrectly diagnose the patient with a new anxiety disorder. Prozac overstimulated so many patients during its clinical trials for FDA approval that Eli Lilly decided to break the rules of the trials by giving tranquilizers and sleeping medications to many of the subjects. When the FDA was informed later on, the agency retrospectively permitted this breach of its own rules. In effect, instead of approving Prozac for the treatment of depression, the FDA approved Prozac in combination with addictive tranquilizers, without ever informing the medical profession or the public about this ruse.[1] Especially when the newer antidepressants are combined with Xanax, the risk of disinhibition and even mania is increased.

Sam eventually sued his doctor and a dispute developed over Sam's condition at the time he went to the psychiatrist. Sam explained to me that he was upset about his physical problems and that he had no prior history of anxiety and depression. Never before had he seen a mental health professional. In deposition, however, Sam's doctor defended his prescriptions by declaring under oath that Sam came to him in a state of severe, long-term anxiety and depression. The doctor's sparse medical record did not mention any serious prior mental problems.

When parties to a conflict have strong interests in promoting their own viewpoints, it can be very difficult to decide who's telling the truth about past events. However, there can be no doubt about what happened to Sam as his treatment continued—and it had little or nothing to do with his mental condition at the time he came for psychiatric help.

Within a few months after starting Xanax, Sam Rudolf gradually became a changed man. He began to spend money excessively in stores and at auctions, and he developed an interest in pornography. After being on increasing doses of Xanax for several years, he met a porn star at a pornography convention and then became friends with her. Mostly, he talked to her on the phone and when she began giving him stock tips, he thought nothing unusual about it. She told him she was getting her advice from a stockbroker boyfriend.

Sam would research her suggestions and sometimes he found reason to follow her advice and sometimes not. Later, he would explain to me that their chats about stocks were a small part of the conversations. He never paid her any money, either for her platonic affection or for her stock tips. There was no evidence that money was exchanged between them.

By now Sam had been taking 6 to10 mg per day of Xanax, plus 40 mg of Prozac for a few years. He suffered from daily emotional ups and downs as each dose of Xanax wore off.

Out of the blue, Sam got a call from the SEC—the Securities and Exchange Commission. Sam was suspected of insider trading. Sam was guileless and readily volunteered to be deposed under oath by the government. He was happy to straighten out any misunderstanding. Unfortunately, he was medication spellbound by a combination of Xanax and Prozac. Neither he nor his lawyer understood that a trap was being set for Sam and that he was too intoxicated to escape it.

As time for the deposition approached, Sam's psychiatrist raised the Xanax dose to 10 mg per day in divided doses. That's the recommended limit for controlling severe panic disorder—which Sam did not have. More than that, the panic disorder studies conducted by the drug company lasted only eight weeks, while Sam had been taking the drug for many years. Upjohn, the manufacturer of Xanax, de-emphasized data demonstrating that patients were actually worse off—more panic ridden than ever—after taking the drug for eight weeks. The company also failed to properly emphasize that many of the patients were unable to stop taking Xanax after only eight weeks' exposure.[2]

According to Sam, his psychiatrist told him that he could occasionally raise the dose if needed to 12 mg per day. Sam never obtained Xanax from anyone except his physician who knew exactly how much his patient was taking. There's nothing in the record to suggest that Sam was using Xanax in a manner inconsistent with his doctor's advice.

Sam's life was falling apart. He was ruining his marriage. His memory was too shot to properly run his business. His insomnia was so bad that he began

arriving at work late in the day or in the evening. A man with conservative up-
bringing and inclinations, he made friends with the porn star, and had no idea
whatsoever that Xanax was disinhibiting him, impairing his judgment and his
impulse control.

Without grasping the full extent of the deficit, Sam did notice increasing
memory difficulties, but his psychiatrist did not think it serious enough to stop
or to reduce his patient's drugs. The doctor seemed to suspect that the antidepressants were causing difficulties and he switched them around a few times. I
have evaluated several tragic cases involving individuals who developed permanent difficulties with memory function, learning, and the clarity of their
thinking after years of exposure to Xanax and other benzodiazepines. In one
case, during a dozen years of exposure to Xanax and Valium, a respected scientist and medical school professor permanently lost his memory function, his
cognitive abilities, and then his impulse control without anyone, including his
several doctors, identifying the cause and stopping the treatment.[3]

At the SEC deposition, Sam was accused of insider trading. He was informed that his friend the porn star was getting her stock tips from a corporate
executive who had insider information. Sam tried to explain that he had no
idea what they were talking about. He didn't know her boyfriend's name, let
alone his job description. Nor did he take all her investment advice and he always researched the options for himself. But Sam was unable to explain all this
clearly or succinctly. The deposition is marred in part by Sam's memory problems but even more by his poor judgment and communication skills. Sam
sometimes could not get his thoughts straight and he seemed unable to verbal-
ize the absurdity of charging him with colluding with a man he did not know
and with whom he had exchanged no communications or money. From my
reading of the deposition, Sam at times did not fully understand the questions
or was unable to gather his thoughts in response to them.

Two months after the deposition, Sam went to a new medical doctor to
evaluate his persisting discomfort in his lower abdominal area and this time
was correctly diagnosed with cystitis. He had not been afflicted with a psychosomatic disorder; he had been suffering from a chronic infection. An antibiotic
easily cured Sam's physical discomfort but by now it was too late—he was already hooked on Xanax, suffering from severe medication spellbinding, and
was in trouble with the law.

No formal charges of insider trading were brought against Sam. Instead he
was charged with perjury in his deposition. I read Sam's pretrial deposition
transcript but I was not given the trial transcript to read so I cannot confirm
the specific nature of his alleged perjury. However, from going over his depo-

sition I was able to determine that he was mentally impaired and medication spellbound, and confused about what was going on at the time.

Following the deposition, Sam's psychiatrist continued him on Xanax and Prozac. In fact, throughout the trial Sam was maintained on an intoxicating combination of high doses of Xanax and Prozac. He did not have the wits to offer an adequate defense and on one occasion was so sedated that he fell asleep at the defense table in front of the judge. According to Sam, the judge recommended that he obtain a psychiatric evaluation before standing trial, but his lawyer discouraged the idea. As I've learned, many attorneys do not realize that psychiatric medications can render a client incompetent to participate in a deposition or to cooperate in his own defense. Sam unfortunately remained spellbound throughout the trial. Indeed, he felt grateful toward his doctor for continuing to prescribe for him during his desperate times.

Sam was sentenced to several years in the state penitentiary. Within a week of landing in jail, Sam's existence became hellish, not because of the prison, but because his brain and body became wracked with pain. He couldn't sleep and suffered overwhelming anxiety. He sweated, trembled, and shook all over. He felt like he was dying of a heart attack.

Inmates of prisons tend to be very familiar with addictive drugs. Many have taken them before incarceration and some continue to obtain them illegally behind bars. A fellow prisoner finally informed Sam, "You're going through withdrawal. You're addicted to Xanax."

Ordinarily prisons won't give Xanax to inmates under any circumstances. The addictive drugs are much too sought after as contraband in jail. Nonetheless, the prison doctor made an exception for Sam. Probably obtaining the Xanax from a prescription written by Sam's original psychiatrist, the new doctor tried to gradually wean Sam. Remarkably, the prison doctor officially diagnosed Sam with "iatrogenic addiction," indicating that Sam's prescribed treatment had caused it. It is very unusual for one doctor to write a diagnosis that impugns the treatment of another doctor, and it is much to this doctor's credit that he wrote this into the record.

The prison doctor tried for five months to withdraw Sam from his Xanax addiction, occasionally making notes in the record indicating the severity of Sam's withdrawal symptoms, such as "Patient complains of chest pain, sweating, anxiety. States symptoms are related to Xanax." The doctor also noted Sam's sleep disturbance. Again, displaying an unusual willingness to call a spade a spade, the doctor wrote, "Anxiety disorder secondary to iatrogenic addiction."

Sam continued to grow worse as the doctor tried to reduce his Xanax and to switch him to other drugs. Sam was described as shaky, nervous, anxious,

and depressed, and finally developed one of the most serious of benzodiazepine withdrawal symptoms: grand mal seizures.

After five months, the state facility decided to transfer Sam Rudolf to a
federal penitentiary in another state where he could obtain more intensive
medical care. After he had been at the new facility for a couple of months, his
psychiatrist wrote in the record:

> Patient says he is doing very well and is still feeling improvement gradually
> with his energy and memory/concentration. He says he is still amazed at
> how he became addicted to benzodiazepines.

Sam remained in the federal medical facility for more than a year as he
gradually withdrew from benzodiazepines. He was discharged to a halfway
house for several months, and then set free.

Sending Sam to a halfway house was unnecessary and humiliating. Sam
didn't need drug rehabilitation because he never sought drugs illegally. He
never stole drugs, hustled drugs from different doctors, bought drugs on the
street, or took drugs in excess of how they were prescribed.

Before Sam began receiving benzodiazepines from a doctor, he was a functioning father and husband and the owner and manager of a thriving business.
He was free of memory problems or other cognitive disorders and indeed was
proud of his mental acuity and memory. Years of exposure to Xanax had laid
waste to his life.

While Sam was in jail, his wife left him and his daughter stopped all contact with him. His wife went to court in a successful effort to take over his
family business that he'd begun with his dad. His father's retirement savings—
the fruits of their family business—were used up in his criminal defense and in
his conflicts with his wife over control of his business. He was destitute and
unable to work. His mental processes were so disordered that he qualified for a
diagnosis of Xanax-induced Persisting Dementia and would never again be
able to work at a physically or mentally demanding job.

A little less than two years after he was released from probation, Sam came
for an evaluation in my office in regard to his malpractice suit against his psychiatrist that had been initiated some time earlier. Sam had all the stigmata of
mild-to-moderate drug-induced dementia. His short-term memory was shot
and he became easily confused. Unbeknownst to Sam, I had overheard him
talking aloud to himself as he stood outside on the sidewalk trying to decide if
he had found my office, and he sounded confused and distressed by the simple
decision.

Sam was in the habit of recording his phone calls in order to remember details on complicated issues such as his legal conflicts with his ex-wife. He played back a phone call for me from earlier in the day that clearly demonstrated his cognitive problems. He had grave difficulty explaining simple matters concerning his medical treatment or legal activities.

Sam had another characteristic of dementia that is often missed by laypersons and physicians alike—inappropriate emotional responses. As he recounted the utter devastation of his life, he did not look or sound depressed. He didn't even sound sad. Instead, he was mildly euphoric, bubbling over with energy and even enthusiasm. He was too loud and leaned too close, both common signs of brain dysfunction impairing social judgment. Hearing Sam talk about his devastated life was like hearing a television car salesman rapping about a tragic disaster.

Although the official diagnostic manual, the American Psychiatric Association's *Diagnostic and Statistical Manual of Mental Disorders,* recognizes Xanax-induced persistent memory problems and dementia, juries are loathe to give money to people unless they suffer from gross physical disabilities, such as a neck twisted badly out of shape or a deforming scar. Despite all the hype about how easy it is to sue doctors, in reality lawyers are reluctant to take cases where the victim is not dead, visibly maimed, or completely disabled. Sam was never going to fully recover from Xanax and he remained completely disabled. Much like Patrick Cunningham (see chapter 2), Sam also suffered from partially disabling painful feelings in his feet and legs, which in my clinical experience may be caused by a Xanax-induced neuritis. But none of Sam's injuries was visible. Sitting at the defense table in the courtroom, Sam looked like a normal person.

When he was called to testify on his own behalf in the malpractice trial, I was concerned that Sam would not make a good impression. The euphoria that I had observed in my office had worn away, leaving him irritable, angry, and controlling. His overbearing style, which is commonly seen in mildly brain-injured people, would not look good on the witness stand.

There was another problem with the lawsuit. Because there was insufficient scientific literature on the subject of Xanax-induced neuritis, the judge prohibited me from testifying about Sam's most agonizing symptom, his painful feet and legs.

At the conclusion of my testimony, the defendant doctor decided to offer a settlement without admitting wrongdoing. This was gratifying but the amount of the offer was relatively small considering the damage done to Sam. As I recall, it was not much above one hundred thousand dollars.

The settlement offer was less than Sam used to make in a good year running his business. It wouldn't pay off his debts and wouldn't rescue his father's spent retirement funds. He didn't want to accept the offer. Sam's lawyer and the judge both advised Sam that it was a good deal; he might lose the case entirely and receive nothing if it went to the jury. I had to agree with them. Reluctantly, Sam accepted the settlement and the trial ended in disappointment for him.

FROM ACUTE TO LASTING DEVASTATION

COMING OFF XANAX frequently produces withdrawal symptoms such as overwhelming anxiety and panic attacks, unbearable insomnia, bouts of dreadful depression, extreme irritability, nausea and vomiting, migrainelike sensitivity to environmental stimulation, shakes, sweating, hallucinations and abnormal sensations, agonizing muscle cramps, and in the extreme, confusion, psychosis, and grand mal seizures. And while Xanax may be more difficult to withdraw from than some other benzodiazepine tranquilizers, all of them can cause these withdrawal symptoms.

Even after going through this tormenting withdrawal, not everyone fully recovers. I have seen people who suffer persistent emotional instability, muscle cramps, and pains in their legs and feet (similar to a peripheral neuritis). Years after stopping the benzos, many people like Sam Rudolf fail to fully recover their mental faculties. Like Sam, their memory remains full of huge gaps for the period of months or years surrounding the drug exposure. They find it difficult to learn new things and to multitask.

As they recover, they become dismayed and then depressed to find out how badly they have wrecked their lives and the lives of loved ones. To make matters worse—much worse—their mental function often fails to fully recover. They continue to forget simple things like phone calls, appointments, and shopping lists, and they cannot multitask or master more complex learning. Their moods remain unstable and often dismal, and they frequently feel embittered and angry. Much like people who never recover from electric shock treatment,* Xanax victims can remain irritable and emotionally erratic years after they have been withdrawn from the tranquilizers.

---

*The brain-damaging effects of modern electroshock treatment (ECT) are discussed in my book *Brain-Discussing Treatment in Psychiatry* (2008).

Addiction from Short-Term Treatment with Therapeutic Doses

Xanax and Halcion are so short acting that withdrawal can take place during the day in between doses. This leads people to take the drug more frequently, encouraging abuse, and outright addiction.

Under WARNINGS, the FDA-approved Xanax label states:[4]

> Even after relatively short-term use at the doses recommended for the treatment of transient anxiety and anxiety disorder (i.e., 0.75 to 4 mg per day), there is some risk of dependence. Spontaneous reporting system data suggest that the risk of dependence and its severity appear to be greater in patients treated with doses greater than 4 mg/day and for long periods (more than 12 weeks).

Notice that the risk begins with doses as small as 0.75 mg per day—well below the typical treatment regimen. Also, notice that the risk increases with "long periods" of treatment and that these are defined as more than twelve weeks in duration—a relatively brief exposure compared to the many months or years that too many doctors consider routine treatment.

The American Psychiatric Association task force report *Benzodiazepine Dependence, Toxicity, and Abuse* (1990) echoes the warnings in the Xanax label, noting that shorter-acting benzodiazepines like Xanax and Halcion have a greater tendency to cause dependence. The task force cites "numerous reports" of physiological dependence caused by both short-acting and long-acting benzodiazepines prescribed by doctors at therapeutic doses. It warns that a worsening of insomnia (called rebound insomnia) can occur after one week of routine doses and that more serious withdrawal symptoms can occur after only four to six weeks of treatment for anxiety.[5] As ominous as this warning seems, it minimizes the problem. Rebound and withdrawal symptoms from Halcion can occur after one or two doses, making people feel agitated and anxious.

The American Psychiatric Association report makes clear that drug dependence (addiction) can take place at routine doses, calling the phenomenon "therapeutic dose dependence." It highlights an eight-month study of Xanax for panic disorder in which, despite careful tapering, "over 90 percent of all patients experienced marked withdrawal symptoms." More than nine out of ten patients had serious withdrawal problems! Furthermore, "26 percent of the patients were unable to stay off their benzodiazepines for longer than one to three days." After routine treatment, more than one-quarter became addicted.[6]

The news is even worse. After a mere six to eight weeks of exposure to

Xanax, patients actually suffered from more frequent and severe panic attacks than before the treatment started.[7]

Withdrawal from Xanax can become so unbearable that some people end up taking small doses indefinitely. Of course, this is not good for the brain and mind.

No Excuse for Persisting Physician Ignorance

Ignorance on the part of physicians about the dangers of benzodiazepines continues to this day, but there is no excuse for it. The bible of psychiatry—the American Psychiatric Association's *Diagnostic and Statistical Manual of Mental Disorders* (2000)—lists numerous drug-induced disorders that confirm the potentially devastating impact of these drugs. This consensus document written by experts in the field lists the following disorders caused by Xanax and other benzodiazepines and sedatives:[8]

Dependence

Abuse

Intoxication

Intoxication Delirium

Withdrawal Delirium

Persisting Dementia [generalized brain and mind dysfunction]

Persisting Amnestic [Memory] Disorder

Psychotic Disorder

Mood Disorder

Anxiety Disorder

Sleep Disorder

The very drugs prescribed for anxiety and sleep problems can cause anxiety and sleep problems. In fact, they routinely do. Many of these reactions are caused by rebound or withdrawal in between individual doses of the drug.

The American Psychiatric Association's Task Force Report on *Benzodiazepine Dependence, Toxicity, and Abuse* (1990) observes that short half-life benzodiazepines are prone to produce "intense discontinuation syndromes." Halcion and Xanax, followed by Klonopin and Ativan, are among the shorter-acting tranquilizers.

The monograph includes a table listing withdrawal symptoms (called discontinuation symptoms). Anxiety, agitation, and irritability are designated to be common. Depression as a withdrawal reaction is common but less frequent.

Psychosis, confusion, paranoid delusions, and hallucinations are listed as uncommon withdrawal symptoms, but they are potentially devastating when they occur.

A LIMITED TRIUMPH OVER XANAX

NOT EVERYONE REMAINS as paralyzed by Xanax adverse effects as Sam Rudolf. Many Xanax-injured people are able to triumph over their disabilities and to live productive and happy lives.

Like Sam Rudolf, dentist Ron Manheim also became addicted to Xanax prescribed by his psychiatrist. Wholly unlike Sam, Ron had a long if intermittent history of drug abuse and dependency before he saw the psychiatrist. His growing problems with alcohol abuse led to his making the appointment. The doctor's notes from the first visit indicate that Ron was painfully honest with him about his drug and alcohol problems:

> For past year, he has had alcohol problem—he gets paranoid when drinking, loses control of behavior, and may drink himself into stupor. Probably some trouble with drugs. Patient has been addicted to narcotics which caused trouble with Dental Board, DEA. Had terrible withdrawal—spent time in three rehabilitation centers.

Ron was up front about his addiction problem and how it had led to difficulties with both the Dental Board and the DEA several years earlier. The psychiatrist diagnosed his new patient with major depression, panic disorder, and "substance abuse—alcohol and drugs."

Within a couple of months of first seeing him, the psychiatrist decided that Ron continued to suffer from panic disorder—frequent episodes of dread with physical symptoms like sweating and palpitations. The diagnosis of panic disorder should not have been made because alcohol abuse with intermittent withdrawal will cause the same or similar symptoms. Panic disorder rarely surfaces for the first time in older patients like Ron whereas paniclike symptoms plague alcoholics as they go through varying degrees of withdrawal on a daily basis.

The Xanax label and multiple publications warn about cross-addiction between Xanax and alcohol. The FDA-approved label makes a direct comparison between the effects of Xanax and alcohol. Under a bold headline in caps entitled DRUG ABUSE AND DEPENDENCE with a bold subhead of "Physical and Psychological Dependence," the warning starts as follows:

Withdrawal symptoms similar in character to those noted with sedative/hypnotics and alcohol have occurred following discontinuance of benzodiazepines, including XANAX. The symptoms can range from mild dysphoria and insomnia to a major syndrome that may include abdominal and muscle cramps, vomiting, sweating, tremors, and convulsions.[9]

The doctor might as well have been prescribing gin for a patient already addicted to vodka. Over a one-year period, Ron inevitably became dependent on Xanax. Eventually, his professional and family life began to suffer, the dental board again became concerned about him, and he voluntarily admitted himself to a rehabilitation center where he was treated for alcohol and Xanax dependence.

Although his exposure was briefer than Sam's, the Xanax had similar harmful effects on Ron. He developed memory difficulties and other cognitive deficits that persisted even after stopping the medication. Early in his rehabilitation hospitalization, attempts at psychological testing were postponed because he was showing so much mental dysfunction from drug withdrawal. Ron's doctor wrote in the chart: "He had neuropsychiatric testing started. The results did show significant impairment from the benzodiazepines. In fact, some of the testing has been put off for a couple of weeks due to the level of impairment." Neuropsychiatric testing involves specialized tests aimed at evaluating mental deficits caused by brain dysfunction.

The history of his twelve months on Xanax remained a jumble in Ron's mind, and I could not rely upon him to give an accurate history of events. Although it would have been to his advantage in his malpractice suit to remember the most painful and humiliating details of the collapse of his dental practice and family life, he simply couldn't. For example, he had no recollection of the many days in which he went into acute withdrawal in the office, became incoherent and unable to function, and had to be given additional Xanax before he could recover.

Ron also suffered permanent neurological damage that affected his peripheral nervous system. In his case it manifested as a partial loss of hand–eye coordination. This deficit was especially noticeable to Ron because of his profession. As a result of the loss of hand–eye coordination, when Ron regained his dental license he was no longer able to carry out complex dental procedures and had to limit his practice. As an ethical professional, he imposed the limits on himself.

I testified that Ron's prior history of opiate and alcohol dependence should have prevented the doctor from starting him on Xanax. Even the label for Xanax warns against prescribing it to people who are addiction prone. I also testified that Ron's drinking problem worsened after his doctor prescribed the Xanax. Because alcohol and Xanax have such similar effects on the brain and mind, people who become dependent on Xanax often abuse alcohol as well. The jurors, however, exonerated the doctor of any wrongdoing in prescribing Xanax. They apparently blamed Ron himself rather than his doctor for the addiction to prescribed medication.

I often warn plaintiffs who hire me as a medical expert in malpractice suits to avoid going to trial if at all possible. The outcomes of trials often seem unpredictable. However, I hoped that Ron's demeanor and determination to keep working at his profession, and his doctor's gross error in prescribing Xanax to a patient with a past history of addiction, would have encouraged the jury to look favorably upon the malpractice suit. Apparently not.

Despite the enormous losses and blows that Ron has suffered, he has remained enthusiastic about life, and thanks God for another opportunity to work as a dentist and to love his family. Unlike Sam, he was not totally disabled, and unlike Sam, he continues to receive loving support from an extended family.

Chapter 13

He Wanted to Do Better in School

IN 2002, MR. AND MRS. BRADLEY traveled from the Midwest to see me in my office in Ithaca, New York. Mr. Bradley was a toolmaker and his wife was a teacher's aide at their son Mike's Baptist school. They had three children, fourteen-year-old Mike and two older sisters, one married and the other going to college. Mike was deceased.

The Bradleys wanted grief counseling and help in understanding what befell their son after starting on a stimulant drug for attention-deficit hyperactivity disorder (ADHD). It was one of the most heartrending interviews of my career. When I phoned them recently, it was as if their anguish remained cemented into place. In many cases involving the death of a child, the family never fully recovers.

Before looking more closely at what happened to Mike, it's important to review concerns about the stimulant drugs currently used to treat children who are diagnosed with ADHD.

THE FDA: MUCH TOO LITTLE, MUCH TOO LATE

THE FDA-APPROVED labels for stimulant drugs, including amphetamine products like Adderall and Dexedrine and methylphenidate products like Ritalin and Concerta, have always been shamefully inadequate. They have misled physicians and parents into believing that these drugs are safer than they are, especially regarding risks of addiction and serious psychiatric side effects such as psychosis, mania, aggression, and suicide. Indeed, in a rare confession of its failure to do its duty, the FDA recently admitted, "Current approved labeling for drug treatments of ADHD does not clearly address the risk of drug-induced signs of symptoms of psychosis and mania (such as hallucinations) in patients without identifiable risk factors, and occurring at the usual doses"[1]—a point I had been making for nearly a decade.

In 2005, the FDA at long last acknowledged that it was receiving an alarming number of reports of adverse psychiatric reactions, including suicidality, for methylphenidate products such as Concerta and Ritalin:

> Post-marketing reports received by FDA regarding Concerta and other methylphenidate products [e.g., Ritalin] include psychiatric events such as visual hallucinations, suicidal ideation, psychotic behavior, as well as aggression or violent behavior.
>
> We intend to make labeling changes describing these events.[2]

The FDA warning was accompanied by a summary of fifty-two adverse psychiatric reactions reported over the prior year for Concerta and Ritalin. The list was dominated by cases of overstimulation (agitation and mania), depression, psychosis, aggression and violence, and suicidal behavior.[3] This is the same array of dangerous effects that the FDA recognized in 2004 to 2005 as those associated with the newer antidepressants. As noted earlier, the similarity between stimulant and antidepressant adverse effects is probably due to the stimulating properties of the newer antidepressants.

Based on new information about an increase in both psychiatric and cardiovascular adverse effects, especially arrhythmias associated with sudden death, the FDA announced plans for a hearing in September 2006, focused on revising the stimulant labels. As the time for the hearing grew near, the FDA's Division of Drug Risk Evaluation issued a lengthy in-house memorandum analyzing reports received concerning "Psychiatric Adverse Events Associated with Drug Treatment of ADHD:"[4]

> The most important finding of this review is that signs and symptoms of psychosis or mania, particularly hallucinations, can occur in some patients with no identifiable risk factors, at usual doses of any of the drugs currently used to treat ADHD. Current labeling for drug treatments of ADHD does not clearly address the risk of drug-induced signs of symptoms of psychosis

or mania (such as hallucinations) . . . A substantial proportion of psychosis-related cases was reported to occur in children age ten years or less, a population in which hallucinations are not common.

The FDA report in March 2006 emphasized that every type of stimulant drug had caused psychosis, and that for each type of drug, there had been reports of rechallenge, where the drug, when administered a second time, once again caused psychosis.[5] The FDA's report also identified stimulant-induced aggression:

Numerous postmarketing reports of aggression or violent behavior during therapy of ADHD have been received, most of which were classified as non-serious, although approximately 20 percent of cases overall were considered life-threatening or required hospital admission. In addition, a few cases resulted in incarceration of juveniles.

Once again, positive rechallenge reports were found for each drug.

Finally, suicide also appeared as a risk. However, except for Strattera, there was less demonstrable causality:

Suicidality has been identified as a safety issue for STRATTERA (atomoxetine), and this information is clearly conveyed in current labeling. A causal association between other drugs therapies of ADHD and suicidality cannot be ruled out on the basis of this review. Further evaluation of this issue is recommended.

ONCE AGAIN, THE FDA PLAYS CATCH-UP

IN PUBLISHING these observations in March 2006, the FDA finally caught up with strong warnings I had issued eight years earlier in November 1998. On that occasion, I was selected by the director's office of the National Institutes of Health (NIH) to be the scientific presenter on adverse drug effects at the government's Consensus Development Conference on the Diagnosis and Treatment of Attention Deficit Hyperactivity Disorder.[6] In preparation for my presentation, I used the Freedom of Information Act (FOIA) to obtain a summary of all adverse event reports for Ritalin sent into the FDA. When I tabulated the results, it became apparent that there were strong signals indicating that Ritalin was causing many psychiatric adverse events.

When addressing the 1998 conference (Breggin, "Risks and Mechanism of Action of Stimulants," 1998), I warned about an unexpectedly high number of reports of stimulant-induced psychosis, aggression, and suicidality. I had found hundreds of psychiatric adverse drug reactions coded in the FDA's summary as agitation, hostility, depression, psychotic depression, psychosis, hallucinations, emotional lability, and abnormal thinking as well as overdose, overdose intentional, and suicide attempt. I then broadened this warning in my scientific review and analysis titled, "Psychostimulants in the Treatment of Children Diagnosed with ADHD: Risks and Mechanism of Action" (1999), and in my book *Talking Back to Ritalin* (2001).

Compared to the FDA and the drug companies, I have limited resources. If I was able to discern the pattern of adverse effects in 1998, then the FDA and the drug manufacturer Novartis with their vast resources should also have been able to do so. After I publicized the problem at the 1998 conference, the FDA and the drug companies no longer had any excuse for failing to conduct their own analyses to confirm my observations. Instead, they delayed for nearly a decade.

ONCE AGAIN, FUMBLING THE BALL

I SPOKE AT THE 2006 FDA hearings on stimulant medication to encourage the agency to seriously consider our seemingly mutual concerns about psychiatric adverse stimulant effects such as suicide and violence. But the FDA was already withdrawing from its previous declarations about the risks associated with stimulants. Except for keeping the already-existing Strattera black-box warning about suicide, the Pediatric Advisory Committee decided not to "scare" parents by adding a black-box warning in the stimulant labels. In reality, the committee members—many with direct ties to the affected drug companies as consultants, speakers, or researchers—did not want to scare their patrons about potential lost profits. The committee did, however, recommend mentioning in the stimulant labels that there have been reports of aggressive and suicidal events in association with these drugs.[7] The committee's recommendations are not binding and the FDA would not even go that far.

In February 2007, nearly half a year after the conference, the FDA finally issued a press release announcing its intention to require label changes indicating psychiatric side effects such as "hearing voices, becoming suspicious for no reason, or becoming manic," but at a rate of only one per a thousand. This rate estimate (0.1 percent) actually made the threat seem less than doctors had previously supposed, since a higher rate of 1 percent had been bandied about for many years.

There is no basis for the FDA's ridiculously low estimate of the risk of psychosis and similar reactions from stimulants. The study that looked most closely at the rates for psychoticlike reactions in children taking stimulants found that nearly 10 percent display these symptoms at some point during treatment.[8] Also, the FDA no longer made any mention of stimulants causing suicide. Once again, the agency grossly failed America's children.

TREATING CHILDREN WITH COCAINELIKE DRUGS

METHYLPHENIDATE (RITALIN, CONCERTA) is a classic stimulant that is almost identical in its effects on brain and mind to other stimulants such as amphetamine and methamphetamine. Dexedrine and Adderall are amphetamines. Methylphenidate and the amphetamines are very similar in their pharmacological effects to cocaine, but because cocaine is shorter acting and more potent, it produces a more dramatic impact and more quickly causes addiction. All the classic stimulants can cause addiction, violence toward self and others, depression, mania, and a broad array of bizarre mental reactions and behaviors.[9]

All but one of the currently prescribed stimulants for the treatment of ADHD are classified as Schedule II narcotics by the Drug Enforcement Administration (DEA). Schedule II includes methylphenidate products like Ritalin and Concerta, and amphetamine products like Dexedrine and Adderall, as well as cocaine, morphine, and other drugs with the *highest* risk of causing dependence and abuse. A complete list of the stimulants is provided in appendix A. The exception, Strattera (atomoxetine), was originally tested as an antidepressant before being tested and approved as a treatment for ADHD, and it is not chemically related to methylphenidate, amphetamine, and cocaine.

Strattera has serious risks of its own. Like so many drugs produced by Eli Lilly, including Darvon, Prozac, and Zyprexa, the company marketed it as potentially safer than its competitors when in reality it can be more more deadly.

Based on a review and analysis of thirteen clinical trials conducted with children, all but one for the treatment of ADHD, the FDA "identified an increased risk of suicidal thinking for Strattera." The FDA could not ignore the data from the Strattera's controlled clinical trials and required the black-box warning, previously quoted in chapter 5.

The same label warning should have been required for all of the stimulants but it was not.

A SPELLBOUND RECITATION

MIKE WAS AN AVERAGE STUDENT, and was not very excited about his studies. He loved the social and athletic aspects of school, and was very heavily involved in extracurricular activities. Like many youngsters, he was motivated to do his schoolwork to keep up his grade average to qualify for playing sports.

It all began very innocently. Mrs. Bradley took her son to the pediatrician for a routine physical exam required by the school for participation in sports. While she remained in the waiting room, Mike privately told the pediatrician that he would like to take the medicine that his friends were taking to help them concentrate on their studies. He wanted to do better.

After the physical exam, the pediatrician accompanied Mike into the waiting room. The doctor explained to Mrs. Bradley, "Your son and I have had a conversation and he wants to do a little better and concentrate a little better in school, and I see no problem with him going on the lowest dose of a medicine called Concerta. It's Ritalin in a timed-release form." Mrs. Bradley asked about any potential side effects and the doctor explained, as best as Mrs. Bradley could recall, "Because this is such a low dose, the worst possible thing would be that within five days your son would be a little bit hyper." But he gave Mike a middle dose, Concerta 36 mg, to be taken once every morning.

Doctors often reassure patients by telling them that a psychiatric drug is being prescribed in such a small dose that it is harmless. In reality, if the dose is sufficient to have any effect on the brain and mind, then it is sufficient to cause mental disturbances. Beyond that, reactions to psychoactive substances are so variable that unusually tiny doses can menace the well-being of some people.

From the viewpoint of his parents, Mike did not need psychiatric medication. He was enjoying his social life, extracurricular activities, and sports so much that he didn't give high enough priority to his studies. He had many friends and delighted in talking and e-mailing them all evening, instead of studying. But the pediatrician reassured his mother that there were no serious side effects and that they would know within a week of taking the drug if it would helpful.

Mike wouldn't have another full week.

Mike's parents didn't know that their son had recently written a school essay that might have set off alarm bells, even before he was placed on medication. The essay was written in response to a discussion question about parents censoring what their children are exposed to on TV, in the movies, or on the Internet. Mike weighed the pro and con arguments in a seemingly rational manner and concluded that parents need to monitor their children's entertainment. In his concluding remarks, Mike described a song about suicide and warned that music like that could encourage a child to hang himself, breaking his mother's heart. It was an oddly abrupt way to end the essay, but probably because it was written in a meaningful context and because Mike showed no signs of depression, it aroused no concern in school.

In hindsight, the essay may have contained a signal that went unheeded. But what happened after the start of Concerta left little room to doubt that the drug played a decisive role in what next occurred.

Mr. Bradley was concerned about Mike taking medications. He had bought a series of books about alternative medicine for himself and had come across arguments against prescribing stimulants to children. He explained to me, "I knew it was mind-altering and I've always been against that. I don't like alcohol because it changes your mind and a person should always be in control of his mind."

Mr. Bradley expressed reservations to Mike about taking the medication, but his son wanted to do better in school. Mike reassured his father, "It'll be all right, Dad." Based on the pediatrician's reassurances that they would know in a matter of days if the medication was working, Mike's parents reluctantly decided to go ahead with it.

His parents decided to start the medication on the coming Monday morning. Meanwhile, Mike had a great weekend. He was the youngest player to make the varsity baseball team at the school, attended his first practice, and got the jersey he coveted with number "1" on it. His sister had a birthday party and Mike enjoyed visiting with the extended family.

On Sunday, Mike developed a mild sore throat and laryngitis. Mom was concerned that he might be getting a cold from practicing baseball on an unusually chilly, damp day. She was also worried that some of the kids at school had viruses. So she kept her son home on Monday, and started him on the Concerta as planned.

That day at home, Mike finished a school project and also completed writing and designing an autobiographical bulletin that he created on his computer. Over the previous weekend, Mike had seen the movie *The Matrix* at a friend's house and asked his dad to watch it with him again. They used the movie as a jumping-off point to talk about differences between New Age and traditional religions. Mike attended Sunday church as well as a Christian school, and had become more religious and spiritual in the past year, especially after attending a church retreat the previous summer.

Mike began to show some signs of increasing fatigue and sleepiness on

Monday and Tuesday after starting Concerta. Stimulants typically make the child lethargic during the day when the drug effect is strongest and then make the child "hyper" at night when drug withdrawal sets in.

Later in the day on Monday, Mike told his mother he felt too tired to stop by school to display a project that he had completed, so she took it over for him. That evening he fell asleep early. His parents never connected these changes with the drug, but in my interviews with them they independently described him as "fatigued" during the last three days of his life.

On Tuesday, Mike stayed home but other than feeling fatigued he seemed fine. His throat was clearing up and he felt well enough to walk a few blocks to the video store to return the movie. That evening he finished an autobiographical booklet entitled, "My So-Called Life." He designated it "Volume 1, Issue 1," clearly anticipating future publications, although he was living his next-to-last day.

The booklet was a cleverly designed and illustrated personal blog filled with everything from wise sayings to a recipe for a "Gram Vanilla Candy Bar Marshmallow Plop." On the cover it said, "My Motto: Life is like a puzzle. If you place a piece incorrectly, you will have a messed-up puzzle." He chatted about his favorite artists, wrote a brief movie review, and also a column about how he was getting ready for the "The Eighth Grade Banquet." In yet another column, he proudly reported on how "I recently joined the Varsity Baseball Team."

In addition to the usual potpourri of early adolescent interests, Mike displayed unusual spirituality, sensitivity, and caring. He addressed one of his columns to his favorite teacher who had recently left to teach in another state. Mike apologized for any embarrassment it might cause but he wanted to tell his teacher how much he mattered: "When you lived up here and taught at my school, I thought of you as my personal mentor. God then led you to teach in Ohio, and it took me a long while to come to grips with that fact. I just know, I will always think of you as my dad." Mike had stamped and hand-addressed this particular copy of his first bulletin in preparation for mailing a copy to his former teacher.

Mike's father told me he felt no competitiveness over his son having a second "dad," explaining it was common in his religious and social community. In this nicely designed and written booklet about the interests in his life, Mike comes across as full of vitality, deeply engaged in many activities, religious, sensitive, and loving.

On Wednesday morning, Mr. Bradley went to physical therapy. Before his father left the house, Mike told him he was going to watch Martha Stewart on television and then take a nap. The nap was unusual but not watching *Martha Stewart*. Mike loved cooking and would share recipes with his grandmother.

When Mr. Bradley returned home from physical therapy, Mike was looking at bedspreads in a catalog. His sister had gone to college and he was moving into her old room. There was no hint of any depression or withdrawal. On the contrary, Mike was filled with future-oriented activities, hardly the viewpoint of someone anticipating death by suicide within a few hours.

Father and son often watched television and movies together and discussed the themes. *It's a Wonderful Life* was a favorite. At some point during the few days he was taking Concerta, Mike also watched and recorded a television show called *Port Charles,* which was about angels. Mike and his dad frequently watched this show together. It featured a teenage girl who had died and been sent back to Earth as angel. This particular segment of the weekly show, according to Mr. Bradley, had a very tender love scene between two teenagers.

Mike was interested in girls and on two occasions over the previous year he had started relationships. Mr. Bradley explained, "Their idea of dating was, 'Meet you at the church.'" The church social group monitored the activities of young people. Mike especially cared about one girl in particular with whom he had spent time at a religious retreat several months earlier. She had not returned his interest and they hadn't seen much of each other for several months.

Mr. Bradley remembered that some time in the past he had explained to his son that in the scriptures human beings do not become angels. That theme would come up in a dreadful monologue that his son would leave behind. Mr. Bradley knew nothing about how stimulants cause overfocusing and obsessions; but he noticed that his son became obsessively focused on themes from the show in his pre-death monologue.

When Mrs. Bradley woke up as usual at 6:00 AM on Wednesday, the third day of Mike's exposure to Concerta, his son was asleep on the couch downstairs. "He does that when he doesn't feel well," she explained to me. She left for work and then Mr. Bradley got up and visited awhile with his son. He recalls chatting about a DVD Mike wanted to buy.

On Monday and Tuesday, both parents were careful to remind Mike about taking Concerta but not on Wednesday. They figured that their son had become accustomed to the routine and they knew that he wanted to take the medication. A pill count would later confirm that the boy had taken the prescribed three doses in three days.

Mr. Bradley returned home from work that afternoon and asked Mike if he had eaten lunch. His son said he hadn't been hungry. Mike was experiencing two common adverse effects of stimulants: loss of appetite and fatigue. Unseen to his parents, he was also in the process of developing a more hazardous stimulant drug reaction: depression with obsessive suicidal preoccupations.

When Mrs. Bradley arrived home from work that evening, she saw nothing amiss. Instead, Mike was very pleased with himself. He told her that, for the first time ever, he had finished his algebra assignment in one session while relaxing in front of the TV. The Concerta was working!

Stimulants work in part by causing obsessive-compulsive behavior, compelling a child to act dutifully and to persist at boring tasks. In Mike's case, the obsessive-compulsive impact of the drug would soon seize his mental processes and mood.

There is no evidence that fourteen-year-old Mike Bradley was depressed at this time—or at any time in the past. He never suffered from mood swings, temper tantrums, sleep problems, nightmares, or gloomy thoughts. He was never tearful. His personal life was filled with many friends and he was close to his parents. He loved music and was planning to form a band with some friends. In addition to sports, singing and acting in school productions, and other social activities, he was practicing on a guitar his parents had bought for him a year earlier. Plus, he had been very busy over the weekend and even during the few days at home when he was feeling tired.

Many drug-induced cases of violence and suicide leave no trace of what the person was actually feeling at the time. This is especially true in regard to children who are less likely than adults to write down their painful feelings. Although Mike displayed no awareness that he was leaving a record for posterity, on Wednesday afternoon he began using his computer to make voice recordings about what was on his mind. When the files were later downloaded, they showed the date and time of day. He began recording at 1:08 PM. He stopped briefly at 1:42 PM for a minute or two. Then he reopened the file, recited a prayer, and closed the file for the last time a couple of minutes later at 1:45 PM.

Mike's recorded voice in the computer file has a monotonous, hypnotic quality. His tone is flat and dreary with a droning quality. His sober tones and deliberate monotone make him sound several years older than he was, almost like a monk reciting prayers. At the same time, he projects an eerie quality with repeated rhyming. Deep sighs and long pauses communicate his stress. He pauses to think for several long seconds and then speaks three or four despairing lines in rhyme. In between rhyming, he intones with the cadence of blank verse.

One of Mike's close relatives who heard the tape responded, "Was he drugged?" But they knew Mike would never use illegal drugs and they had no idea that a psychiatric medication like Concerta could have made him sound drugged. The family would not make the connection between Concerta and their son's death until almost two years later when they read news accounts about the 2004 FDA hearings on medication-induced suicide in children.

Mike's dreadful monologue is devoted to ruminations about life and death that focus on his unrequited love from a classmate whom he had dated briefly several months earlier. He doesn't directly mention suicide but he hints at it when he says that he would like to come back as an angel to watch over her, quickly adding as a Christian that he knows humans don't become angels.

Did this failed relationship cause Mike's abrupt onset of profound sadness? It seems unlikely. There's no evidence of his ruminating sadly about the relationship or about anything prior to taking the medication. Until starting Concerta, he had maintained a busy activity schedule that he greatly enjoyed. Keep in mind that he seemed as happy as a lark a few days earlier about making the team.

The Mike who reveals himself through the distortions of drug intoxication is an intelligent, sensitive, earnest, responsible, caring boy caught in the compelling grip of something he doesn't understand—medication spellbinding that is driving him into obsessive despair.

Mike seems to be anticipating graduation in four years and then college together with the girl as he recites in a slow, deliberate tone punctuated with rhymes:

> *Going through the ceremony together the same year*
> *Throw up our hats and shout with cheer*
> *Then after that pause*
> *Four more years to learn*
> *During that course [pausing]*
> *Your heart I will earn*
> *Soon after we would be as one*
> *Together through the shit and fun*
> *And there's one thing I know for sure*
> *During that course there's one that would never, never happen*
> *There'd never be need for divorce.*

Then with heaviness in his voice, he concludes that all these hopes will never materialize, and his last words repeat a familiar prayer:

As I lay me down to sleep
I pray the Lord my soul to keep
If I die before I wake
I pray the Lord my soul to take.

Mike sounds spellbound as he recites the prayer in a slow, solemn cadence. If we didn't know the tragic outcome, we might be tempted to think he was trying to act as if he were under a spell. After he finished the prayer, there were no further sounds and the recording ended.

Mr. Bradley found his son less than half an hour after his last voice entry into his computer. The boy was kneeling with a cord looped around his bunk bed and his neck. During his death throes, he could simply have stood up to end the hanging. He must have held himself off the ground until becoming unconscious.

The original coroner's report found no methylphenidate in Mike's blood. A graph in the *Physicians' Desk Reference* shows the amount of Concerta that remains each day after a single dose. By twenty-four to forty-eight hours the curve approaches zero with almost no Concerta remaining in the body. Based on this data indicating how rapidly Concerta is excreted from the system, I concluded that routine tests such as those conducted for autopsy would not necessarily detect any of the three doses. I had already urged the family to request the coroner to freeze samples of their son's blood and now I suggested that they ask the coroner to send a sample to another lab to check for traces of Concerta. It was important that officials handle the transfer to avoid any concern about tampering by the family or other interested parties. It's called the chain of custody—it must remain intact from one authority to another, and it did. The new laboratory analysis found traces of Concerta, confirming that Mike had recently taken the drug.

Mike had been taking Concerta 36 mg, a slow-release form of methylphenidate, the same chemical in Ritalin. Slow-release drugs are embedded in a matrix that dissolves over a period of hours, so that the active chemical is absorbed more slowly into the body. Presumably the effects and side effects are very similar to those of the drug when taken in ordinary single doses. The hope is that the slow-release version provides a "smoother" dose level throughout the day than taking three or four single doses. The slow release might also produce a less acute or intense withdrawal syndrome. Unfortunately, in comparison to these speculations, there is one unquestionable risk to slow-release drugs that is never discussed by drug advocates. If adverse effects develop, the drug is going to remain longer in the body before it is deactivated and or excreted, thereby prolonging any harmful reactions.

SUICIDE AS AN AMPLIFICATION OF THE DRUG'S "THERAPEUTIC EFFECT"

DEPRESSION AND SUICIDE are not side effects as much as they are primary effects of stimulant drugs. Depression and suicide are simply exaggerations of the same effects that seemingly make the child look more "normal" by reducing spontaneity and enforcing obsessive-compulsive responses.

When normally rambunctious chimpanzees are given stimulants, they will stop socializing with their fellow chimps, stop exploring their environment with any gusto, and stop trying to escape confinement. This is the apathy or relative disinterest in life in general that the drug causes in humans as well. It's the same drug-induced effect in children that often becomes amplified into sadness and even depression.

When given to our nearest primate relatives, the chimpanzees, the stimulants also cause the animals to narrow or constrict their focus. They no longer yearn to do the things that normally interest and excite them. Instead, they focus narrowly on tasks that ordinarily would have been too boring to capture their attention. They compulsively pick at their skin, play with a pebble, pace a corner of the cage, or simply stare blankly ahead. Literally dozens of carefully conducted animal studies show how the chimps become apathetic and compulsive when given stimulants like Ritalin and Adderall. These studies then shed light on the results of dozens of human studies showing how the children become less social, more listless, and more compulsive, as well as outright depressed.[10]

No wonder these drugs have been viewed as a blessing by overworked, stressed-out teachers and parents. Just as they make "good" caged animals, they make "good" classroom children. A previously rambunctious child becomes relatively apathetic and compulsively follows instructions. It happens with the first dose and looks like a miracle in the classroom. The classroom teacher has no idea that he or she is witnessing a manifestation of drug-induced mental impairment. The teacher only knows that the child is better behaved, obedient, and much less demanding of attention.

On occasion, researchers from the stimulant/ADHD lobby give some recognition to the hazards of the drugs. In 1992, a team of experts was selected by the U.S. Department of Education to survey the entire scientific literature on stimulant drugs for children.[11] Although they favored the use of stimulant drugs, they nonetheless made a sobering observation: "Cognitive toxicity may occur at commonly prescribed clinical doses of stimulant medication." Cognitive toxicity means a deterioration of mental functions related to thinking such as learning, attention, and memory. Based on their extensive review, they summarized:

> In some disruptive children, drug-induced compliant behavior may be accompanied by isolated, withdrawn, and overfocused behavior. Some medicated children may seem "zombielike" and high doses which make ADHD children more "somber," "quiet," and "still" may produce social isolation by increasing "time spent alone" and decreasing "time spent in positive interaction" on the playground.

Notice that the authors go so far as to call it a "zombielike" effect at higher doses. Consistent with the brain-disabling principle of psychiatric treatment,[12] a more subtle degree of zombie effect makes children seem to behave better and so it is called therapeutic, but a more obvious zombie effect becomes an embarrassment to adults and so it is called toxic.

How many children show signs of this cognitive toxicity? These experts concluded that the adverse reactions occur in "40% or more of the typically treated cases." Almost half of routinely treated children show toxic mental symptoms! The overall effect does not improve learning but impairs it.

Two other experienced researchers described the stimulant-induced mental deficit as occurring "in the realm of complex, higher-order cognitive functions such as flexible problem-solving and divergent thinking."[13] That is, children are being forced to overfocus on repetitive, rule-following tasks at the expense of their ability to think and to learn.

The frequency of these stimulant-induced mental dysfunctions confirms my point that they are in fact the "therapeutic effect." Understandably, adults can feel relieved when a child becomes less troublesome and more obedient, so I don't blame stressed parents and teachers who have been bamboozled by false promises of "correcting biochemical imbalances." I do blame my colleagues in psychiatry, the experts who should know better, for promoting the use of medication to subdue and control children. It is no exaggeration when I call this medical manipulation a form of technological or pharmacological child abuse.

The use of the term "zombielike" was striking and occurs elsewhere on occasion in the scientific literature. Few if any have done more to advocate stimulant medication for children than Peter Jensen, formerly at NIMH and now at Columbia University. Nonetheless, in a widely read psychiatric textbook, Jensen and a coauthor describe the "zombie" effect sometimes caused in children by stimulant medication. They relate it to a "pinched, somber expression" and a "constriction" in feeling and spontaneity.[14] They say that the effect is "harmless in itself but worrisome to parents, who can be reassured."

Like most drug-induced impairments of the brain and mind, the zombie effect occurs along a continuum. In relatively mild cases, children lose the brightness of their personalities. Their spirit is dampened and their responses are less spontaneous. They are less troublesome and less delightful. "My child just didn't seem like himself anymore. I hardly knew him," parents have often told me, adding, "Sure, he was easier to be around, but it made me sad, because I'd lost him in the process."

Most children taking stimulants will become abnormally obsessive and compulsive. I have found only one study that focused on these effects, an NIMH research project that aimed at evaluating the rate of stimulant-induced obsessive-compulsive disorder in children.[15] The findings were shocking: More than 50 percent of children treated with methylphenidate and amphetamine developed varying degrees of drug-induced obsessive-compulsive disorder. This incredibly high rate of drug-induced obsessive-compulsive disorder once again confirms the brain-disabling principle that the adverse effects are the very same effects that are being called therapeutic.

Some of the obsessive reactions in the NIMH study were severe, for example, a child who raked leaves for seven straight hours and then waited for individual leaves to fall off the trees to rake some more. Typically, the stimulant-treated youngsters played their games or other activities in a compulsive, difficult-to-interrupt manner. In school activities, they would bear down hard enough on their pencils to tear their papers. They would repetitively erase and worry over insignificant details. To the teachers, these children undoubtedly seemed to be trying harder, when in reality they were driven by drug-induced spellbinding of a pernicious but subtle variety.

Young Mike Bradley's voice recording made moments before his death gave us a rare window into the mind of a stimulant-treated child shortly before committing suicide. Mike sounds robotic. His tone of voice is monotonous and he articulates very slowly.

One dose of stimulant can make children overfocus on tasks of little intrinsic merit or interest, even to the point that it becomes difficult to make them stop.[16] A number of studies show that half or more of children become sad and depressed while taking these drugs. One widely used psychiatric-drug handbook summarized the scientific literature as demonstrating that methylphenidate causes drowsiness in 5.5 percent of children, confused and dopey feelings in 10.3 percent, and depression in an astounding 39 percent.[17]

Why then do so few doctors and researchers recognize these extremely common harmful stimulant effects? To start with, they don't want to find these telltale signs of drug-induced brain dysfunction in the children they treat and, therefore, they don't look for them. When they do notice them, they interpret them positively, seeing the children as less distracted by socializing and playing, and more obedient and hardworking. Finally, when the obsessive-compulsive symptoms, or the apathy about life in general, become very severe, the doctor rarely takes responsibility by admitting that the drug is disabling the child's brain and mind, and is making him compulsive and depressed.

Of course, not all children on stimulants show visible signs of apathy and compulsiveness—but to the degree that the drug is working, it does so by causing these effects. But the drug-induced apathy and compulsiveness is uneven and often lasts only a few weeks. That's why studies uniformly show that the "therapeutic" effect of these drugs is limited to a few weeks. The brain tries to compensate for the toxic drug effect, producing a complex, unstable condition in which the child is sometimes more subdued and, as the effect wears off, more hyperactive and mentally dispersed.

When a child displays no noticeably harmful drug effects, does that mean the drugs have indeed done no harm during months or years of exposure? No. Drugs can cause many serious adverse effects that are not immediately apparent. For example, growth suppression of height and weight is a documented side effect of stimulant drugs. Sometimes, the medicated child will appear underweight and shorter than expected, but often it's difficult to tell. If a child would normally have been taller than average, no one will suspect a harmful drug effect when he only grows to an average height. But each time I've withdrawn a child from prolonged stimulant therapy, the child has experienced an enormous spurt in height and weight, indicating that the drug was suppressing growth. If the drug has been suppressing gross body growth, what has it been doing to the more subtle development of the brain and mind? We already have some of the answers from animal studies. Relatively short-term, low-dose animal studies involving clinical doses of stimulants demonstrate lasting and probably permanent abnormalities in brain neurotransmitters.[18]

WITHDRAWING CHILDREN FROM STIMULANTS

ALTHOUGH SOME CHILDREN "crash" in an ominous fashion when abruptly removed from long-term treatment, many times I've gradually withdrawn children from these medications with little or no change in their outlook or behavior. The parents and child alike had been afraid that the drug was necessary, when in fact it was never missed once it was stopped. After being withdrawn from the drug, the children often need nothing more than a little coaching on how to concentrate in school and tutoring in their weakest subjects. If they are "hyperactive" or "impulsive"—other signs of so-called ADHD—then they need better discipline from their parents and a better personal understanding of how and why to learn self-control.[19]

There is no evidence that ADHD is a brain disease or even a medical disorder. It is not associated with any biochemical imbalances. Studies that supposedly show brain shrinkage in children diagnosed with ADHD are in fact showing stimulant drug damage.[20]

It will never be possible to find a biological basis for ADHD. If we examine the criteria for diagnosing ADHD, it becomes apparent that the "symptoms" are nothing more than a list of items that require extra attention from parents and especially from teachers. According to the official diagnostic manual of the American Psychiatric Association (2000), the behaviors, all of which annoy teachers and demand their attention, include the following: "often fidgets with hands or feet or squirms in seat," "often leaves seat in classroom," "often runs about or climbs excessively," "often talks excessively," "often blurts out answers before questions have been completed," "often has difficulty waiting turn," and "often fails to give close attention to details or makes careless mistakes."

The diagnosis has obviously been tailored to the need for control in the classroom. A drug that crushes spontaneity and enforces obsessive focusing will quickly suppress many or all of these behaviors, at least for a time until the drug is no longer effective.

Meanwhile, if a child does in fact display many of these traits, the causes can be infinite from inadequate teachers and boring classrooms to an unusually imaginative and energetic child struggling with the humdrum conformity of an ordinary schooling. Especially in severe cases, it could even be caused by myriad physical disorders, from chronic fatigue and poor nutrition to head injury. Because the list of symptoms or behaviors does not by itself tell us that there is anything wrong with the child, and because children are so responsive to their environments, and to parenting and teaching, the list of ADHD symptoms cannot be viewed as a disorder.

In my experience, so-called ADHD symptoms, when genuinely troublesome, usually reflect inadequate disciplinary training at home. Often, parents have lost confidence in their moral authority or are trying to impose confusing and contradictory rules on the child. They have usually been told by "experts" that their child has a biological disorder and therefore there's no need to improve their parenting stills. As I describe in *Talking Back to Ritalin* (2001) and in *The Ritalin Fact Book* (2002), it can be relatively easy to help parents develop a consistent program of discipline combined with generous amounts of unconditional love. Parenting groups, often offered at relatively low cost by community services, can be very helpful.

In every case in which I have gradually withdrawn stimulants from a child diagnosed with ADHD, the child has done better without the drugs. Often the child's improvement has been spectacular. But there is a caveat: In every one of these instances, the parents have been very cooperative with me and worked on improving their parenting skills. Often the teachers have also been willing to try new approaches to the child.

Improvement in the child's life requires that parents take charge of family life in a more positive fashion. Ultimately, the parents, not the therapist, will determine how well their children develop. The therapist is a coach but the parents and teacher are the players.

Because the children have been convinced they have no control over themselves, it is important to approach them as moral beings who can understand right and wrong, and make good decisions. As long as the children are old enough to talk, I carry on conversations about them about how good it is control oneself, to be nice to little brothers and sisters, and to get along with Mom and Dad. With the littlest children, games, drawings, or parables can be used to communicate the benefits of improved conduct. I'm not talking about elaborate or lengthy play therapy, but about the simple illustrative techniques that many parents spontaneously use to teach moral lessons at bedtime and when playing with their children.

While the parents work on improving how they relate to their children, their children learn to become self-disciplined. No child can do this while believing he is an "ADHD kid" who needs drugs to control his behavior.

The challenge is more difficult when a child has greater problems than so-called ADHD and displays a great deal of emotional disturbance. The challenge becomes even greater when the youngster has been exposed to multiple medications over many years, fouling up his normal brain chemistry. In these desperate situations, the parents themselves are often suffering from serious emotional problems, as well as conflicts between each other, that impede helping the child. In these cases, intensive and lengthier treatment for the whole family may be required.

DO STIMULANTS BENEFIT CHILDREN?

IN PUBLIC, "experts" almost uniformly tout the stimulants as an unmitigated boon to parents and children. However, they sometimes admit to a different story when communicating to their colleagues. A review in the American Psychiatric Publishing's *Textbook of Psychiatry* concluded:

> Stimulants do not produce lasting improvements in aggressivity, conduct disorder, criminality, educational achievement, job functioning, marital relationships, or long-term adjustment.[21]

An NIMH publication concluded "the long-term efficacy of stimulant medication has not been demonstrated in *any* domain of child function"[22] and another group of mainstream researchers confirmed there is no "long-term advantage" to taking stimulants.[23] One of the most thorough reviews was sponsored by the U.S. Department of Education. It came to conclusions that would startle most people who have been exposed to pro-drug advocacy.[24] The following is taken verbatim from the report:

- Long-term beneficial effects have not been verified by research.
- Stimulant medication may improve learning in some cases but impair learning in others.
- Teachers and parents should not expect significantly improved reading or athletic skills, positive social skills, or learning of new concepts.
- Teachers and parents should not expect long-term improvement in academic achievement or reduced antisocial behavior.

More recently, a thirty-six-month-long multicenter study financed by NIMH concluded that there were no demonstrable long-term positive effects from stimulant drugs.[25] The same series of studies also reconfirmed that the drugs stunt growth.[26] These results were recorded despite the extreme pro-drug bias of the researchers.

Why do doctors continue to prescribe these drugs and why do parents and teachers so often go along with it? Initially the suppressive effects of the drug on behavior seem like a relief to parents and teachers alike. Because the drugs are spellbinding, the children are unable to perceive and to complain about being suppressed. After a while when the child's condition begins to deteriorate, the prescribing doctors almost never attribute it to the drugs but instead increase the dose and add new drugs—leading us into the next tragic story. Many times, when children seem to improve while taking stimulants over months or years, they have simply matured—despite the drug-induced mental impairments.

Millions of children are having the spiritual stuffing knocked out of them by stimulant drugs. Most of the time this effect is subtle. You may have to look hard to see that the sparkle is gone from the eye and twinkle is gone from the smile. But sometimes the apathy turns into severe depression and the compulsiveness becomes overwhelming, driving the children to suicide as in the tragic case of Michael Bradley.

Chapter 14

Spellbound by Ritalin Addiction

ADDICTION IS AMONG THE MOST spellbinding drug phenomena. It can be the most beguiling, the most destructive. Whereas spellbinding often occurs abruptly after a few doses or during dose changes, the development of addiction can take place gradually. Slowly and subtly the drug effects creep up and take over before the individual realizes that drug dependence and abuse has laid waste to his or her life.

To those of my colleagues who continue to believe that stimulants like Ritalin, Concerta, and Adderall taken in prescribed doses cannot lead to addiction, I propose this short summary of the life of Willow Barlow:

Born December 9, 1975
Died February 27, 1999
Ritalin Addict

IT ALL BEGAN WITH ADHD

WILLOW'S MOTHER thought her daughter was a little hyperactive. Willow "liked toys with a lot of motion," she explained to the doctor. In addition, Willow's kindergarten teacher thought the child was a somewhat slower learner. So at the age of five and one-half years, Willow was sent for neurological evaluation.

According to official diagnostic standards, children under age six are too young to be diagnosed with attention-deficit hyperactivity disorder (ADHD).

But after evaluating Willow, the neurologist wrote, "I really feel that Willow fits into the attention deficit disorder category with potential for learning disability." It was another way of saying, "The kid needs drugs."

As so often happens, being diagnosed would shape a lifetime. For Willow it became her first step into a brief and terminal career as a psychiatric patient.

After the neurologist started Willow on the stimulant Ritalin, Mrs. Barlow dutifully gave her daughter the drug for several months until she could no longer tolerate seeing her child look and act like a "zombie." When the drug seemed to reduce her daughter to a shell of herself, Mrs. Barlow stopped taking her daughter to the doctor and Willow did well for several more years without psychiatric interventions.

ACUTE EFFECTS VS. ADDICTION

BEFORE CONTINUING with Willow's story, it's important to distinguish between the acute behavioral effects of stimulant intoxication and the longer-term hazards of abuse and addiction.

Even at routine doses, stimulants can have direct toxic effects on children and adults. Some people are driven into psychosis and much more commonly they are made apathetic and depressed, the zombie effect that Willow's mother observed. The stimulant drugs can also cause anxiety and agitation.

As noted in an earlier chapter, with the exception of Strattera, all stimulants can cause addiction. The addiction process can be jump-started by the dangerous and potentially lethal practices of inhaling or snorting stimulants such as Ritalin, amphetamine, and cocaine, or by taking them intravenously. By contrast, when Ritalin and the amphetamines are taken orally, and especially when they are prescribed in recommended doses, the addictive process is usually slower with many warning signs along the way.[1] That's what happened in Willow's case.

WILLOW IN HER TEENS

WHEN WILLOW REACHED HER TEENS, she ran into increasing emotional difficulties. Like many children, she needed more attention and more skilled approaches than her public school was offering, and she grew to hate school. To improve her daughter's learning environment for a few months a year, Mrs. Barlow sent her to a special summer school for children with learning problems, where Willow felt happy and thrived. Willow wished she could go to the special school year round but it was too costly.

At about this time in her early teens, Willow's much older pregnant sister and her husband came to stay with Willow and her parents until they could afford a home of their own. Having enjoyed life as the only child in the home, Willow now had to contend with sibling competition. Although her mother believes that the medical records exaggerated what she had told the doctor, Willow may have also made threats about harming the unborn baby. In her competitive need for her attention, Willow's reactions were more characteristic of a child much younger than age thirteen; but her mother asserts that she never felt that Willow would hurt the baby.

Feeling overwhelmed by family pressures and conflicts, Mrs. Barlow brought Willow back to the neurologist who had diagnosed her with ADHD as a small child. The neurologist started Willow on one of the older antidepressants and soon referred her to a psychiatrist. Willow was almost fourteen when she arrived at the psychiatrist's office.

Willow's psychiatrist treated her for the next nine and a half years, switching her from one medication to another, never offering her a drug-free respite, and eventually trying several different antidepressants including Prozac, Zoloft, and Wellbutrin. As commonly happens when children are exposed to multiple psychiatric drugs, Willow continued to get worse.

Perhaps concerned about dangerous cardiovascular effects caused by antidepressants in children, particularly cardiac arrhythmias, the psychiatrist decided to switch medications. The medical record shows that Mrs. Barlow informed the doctor that Ritalin had previously caused her daughter "severe sleep disturbances and weight loss despite low to moderate doses," as well as emotional flattening. Nonetheless, the psychiatrist decided to try the teenager on Ritalin again.

WILLOW SHOWS SIGNS OF ADDICTION

WITHIN MONTHS OF RESTARTING Ritalin at the age of fifteen, Willow became much more difficult to handle at home and school. The medical record is peppered with reports of worsening behavior. She developed mood swings and became progressively more depressed. As in most cases I have evaluated, the doctor seemingly gave no thought whatsoever to the possible role of medication in Willow's steadily deteriorating condition.

Within Willow's first year back on Ritalin, an ominous signal was recorded in the office telephone log. Mrs. Barlow told the nurse that her daughter had purposely taken extra Ritalin pills that morning. On another occasion, according to the psychiatrist's record, Mrs. Barlow also reported that Willow was "demanding Ritalin." This was another expression of addictive behavior but the psychiatrist continued prescribing Ritalin "for ADHD," often along with Prozac.

ADDICTION WARNINGS

Willow's doctor should have shown more appreciation for Ritalin's addictive potential. The Ritalin label contains the following black box:

> ### DRUG DEPENDENCE
> Ritalin should be given cautiously to patients with a history of drug dependence or alcoholism. Chronic abusive use can lead to marked tolerance and psychological dependence with varying degrees of abnormal behavior. Frank psychotic episodes can occur, especially with parenteral abuse. Careful supervision is required during withdrawal from abusive use, since severe depression may occur.

> AMPHETAMINES HAVE A HIGH POTENTIAL FOR ABUSE. ADMINISTRATION OF AMPHETAMINES FOR PROLONGED PERIODS OF TIME MAY LEAD TO DRUG DEPENDENCE AND MUST BE AVOIDED. PARTICULAR ATTENTION SHOULD BE PAID TO THE POSSIBILITY OF SUBJECTS OBTAINING AMPHETAMINES FOR NONTHERAPEUTIC USE OR DISTRIBUTION TO OTHERS, AND THE DRUGS SHOULD BE PRESCRIBED OR DISPENSED SPARINGLY.

The more recently updated labels for Dexedrine and Adderall contain a stronger black-box warning written in caps and placed at the very top of the label, plus additional warnings in the text of the label. Here is the Adderall label's black-box warning:

There is no valid reason why the Ritalin label contains a much weaker addiction warning than the Adderall label. The FDA has been lax in forcing drug companies to update older labels. By contrast the DEA has repeatedly warned that Ritalin has the same abuse potential as amphetamine.[2] Numerous textbooks make the same observation, including the chapter on stimulants in Graham Dukes's encyclopedic textbook, *Meyler's Side Effects of Drugs* (1996), which observes, "Methylphenidate shares the pharmacological properties and the abuse potential of the amphetamines."[3]

When it came to how Willow's doctors behaved, the more ominous warnings in the Adderall label proved no more discouraging to them than the weaker Ritalin label. Her psychiatrist, and the family doctor who followed, tried Willow both on Adderall as well as Ritalin, but Willow preferred the Ritalin, probably because it was being given in higher doses.

At age sixteen, Willow remained on Ritalin and Prozac, and began to seriously abuse alcohol. Both Ritalin and Prozac can overstimulate children and adults, causing them to start drinking alcohol or to increase their alcohol intake as a method of calming themselves down. Because the stimulants are very spellbinding, those addicted to the drugs rarely appreciate that they are drinking alcohol to control adverse stimulant effects—they just know that the drinking is somehow helping them feel better.

A little more than two years after restarting Ritalin, Willow's psychiatrist described her for the first time as suffering from "multiple substance problems." Willow was "sniffing paint thinner, spray paint, and cement glue"; she was drinking; and she was abusing Ritalin. She also began to smoke cigarettes and then marijuana. Ritalin had become her gateway drug to multiple substance abuses—but her psychiatrist, not grasping the role of Ritalin in her growing abuse of multiple chemicals, continued to prescribe Ritalin even as she diagnosed Willow with "substance abuse" and encouraged her to go to Alcoholics Anonymous meetings.

This was an opportune time for Willow's psychiatrist to make a definitive intervention in her young patient's life. Willow needed to be tapered from Ritalin under close supervision and she need rehabilitation to stop abusing multiple nonprescription drugs. If necessary, Willow should have been placed in rehab in a hospital or residential setting. Instead, the psychiatrist began spacing Willow's appointments at five-month and then seven-month intervals, at the same time continuing to write her prescriptions for Ritalin.

As the doctor's telephone records confirmed, Willow became a Ritalin binge addict. The prescriptions provided for 40 mg per day of the stimulant but Willow would take large amounts in a single dose. As a result, Willow's mother tried to take control of Willow's pill supply, causing conflict between them. Willow was transforming from a unique human being to a stereotypical addict—a six-year plunge into drug hell while her mother desperately tried to manage the situation.

At age seventeen, Willow swallowed five sustained-release (long-acting) Ritalin pills at once. The doctor's telephone log recorded, "felt suicidal, mood swings, felt violent, irritable, general malaise . . ." This is a classic description of episodes of withdrawal or "crashing" in between Ritalin bingeing. The DEA seems to have been warning us about Willow's destruction when the agency wrote:[4]

> Like amphetamine and cocaine, abuse of methylphenidate can lead to marked tolerance and psychic dependence. The pattern of abuse is characterized by escalation of dose, frequent episodes of binge use followed by severe depression, and an overpowering desire to continue the use of this drug despite medical and social consequences.

The DEA went on ominously, "The high percentage of attempted suicides [among Ritalin abusers] is consistent with the high frequency of depression associated with stimulant abuse."[5] Willow's doctor was also continuing to prescribe Prozac, probably adding to worsening emotional instability.

As Willow continued to deteriorate, Mrs. Barlow called the doctor to explain that her daughter had located a handgun in the house but had promised she would not do "anything to hurt her mother." According to Willow's parents and confirmed by the medical record, the doctor did not call for an immediate intervention, such as a plenary session in the office with the entire family, or an evaluation at the admitting office of a rehabilitation clinic, but she did instruct the parents to remove the gun from the house. According to the family, Dad dismantled the pistol, rendering it unusable, without disposing of it.

Continuing on her stereotypical addict trajectory, Willow turned to crime to obtain drugs, breaking into a neighbor's house to steal Ritalin, and in the process stealing a Rolex watch. Willow's mother dutifully reported this on the phone to the psychiatrist who continued to enable the Ritalin abuse while failing to react as if the youngster's life was at stake.

The failure of many doctors to grasp the drug's toxicity and abuse potential is in part a testimonial to the success of the manufacturer, Novartis, in convincing the medical profession that Ritalin is "mild" and relatively harmless. In fact, the misleading description of "mild stimulant" remains in the FDA–approved label to this day.

Willow was now nineteen years old and like any addict her life was falling apart. She couldn't stay in school at the community college. She couldn't hold down a job. She lived at home and fought with her mother over the control of her medications.

Willow's psychiatrist now decided to stop her Ritalin and she wrote one last prescription for a thirty-day supply, forcing her patient to go "cold turkey" when the medication ran out. Meanwhile, she continued to prescribe other kinds of psychiatric drugs during a four-month period without seeing Willow in the doctor's office. At home, Willow deteriorated into severe withdrawal.

A few months after Willow ran out of Ritalin, her psychiatrist received a phone call from the local pharmacist. Willow had tried to fill a prescription for Ritalin that didn't look right to the pharmacist. Most likely, Willow had stolen one of the doctor's prescription pads sometime in the past, and now she had forged a Ritalin prescription. It was typical addict behavior but the doctor treated it like a criminal offense. In a medical note that communicated her personal outrage, the psychiatrist recorded how she had informed Willow's mother on the phone that her daughter had committed a "felony." In the medical record, the doctor referred to Willow's "sociopathic" behavior, in effect calling her a criminal type. In reality, Willow was suffering from addiction to Ritalin with all of the typical negative behaviors.

Mrs. Barlow became afraid to take her daughter back to the psychiatrist. Instead she implored an internist—a man who knew Willow's dad—to undertake the care of her daughter. Although the internist diagnosed Willow with ten disorders including ADHD, anxiety, depression, fatigue, insomnia, and substance abuse (marijuana only), for the next year he prescribed Ritalin to her "for ADHD."

Addiction experts know that it is futile to diagnose underlying psychiatric disorders such as ADHD, depression, or anxiety when a patient is abusing drugs. Drug abuse or dependence with its cycles of intoxication and withdrawal mimics every possible psychiatric problem from manic-depressive (bipolar) disorder and brief psychosis to anxiety disorder and sociopathic personality disorder. Any coexisting or underlying mental problem cannot be realistically assessed until the drug abuse or dependence has been adequately treated. In the process of drug rehabilitation, a new person often emerges—a more emotionally stable, rational, and likeable human being who no longer fits into any psychiatric diagnostic category except "substance abuse, in remission."

Mrs. Barlow did not tell the full story of her daughter's desperate straits to the new doctor. Understandably, she was reluctant to inform him, "My kid's an addict and a potential felon. Hide your prescription pad." She wanted her daughter to receive help and no one had told her how to go about it—by properly diagnosing Willow with drug dependence and guiding her into a drug treatment program for supervised withdrawal.

Meanwhile, the signals of Willow's addiction began to pile up in the internist's office telephone records. On more than one occasion, Mrs. Barlow made clear to the new doctor that she was fighting with her daughter over the control of the drugs. A particularly poignant phone memo by the doctor's staff read: "I spoke with Willow's mom today and she is very upset and thinks her daughter may have taken all 180 [Ritalin] tabs within three days and may need blood drawn."

Willow continued to binge on the pills, on at least one occasion obtaining extra doses by claiming that the original prescription had failed to arrive by mail. Once again, these desperate signals brought no definitive medical response, and no end to the prescription of stimulants. Like the psychiatrist who had addicted Willow, her new doctor went months at a time without seeing her.

The doctor finally recognized that his patient was abusing her medication but apparently he did not know how to respond to the situation. He kept on prescribing, now at the rate of 60 mg per day of Ritalin. This is the very high end of recommended doses. Most children and young adults in their early twenties like Willow are treated with half that amount, or even less.

After one year, the internist gave up. He wrote Willow a one-month prescription for Ritalin and told Mrs. Barlow that he wouldn't refill it in less than a month even if Willow used it all up.

Mrs. Barlow was now frantic. As far as I can ascertain, no one had confronted her and her daughter with the obvious reality that Willow needed immediate admission to a hospital or rehabilitation unit. Instead, Willow's mother took her daughter to two more doctors who provided additional prescriptions.

Using the pharmacy records, I was able in retrospect to add up all the Ritalin that Willow received during this one-month period—the last thirty days of her life. Willow acquired 640 pills for a total of 6,500 mg of Ritalin. Even at the very high dose of 60 mg per day, this would have been enough for 108 days.

In the last week of her life, Willow was fired from a job that she held briefly. Sometimes personal losses will push an addict over the edge, but Willow seemed to bounce back quickly. In another stressful event that occurred the evening before her death, Willow feared that her boyfriend was standing her up on a date, and she wrote a brief note threatening to kill herself. When her boyfriend showed up for the date, Willow's mood transformed, and they happily went shopping together. That night, Willow bought several personal items at the drugstore, acting like a woman with no immediate plans to die.

No one will ever know exactly what happened the next day. Reconstructing the scene as much as possible, Willow had gotten high by taking a huge amount of Ritalin. Probably frantic to avoid an equally huge withdrawal crash, she went tearing through bookshelves in a spare room at her home looking for Ritalin that she or her mother might have hidden in the past. Instead she found a pistol. According to her parents, the gun had been hidden there so many years earlier that no one remembered its existence.

Willow took the pistol into her bedroom where she shot and killed herself. A sample of her blood taken at autopsy showed almost one hundred times the usual therapeutic level of Ritalin. If Willow had not shot herself, she might have suffered a cardiac arrest caused by stimulant toxicity.

ADDICTION AS A CAUSE OF DEATH

DRUG ADDICTION, now called dependence in the official diagnostic manual, is the most frequent identifiable factor in the suicide of young people. The suicide can result from an impulsive action during acute intoxication or from the grinding effects of abuse and addiction.[6] Willow's story is another testimonial to these sad truths. Willow was in the midst of an acute intoxication with extremely high blood levels of Ritalin but she was also suffering from the roller coaster of chronic addiction with its inexorable ruination of her life.

Unlike fourteen-year-old Mike Bradley, Willow was not an example of stimulant-induced suicide. In Mike's case, the youngster had become depressed while taking routine doses of stimulants without the complicating factor of severe drug addiction. Willow's story is about emotional ravages of chronic polydrug addiction in which the stimulant Ritalin was the gateway drug and the main offender. Willow has been gone for several years but her mother and father have not recovered.

RITALIN AS A GATEWAY DRUG TO STREET DRUGS

AS ALREADY DESCRIBED, with the exception of Strattera the Drug Enforcement Administration (DEA) has placed all the drugs used to treat ADHD in Schedule II, the category of most highly addictive medications. Cocaine and morphine are also classified in Schedule II. By contrast, most sleeping pills and tranquilizers, such as Valium and Xanax, are placed in Schedule IV, indicating that the DEA considers them less likely than the stimulants to cause dependence and abuse.

The Ritalin in Willow's case was prescribed in much too cavalier a manner, enabling Willow to repeatedly binge with the drug. If an individual is given routine doses of Ritalin or other FDA-approved stimulants with appropriate monitoring, there's much less likelihood of addiction. Many children, for example, stop taking their stimulants every weekend, on holidays, and for the entire summer without any noticeable withdrawal effects or even mild dependence. Although there are exceptions, if a physician prescribes within accepted standards of care there's little likelihood of a child developing severe abuse and dependence *during the treatment process*. However, the long-term effects are more menacing. The routine use of Ritalin in childhood for the treatment of ADHD predisposes the individual to abuse cocaine in young adulthood.

Prescribed even in relatively small clinical doses, stimulants have a long-term and persisting impact on the brain. Stimulants change the way the brain functions, inevitably modifying the growing brain in ways that can become irreversible. Many animal studies confirm that even short-term clinical dosing causes long-term and probably irreversible changes in the brain, including the sort that lead to abuse and dependence.[7]

The most sophisticated, longest follow-up study of children treated with Ritalin has shown that they suffer from a several-fold increased risk of using cocaine as young adults.[8] The studies were conducted over many years by Nadine Lambert who compared children diagnosed ADHD who were treated with Ritalin to children diagnosed ADHD who received no drug treatment. I have been a medical expert in two cases in which young boys turned to cocaine after their prescribed Ritalin was stopped. In each case, the individual was convicted of murder in his teens during a period of post-Ritalin cocaine abuse.

The delayed addictive effects confirm that stimulants can cause long-lasting abnormalities in the brains of children. We cannot with impunity bathe the growing brains of our children in toxic substances.

Remember again that the adverse effects of psychiatric drugs occur along a continuum from barely perceptible to severe and overwhelming. Severe drug toxicity and spellbinding represent the extreme end of a continuum of mental impairment that is sufficiently subtle to go unrecognized even as it adversely affects the life of anyone who takes psychiatric drugs.

For every one of the more extreme and horrifying outcomes described in this book, there are untold numbers of people who are suffering similar reactions of a lesser degree or intensity. Instead of becoming depressed and suicidal, they feel "down," apathetic, or perhaps saddened—life loses its luster and nothing seems to matter much anymore. Instead of killing themselves, they worry a great deal and feel that life isn't worth living; they withdraw from others or stop taking good care of themselves. Or instead of becoming murderous, they become more irritable and aggressive, distressing their friends, loved ones, and coworkers. And all these people will be too medication spellbound to realize what is happening to them.

Chapter 15

Parents Forced to Drug Their Children

WHEN CHILDREN ARE SNOWED under with psychiatric drugs, their spunk and determination often won't let them cave in to adults whom they see as treating them unfairly. They fight back heroically to maintain their dignity and sense of self, but because of their drug-drenched brains and youthful immaturity, they are unable to resist rationally or effectively. Often, these courageous warriors are among our best and brightest—the spirited ones who if properly guided could contribute the most to society. Instead, their drug-driven outbursts of anger and suicidality are viewed as signs of a worsening mental disorder and so they are given more and more of the suppressive chemicals, robbing them of their potential.

When stimulants, antidepressants, and tranquilizers fail to subdue the rebellious ones, eventually they are given "antipsychotic" drugs such as Risperdal, Zyprexa, and Seroquel. By shutting down the function of the highest centers of the brain, these drugs can produce an actual chemical lobotomy and a chemical straitjacket from which no adult or child can escape.[1] Given sufficiently toxic doses of these drugs, any child can be rendered docile.

Most parents don't easily go along with this prescription for crushing their children. They are duped into going along with the process, often against their better judgment. Other parents become so frustrated and even outraged at their children that they seek out doctors who are willing and even eager to drug children. Still other parents—the ones described in this chapter—find themselves being forced into participating in medical child abuse.

A VERY GENTLE FATHER FIGHTS BACK

ABOUT ONE YEAR AFTER Reggie Thompson's mother divorced her husband, she took her three-and-one-half-year-old son to a pediatrician, explaining that he had been biting and scratching people and saying he hated them. The pediatrician's medical notes indicated no interest in the potential causes of this behavior either in the stresses of divorce or in inadequate parenting practices. As often occurs in divorces, especially when the husband wants to avoid a fight in court, Mrs. Thompson was awarded sole custody. Knowing that her former husband would probably disapprove of diagnosing and medicating their son, she did not invite him into the treatment process.

Reggie was referred to a specialist who diagnosed ADHD, a label that's not supposed to be applied to children under age six. The doctor prescribed Ritalin, a drug that's not approved for children younger than six. At the time, many drug companies were pushing medication for younger and younger children, a practice that would soon be drawing criticism even from within establishment medicine.[2]

Reggie's father saw nothing at all the matter with his son. According to Mr. Thompson, Reggie was behaving normally with him throughout this period of time when his mother was taking him to doctors to have him drugged.

Reggie's mother reported to the doctor that his behavior initially calmed down on the Ritalin, but within months, his behavior worsened, and she took her son to a university clinic where he was put on amphetamine in the form of Adderall or Dexedrine. The clinic defied common sense and good medical practice by filling prescriptions over periods of nearly six months without seeing Reggie. During this time, Reggie continued his downhill slide, developing self-punishing behaviors, "biting self," and being "mad at himself," that are common adverse reactions to stimulants.

Reggie was switched back to Ritalin and given very large doses of 80 mg per day. Then the "mood stabilizer" Tenex (guanfacine) was added. Tenex is an antihypertensive agent that can have dramatic sedative effects in children, so doctors have used it to subdue the behavior of children. Unfortunately, the combination of Ritalin and Tenex can cause cardiac arrest and should never be used. Meanwhile, according to Mom's reports in the medical records, Reggie's moods and behavior grew increasingly uncontrollable.

One of Reggie's doctors noted that stimulants can depress children but he nonetheless failed to stop prescribing the drugs. At age nine, yet another psychiatric evaluation obtained by his mother noted that Reggie had not done well during his six-year exposure to various medications. But the doctor did not give the boy a drug-free trial to see how he would do when his brain was free of intoxicating chemicals. Instead, the psychiatrist did what so many modern doctors do—he raised the medication ante to the next horrific level and prescribed Reggie the adult antipsychotic Risperdal.

Risperdal was not at the time approved for children, let alone for nine-year-olds, although the FDA has recently approved to treat severe irritability associated with autism and psychosis in older children and teens. The FDA seems to have forgotten that Risperdal, like all antipsychotics, flattens emotions, reduces empathy, and enforces social withdrawal from others—exactly the problems already faced by all autistic children and by many disturbed adolescents. Nothing is more likely to worsen autism or social withdrawal more than a potent lobotomizing agent like Risperdal—not to mention the drug's other hazards, such as diabetes, pancreatitis, and tardive dyskinesia.

Efforts by the manufacturer to promote Risperdal as relatively benign led to its widespread use in children long before the FDA gave limited approval for its use in this age group. In the past few years, I've evaluated many heartbreaking cases of tardive dyskinesia in children caused by Risperdal. Now that the FDA has given the green light to treating children and teens with the drug, the coming years will see increasing numbers of children afflicted with the disfiguring and potentially disabling disorder.

After three months on Risperdal proved no help, the doctor switched Reggie to yet another highly promoted adult antipsychotic, Zyprexa. When Reggie continued to get worse, lithium—an adult mood stabilizer—was added to the regimen. Although overall Reggie's case is typical of how children start on stimulants and end up on antipsychotic drugs, he was one of the youngest children I've seen on lithium, a chemical so dangerously spellbinding that blood levels have to be drawn at outpatient labs to make sure that the patient isn't becoming toxic without anyone realizing it.

Although there was no evidence for manic behaviors in the medical record, Reggie was given the diagnosis of bipolar disorder. Diagnosing bipolar disorder in children has become common in recent years among those physicians who push medication for children. Psychiatrists like Harvard's Joseph Biederman work closely with drug companies and constantly defend and promote their products. Diagnosing children as bipolar opens up a huge market for a wide variety of drugs that are used to treat adult bipolar disorder, including neuroleptics, antidepressants, tranquilizers, and mood stabilizers. Even the corporation-friendly *Wall Street Journal* voiced concern about the increase in diagnosing and treating small children and felt constrained to mention Biederman's financial relationships with drug makers.[3]

The promotional efforts of drug advocates have been phenomenally successful. A recent survey found that the diagnosis of bipolar disorder in children and youth under age nineteen had escalated *forty* times between 1994–1995 and 2002–2003.[4] Over 90 percent of the children received psychiatric drugs with more than 62 percent receiving them in combinations. Mood stabilizers like lithium and Depakote were prescribed to 60.3 percent of the youngsters, and antipsychotic drugs to 47.7 percent. As confirmation of how callously children are medicated, the same survey found that only 33.7 percent of adults diagnosed with bipolar disorder were given antipsychotic drugs. The study also confirms the regularity with which children are treated as badly as Reggie.

Nine-year-old Reggie was now taking stimulants, antipsychotics, and mood stabilizers in a cocktail sufficient to level a giant adult. It's a miracle that he could stay erect. But he could not maintain his sanity. Intoxicated by psychiatric drugs, Reggie for the first time began to display multiple severe psychiatric symptoms. A checklist by one doctor included for the first time "periods of extreme sadness," "elevated or irritable mood greater than one hour per day," "elevated and irritable mood greater than two days," "depressed mood greater than one hour/day," "paranoid thinking," and "bizarre behavior." All of these symptoms commonly occur as a result of severe overmedication.

Reggie's mother and the psychiatrist admitted the boy to a mental hospital. The hospital records were never released, but according to Reggie and his father, Reggie had a difficult time. Heavily medicated, he was placed in solitary confinement, for exactly how long Reggie cannot tell. At this point, a proper medical intervention would have removed the child from all his drugs. Instead, the hospital doctors escalated the drugging. Reggie was discharged with continued Zyprexa. Lithium was changed to another adult mood stabilizer, Depakote. He was also placed on a long-acting form of stimulant called Concerta (methylphenidate). Topping off his toxic cocktail, Reggie was given Topamax (topiramate), an anticonvulsive drug that doctors have been cavalierly experimenting with as a psychiatric mood stabilizer. This heavy regimen of toxic substances was inflicted on a seventy-pound nine-year-old.

After trying to avoid a legal battle with his wife for six years, Reggie's father decided that he could no longer remain on the sidelines. He could see that the hospitalization and the massive drugging were destroying his son. He went to court and the judge allowed him to bring his son to me for a second opinion.

My first concern was the effect of antipsychotics on the boy since they frequently cause tardive dyskinesia. As discussed in chapter 8, tardive dyskinesia is characterized by disfiguring and disabling abnormal movements. The out-of-control movements can occur in any muscle in the body that is usually under voluntary control such as the muscles of the extremities, back, torso, and shoulders, and more commonly, the face, eyelids, mouth, tongue, and neck. Voice, swallowing, and breathing can be impaired. Unless caught early, tardive dyskinesia usually becomes permanent. Cases vary from barely perceptible to wholly out of control so that the individual can barely stand or walk.

When I met with Reggie, I performed a complete evaluation for tardive dyskinesia and found that when his tongue was resting in his open mouth, it spontaneously curled back into his throat, quivering and cupping at the edges. This is a classic early manifestation of tardive dyskinesia and not something that can be faked. Reggie and his dad also reported occasional jerking movements of his arms. This is also a common early sign of tardive dyskinesia. Because tardive dyskinesia symptoms typically wax and wane from moment to moment, hour to hour, and day to day, it was not surprising that the jerking movements were not present on the day of examination.

At the conclusion to my report to the court, I made the following suggestions:

1. First and foremost, Reggie must be immediately removed from Zyprexa before his early signs of tardive dyskinesia develop into a lifetime, untreatable, disfiguring, or disabling neurological disorder.
2. Reggie should be removed from the care of his current physicians.
3. Reggie's care should be immediately turned over to his father.
4. Reggie should be temporarily homeschooled by his father with help from other family members while he is withdrawn from psychiatric drugs.
5. Under no circumstances should Reggie be hospitalized or placed in residential treatment of any kind.
6. Establish an immediate medical program to withdraw Reggie from Zyprexa.

After reviewing my report, the judge requested another opinion from a local physician not involved in treating Reggie case. In a show of courage the doctor broke with the local physicians who were drugging Reggie and confirmed my diagnosis, in effect verifying that Reggie's ongoing treatment was a disaster.

The judge followed my recommendations. He awarded custody to the father and empowered me to supervise the drug withdrawal. With the help of a sympathetic local pediatrician and a local therapist, I was able to guide Reggie's withdrawal from the cocktail of drugs. Reggie's gentle and devoted father consulted with me by telephone throughout the process, mostly to obtain confirmation and assurance that he was properly handling the emotionally rocky process of withdrawing from the drugs.

Reggie's tardive dyskinesia was caught at a very early stage and disappeared some time after the drugs were stopped. I had several follow-up phone contacts over the next months and Reggie continued to thrive.

STATE DOCTORS GANG UP ON A FAMILY

THE LITTLE FAMILY, hardworking, poor, and uneducated, lived in a small town in the Appalachian Mountains. It was a huge leap for them to take on the state authorities but they saw no alternative.

The conflict with the state began when the school referred their twelve-year-old son, Buddy, to a county clinic for help with behavior problems in school. At the clinic he was prescribed multiple psychiatric drugs but no counseling or parenting guidance was provided. When Buddy's behavior worsened on the cocktail of medications, the clinic insisted on hospitalizing him.

In the long-term residential facility, Risperdal was added to Buddy's drug regimen and he began deteriorating into a child his parents could barely recognize. He was terrified by his surroundings and stupefied by the drugs. He talked vaguely about being sexually abused. Mr. and Mrs. Little felt in danger of losing their son forever.

After their frantic efforts failed to get support from local physicians, the family found me and I wrote a letter to the state authorities confirming that I was willing to see Buddy for a second opinion. The authorities refused, claiming the boy was too sick to leave the hospital, even in the care of his parents, and threatened to bring an action to take Buddy away from his mother and father and to make him a ward of the state.

Based on the parents' description of Buddy, some of his medical records, and a videotape of Buddy taken at home, I became gravely concerned that the boy was developing tardive dyskinesia. I wrote a brief report for the local court stating:

> If drug treatment is not discontinued immediately, the danger grows that the tardive dyskinesia will become irreversible, severe, disfiguring, and disabling. For that reason, I requested the opportunity to conduct an emergency evaluation of Buddy Little. His current treating physicians in the state facility have refused to allow Mrs. Little the opportunity to bring him to me.

I also brought up Mrs. Little's concern that her son had been sexual abused in the facility:

> The Post-Traumatic Stress Disorder associated with sexual abuse in a young boy can lead to hallucinations and even to schizophrenialike disorders. When this happens in an institution, the result is invariably a deterioration of the child's condition while he remains in the institution. Even if the institution could be made safer, and the child protected, the continued psychological threat posed and the psychological association between the sexual abuse and the institution in which it took place would cause further deterioration in his condition.
>
> Overall, his medication regimen is inappropriate and probably negligent. Risperdal and Wellbutrin, as already mentioned, are not even FDA-approved for use in children.* In addition, polypharmacy such as this is not indicated in his case and is generally inappropriate in children.

I concluded, "In my extensive forensic experience, this sounds remarkably like a situation in which the treatment is doing more harm than good."

The court empowered Mr. and Mrs. Little to bring their son to me for a face-to-face evaluation. In my office, I was immediately struck by how normal he seemed. I wrote in my notes:

> He is completely oriented. Has a good sense of humor. Got sad and even tearful at appropriate times when talking alone with me. Was full of normal energy otherwise. Was very respectful, and even loving toward me, and tremendously grateful for my caring attention to him. He was enormously relieved to find out he wasn't crazy.

Based on my recommendation, Mr. and Mrs. Little again asked the state to release their son into their care. Instead the state officials decided to make an example of the obstreperous Little family. They went to court, demanding to keep Buddy involuntarily hospitalized at the state facility.

I testified by telephone on behalf of the parents against the combined might of the state hospital director and the commissioner of mental health for the county, both of whom appeared in court to insist on their right to incarcerate and to drug the child against the will of his parents and against the ad-

---

*As noted earlier in the chapter, Risperdal is now approved for children under limited circumstance.

vice of their personally chosen psychiatric consultant. Because the parents came from a disadvantaged background, I'm sure these authorities expected to carry the day.

Based on my testimony, the parents won, and the judge permitted me to supervise the removal of Buddy from medication. This was accomplished long distance on an outpatient basis with the help of a local therapist who worked with the boy and his parents during the withdrawal. It took Buddy many months to gradually recover from the medication adverse effects but he has continued to improve and is doing well.

TRYING TO PUSH AROUND THE WRONG FAMILY

When her son Michael was in first grade, Patricia Weathers (her real name) was told to put him on stimulant medication or the school would transfer him to another special education school. Soon after starting Ritalin, Michael became depressed and withdrawn and began compulsively chewing on objects. Of course, Mrs. Weathers did not know that stimulant drugs can produce depression, withdrawal, and compulsive behaviors. Instead, the school psychologist informed her that her son had "bipolar disorder" and referred her to a psychiatrist.

The psychiatrist agreed with the diagnosis and prescribed an antidepressant, telling Mrs. Weathers, according to her report, that it was a wonder drug for children. In reality, giving antidepressants to someone who tends to get manic is like pouring gasoline on a fire, but in Michael's case, as in every child I have seen in recent years, there was no justification for a diagnosis of bipolar disorder.

Mrs. Weathers, who is now president of www.ablechild.org, an organization devoted to "label- and drug-free education," testified before an FDA panel in 2004. Because I have reviewed her son's school and medical records and interviewed him and his mother, I can verify her testimony at this public hearing:[5]

My activism began after my son's school coerced me to place him on Ritalin, a drug that caused him to become extremely withdrawn. The school psychologist and psychiatrist then diagnosed him with social anxiety disorder and recommended Paxil as a "wonder drug for kids."

On Paxil [at the age of nine], Michael began hearing voices in his head, drew violent pictures, and even attacked me. I could no longer recognize my own son. He pleaded with me at one point, "Mom, make it stop." I finally realized that it was the Paxil that put him in a drug–induced psychosis so naturally I removed him from the drug.

Mrs. Weathers went on to describe how the school called Child Protective Services (CPS) to charge her with child neglect because she had removed her son from Paxil, and how CPS then tried to force her to continue medicating Michael.

I evaluated Michael at the age of ten years old in April 2000. At the time, Mrs. Weathers had already freed herself from the government's grip and had become an effective national advocate. She now asked me to help her son obtain proper services from his school. In my report to the school, I emphasized that his worst behaviors in school had been caused by his prescribed medications:

> Soon after starting on Paxil, Michael began to hear voices in his head. Under the influence of the voices, for example, he climbed out a window in his home and rode his bike ten miles to his father's house. . . . He developed insomnia and nightmares on Paxil.
>
> On December 3, 1999, during his period of recovery from Paxil, Michael was upset at school and explained that he had heard a voice in his head. During this time, his physician recommended hospitalization and antipsychotic drugs without actually seeing him. At the time, Michael was taking Dexedrine and recovering from Paxil, which he had stopped less than five weeks earlier.
>
> The voices began to subside when he came off the Paxil but lasted for at least five weeks following discontinuation of the drug. Both the rapid onset and the lengthy recovery time are typical of adverse reaction to this class of drugs. Some drug reactions last many months or more.
>
> Michael is much improved since stopping the Paxil and no longer has any signs of a serious mental disorder. He has no hallucinations. He has grown three clothing sizes since discontinuing medication. The differences in his physical health are readily apparent to those who know him.

According to Mrs. Weathers, at the time that Michael was suffering from medication madness, his psychiatrist and the school psychologist told Mrs. Weathers that Paxil could not have caused Michael's acute emotional disturbance. The doctor wanted to hospitalize him for even more intensive medication. When Michael's parents refused orders from the school and the doctor, and stopped giving the drug to their child, that's when the school reported the family to

Child Protective Services. Yes, schools in the United States have reported parents for "child neglect" because they have refused to medicate their children! Fortunately, Mrs. Weathers fought back vigorously and won, but at great cost to herself and her child.

BEWARE MENTAL HEALTH SCREENING

MY EXPERIENCE WITH PARENTS being forced to drug their children has been limited to particular circumstances exemplified in this chapter: overzealous school psychologists unleashing child protective services upon parents who refuse to knuckle under pressure to drugging their children; overzealous state hospital doctors attempting to seize control of a child from his drug-resisting parents; and most commonly, divorced parents going to court to compel their ex-spouse to drug their child.

There is no central database to document how frequently the coercion of parents occurs but it seems to be on the rise. I receive a large number of calls from parents whose ex-spouses want to enforce the drugging of their children. There have been signs of a healthy backlash against schools coercing parents to drug their children with recent legislation in many states placing limits on what teachers and schools can recommend and prohibiting coercion.

Meanwhile, the nation is rapidly rushing toward something far more menacing—the systematic "mental health screening" of schoolchildren and even infants. The federal government's New Freedom Commission supports both Early Mental Health Screening in the schools, and the Texas Medication Algorithm Project, a pharmaceutical company attempt to enforce guidelines necessitating the use of its products. Because most children will be referred for medical evaluation, virtually assuring the prescription of psychiatric drugs, the country is being threatened by what Alaskan attorney Jim Gottstein, director of PsychRights, has called a drugging dragnet.

Minnesota pediatrician Karen Effrem has been leading the fight against proposed "TeenScreening" in our schools—only to find that her own state is moving toward "toddler screening," and even "infant screening."[6] In Minnesota, legislation has been introduced calling for "socioemotional" screening of toddlers before admission to kindergarten, and Minnesota governor Tim Pawlenty has endorsed a plan put together by state and private agencies based on federal programs to "assure that all children ages birth to five are screened early and continuously for the presence of health, socioemotional, or developmental needs . . ."

Karen Effrem, along with many international reformers in the mental health field, is on the board of directors of the International Center for the Study of Psychiatry and Psychology. She often presents at the annual conferences of the group. Given that our children need attention to their real educational and family needs, and not diagnosing and drugging, these mental health screening programs are worth fighting against! Information about them can be obtained on www.icspp.org.

As "ToddlerScreening" and "TeenScreening" take hold, they will become a psychopharmaceutical steamroller.[7] Even without these latest impositions on our children, millions are being pushed into becoming lifetime consumers of psychiatric drugs. The engorged psychopharmaceutical complex is spreading its tentacles over family and school alike.

Throughout America and indeed in every Western society, psychiatric medications are breaking the spirits and the brains of our children, while insufficient emphasis is being given to the necessary improvements in their educational and family life. Recent years have seen the beginning of a cultural shift. Enlightened people are beginning to realize that we are massively over-drugging our children. I hope that some day our society will realize that drugs are *never* the answer to a child's emotional problems and that pro-drug physicians and drug companies have been perpetrating massive child abuse.

Chapter 16

This Is Not My Daughter

THE "ANTIPSYCHOTIC" MEDICATIONS like Zyprexa, Seroquel, and Abilify have their primary or "therapeutic" effect by causing severe apathy and indifference. The personality and self-determination of the individual are subdued and, in some cases, nearly snuffed out. These drugs may render people unable to care about themselves and about life. I have described these lobotomizing effects as "deactivation," a general crushing of spontaneity and autonomy with the production of apathy and docility.[1] Although the emphasis of this book is on obvious clinical effects, a variety of scientific studies show the existence of corresponding drug-induced damage to brain structure and neurons.[2] The so-called mood stabilizers like lithium and Depakote have similar but sometimes less overwhelming effects, and they, too, can damage the brain.

IT SEEMED TO HELP HIS ALLERGIES

BECAUSE ANTIPSYCHOTIC DRUGS are often given to very distressed or disturbed patients, healthcare providers can easily blame their harmful effects on the patient's "mental illness." The subdued, withdrawn demeanor of most psychiatrically hospitalized patients is not due to their psychological condition as much as it is due to their medication.

Sometimes, unintended experiments involving normal individuals can help to demonstrate the inherently subduing effects of these drugs on people regardless of their prior mental condition. Jeb Ingram's pediatrician phoned in a prescription for ninety tablets of the antihistamine Zyrtec[3] to help the fourteen-year-old with his allergies. By mistake the pharmacy dispensed ninety tablets of the potent adult antipsychotic drug Zyprexa at the recommended adult dose of 10 mg per day.

Zyprexa is an antipsychotic drug that blunts mental function and can cause tardive dyskinesia, Parkinson's disorder, diabetes, pancreatitis, obesity, and numerous other problems, some of them life-threatening. Over the next eleven months, Jeb took the Zyprexa as needed for his allergies. He consumed eighty-seven tablets or a little more than two per week. Zyprexa is a particularly "dirty" drug in that it affects multiple neurotransmitter systems. Among its actions, it has potent antihistaminic effects. Zyprexa seemed to provide Jeb some relief from his allergies, misleading him into thinking he was taking the right medicine. Perhaps sensing they were too strong, Jeb ended up breaking them in half and may have been taking them at the rate of 5 mg several times a week.

The pharmacy error was not discovered until the prescription had been nearly used up. When Jeb and his grandmother went to pick up the new prescription, the boy noticed that the "new" Zyrtec pills didn't look like the "old" ones.

In reviewing the medical records and depositions in the legal case against the pharmacy and through evaluating Jeff with his family, I found that the most obvious adverse effect on the boy was fatigue. Despite taking the drug only twice a week, Jeb became tired all the time. He fell asleep heavily at night and had difficulty getting up in the morning. He fell asleep in class on occasion.

Jeb lost interest in his schoolwork. A very bright child, he was distressed when he got a C in English for the first time. He no longer looked forward to going to school and began to stay home more often because he wasn't feeling well. His mind didn't seem as sharp and his memory was not as good. He also lost his usual emotional composure. His family described mood swings, fits of irritability and anger, sulking, and diminished cooperativeness. At times he talked about getting "really scared" and "having a bad time."

Mom in retrospect realized that her son had lost his sparkle and seemed to have a "haze" over his eyes. In general, he was less friendly and less social.

Jeb also had episodes when he would become wobbly when trying to stand up for the first time in the morning. This is called orthostatic hypotension—an abrupt drop in blood pressure on standing up—another Zyprexa effect. He also got dizzy at times during the day and would end up supporting himself against a wall or he'd find himself slumping over in his chair. Jeb would feel as if he were "blacking out" without actually losing consciousness. On one occasion, a friend noticed and reported it to a teacher.

Jeb's temperature regulation was also thrown off and he would feel too hot or cold with relatively slight variations in temperature. Heat intolerance in particular is a well-known effect of antipsychotic drugs, notoriously causing death by heat stroke in state hospitals and tenements that lack air-conditioning. Both hypotension and heat intolerance are caused by drug-induced dysfunction in the autonomic nervous system that governs physiological activities. He had stomachaches and took Tylenol for headaches.

Jeb was not completely disabled by these symptoms. He continued to go to school and to have friends but his social life was dampened. He ran track but his grandmother described him as "getting red as a beet" and having leg cramps when she watched him compete.

Jeb's parents noticed an occasional tic in his eye but initially reported no other potential abnormal movements that looked like tardive dyskinesia.

On several occasions Jeb's mother called the pediatrician's office and was told by the staff that Zyrtec could cause fatigue and that it was nothing serious. She also began to see other symptoms, including emotional volatility, and was told by the doctor's office that the antihistamine could *not* cause them. Of course, no one imagined Jeb was taking an entirely different and far more toxic drug.

All of Jeb's many new symptoms are recognized adverse reactions to Zyprexa and to other antipsychotic drugs. But reviewing the myriad symptoms, it's apparent how confusing they could be to a parent. Almost all of them could be mistakenly attributed to the onset of adolescent emotional mood changes! If most of them hadn't cleared up within weeks and months of stopping the drug, one might have wondered if Jeb wasn't suffering from depressed and anxious feelings in his early teens.

Now imagine if a child has already been labeled with a psychiatric diagnosis—any psychiatric diagnosis—and prescribed Zyprexa. Would the doctor have realized the drug was causing the escalation in emotional problems? In almost every case I've seen, including Reggie Thompson, and Buddy Little in the previous chapter, doctors have attributed adverse drug reactions to the child's worsening psychiatric condition rather than to the medication.

I evaluated Jeb in my office two years after he stopped taking the Zyprexa. He had improved enormously. He no longer had the "haze" over his eyes. He was bright and cheery. He was no longer fatigued and didn't suffer anymore from fits of irritability and feeling sick. His stomachaches, headaches, dizziness, and blackouts were gone.

Nonetheless, Jeb continued to suffer from persistent problems that are almost certainly residual drug effects. He easily forgets things, has to be given lists, and must study harder than he used to. His mother and grandmother explained that Jeb previously had a "photographic memory." In addition, as I wrote in my report on the case, he had "some continued personality changes, but to a lesser degree, including a tendency not to listen and to be uncooperative, to get unaccountably irritable, and sometimes to have tears that he cannot explain. It is difficult to separate this from a normal adolescent developmental stage, but it was worse during the exposure to Zyprexa, indicating a probable connection."

Jeb continued to have occasional twitching of one eye. He had occasional neck spasms, pulling his head to the right, probably a relatively mild form of tardive dyskinesia called tardive dystonia. The family had noticed it while he was taking Zyprexa but attributed it to nerves or to shakes. Hopefully these mild residual symptoms of tardive dyskinesia will fully remit with time.

Jeb's subtle personality changes and memory problems seemed especially serious to me. I wrote in my report, "Even a slight degree of personality change is significant. Personality instability in the form of irritability relates to the individual's entire identity. Increased irritability, while somewhat acceptable in an adolescent, will become an increasing problem if it persists into young adulthood. It can disrupt marital and work relationships."

I concluded that it would take years to determine the long-range effects of Jeb Ingram's eleven-month exposure to Zyprexa at age fourteen. In reality, drug-induced personality and memory problems, however slight in their appearance, can plague a person for a lifetime without being adequately identified or measured.

SPELLBOUND BY ANTIPSYCHOTIC STABILIZING DRUGS

AS I DOCUMENT in great scientific detail in *Brain-Disabling Treatments in Psychiatry* (2008), all antipsychotic drugs clog the brain and mind by performing a chemical disruption of frontal lobe function, the equivalent of a pharmacological lobotomy. Patients become more docile, less expressive of their distress, and less troublesome because their frontal lobes have been rendered dysfunctional. These agents spellbind so profoundly that many patients walk about helplessly in a state of passivity induced by cerebral dysfunction.

Almost all the neuroleptics, including newer ones like Risperdal, Zyprexa, Abilify, and Seroquel, block the function of neurons (brain cells) that require the neurotransmitter dopamine for their activation. From their origin deep in the brain in the basal ganglia, nerve trunks activated by dopamine reach upward into the frontal lobes and into the emotion-regulating functions in the limbic system. They also reach lower into the brain to the energizing functions in the reticular activating system of the brain.[4] When these functions are blocked, the human being's emotional and motivational system is vastly reduced. The overall impact is a dose-dependent apathy or indifference to everything and anyone. In more sensitive patients or at higher doses, these drugs make people grossly zombielike.

ZYPREXA ZOMBIE

IN DESPERATION and as a last resort, the parents of twenty-three-year-old graduate student Regina Dawson brought her to my office for an evaluation. A week earlier they had arrived from out of town for a brief visit and had been aghast at their daughter's condition. She was taking Zyprexa.

Regina's grades were falling and she was having trouble completing assignments, alerting her parents for the need to make an emergency visit. What they found was far, far worse than anticipated. Regina was living in squalor in her apartment and becoming morbidly obese. The worst change was the blunting of her personality. This previously lively, intelligent, and athletic young woman now looked, in her dad's words, like a zombie. Her expression was flat, her movements slow, her initiative almost nil. She couldn't connect emotionally to her parents or anyone else.

No one had diagnosed Regina as schizophrenic and it was unclear why she had been put on an antipsychotic. I would later find out that she was having very disturbing nightmares and experiencing dangerous sleepwalking episodes that terrorized her and sometimes put her in vulnerable circumstances, problems that would require help as she became drug free. Zyprexa provides heavy sedation and the doctor probably hoped to suppress both the nightmares and the sleepwalking.

Mr. Dawson was a wealthy businessman who was determined to use his resources to rescue his daughter from her desperate plight. Within days of arriving in town, he and his wife had taken Regina to a well-connected professor of psychiatry they found on a "Best Doctors" list. The doctor had examined Regina and told her parents *not* to be concerned about the "routine medication effects" of Zyprexa. According to her parents, he explained that Regina's treatment with Zyprexa was entirely appropriate, indeed state of the art, and that she should continue in treatment with her original doctor. He sent them off without a follow-up appointment.

Flabbergasted, but as yet undaunted and profoundly motivated by his concern for her daughter, Regina's father drew on the determination that had made him a success in business. He would find the very best expert on "mental illness" and antipsychotic medication in all of the Washington metropolitan area. He found him at the National Institute of Mental Health (NIMH) in the great redbrick clinical center building that dominates the sprawling government campus. The highly touted, much-published specialist looked at Regina and repeated, almost word for word, what the university professor had said. Regina was getting the best possible treatment with the latest and safest drug, and she should continue in treatment with her prescribing doctor.

A lesser man than Regina's father would have given up but he kept looking until he came across my name and then one of my books. In his mind I was the last hope.

Dad and Mom entered my office while Regina—spellbound by Zyprexa— followed along in a docile fashion. Regina murmured something about not liking be dragged around from doctor to doctor, and that was it. Her words were uttered with fatiguing effort, her expression was flat, and she made no eye contact. It was instantly apparent that she was drugged into near oblivion.

While Regina sat passively in my office with a dull expression on her face, her grief-stricken parents explained to me that a few months earlier during summer recess their daughter had been full of life, playing tennis, joking around, and generally being herself. Previously meticulous about her appearance, Regina showed no concern about her huge weight gain and puffy face. Her parents pleaded with me to believe that this was not their daughter—not the sparkling and even brilliant Regina that they knew and loved.

"This is not my daughter," Regina's father protested.

By the end of the session, Regina was feeling a ray of confidence that maybe her parents and I were correct in assessing her as suffering from a dangerous and disabling degree of Zyprexa toxicity. She hesitantly agreed to come for regular therapy.

It took many months to withdraw Regina from the Zyprexa. Every time we reduced the drug a little more, she teetered on crashing into a more horrible state of apathy and depression. I had to work with her family support system and to be constantly available for emergencies. I have come across this kind of Zyprexa "crashing" withdrawal reaction on other occasions as well but have no explanation for how the drug produces a withdrawal reaction so similar to its direct effect.

When she was finally drug free, Regina landed on an emotional roller coaster. It would have been easy for me to diagnose her as "bipolar"—nowadays nearly all psychiatrists would have—and to start her on lithium or some other mood stabilizer. But I knew her brain was going through withdrawal, and we wouldn't know Regina's real emotional condition until we'd gotten through it.

I wish there were a residential sanctuary where people like Regina could go to be safe and to be supported by caring therapists. Unhappily, there are few if any places in the world today where a disturbed and distressed human being can recover without being further drugged. Even detoxification centers for alcoholics and drug addicts tend nowadays to switch their patients permanently to other psychoactive medications, never permitting them to experience a drug-free brain and mind. After careful consideration, Regina, her family, and I decided to continue with the somewhat risky endeavor of treating her as an outpatient in my private practice.

Over a period of several months, Regina gradually began to find her drug-free self. For Regina it was like coming out of a coma that she'd mistaken for an awful version of reality. She emerged to be the young woman her parents had told me about—extremely intelligent, motivated, full of humor, and daring. Now, several years later, I continue to hear on occasion about how well she continues to do.

A WOMAN NEARLY DESTROYED BY ANTIPSYCHOTIC DRUGS

NOT LONG AGO, a very lovely woman in her early sixties came to me for a consultation concerning that dreadful, irreversible adverse drug effect called tardive dyskinesia. Mrs. Angela Dignity had been exposed to numerous older antipsychotics over a period of many years, including Mellaril, Trilafon, Thorazine, Stelazine, and Asendin, a drug marketed as an antidepressant that is, in fact, a very dangerous antipsychotic agent. Her last psychiatrist kept her on antipsychotic drugs for approximately seven and one-half years. She also received Zyprexa. She was at times prescribed other types of drugs but most consistently she was exposed to antipsychotic agents.

From reviewing the medical records and interviewing her and her family, it is apparent that from the beginning Mrs. Dignity's symptoms were mainly mild depression, some anxiety, and insomnia. She voiced concerns and fears about her husband in a marriage that otherwise seemed close and loving.

Under no circumstances should Mrs. Dignity have been exposed to a single day of antipsychotic drugs. She probably would have prospered with couples counseling for herself and her husband—something her psychiatrist never offered or suggested to her.

For the last five years of her psychiatric treatment, the antipsychotic medications wore her down to such an extent that her husband and children grew
concerned about her. She was zombielike for much of the time, no longer enjoying reading, television, or socializing with her loving family. Although she
was a very industrious person, she was unable to cook, do the dishes, or even
housekeep while taking the medications. As the children testified, "Dad did
everything for her." Trying to defend her pride, she protested, "I did some of
the dusting."

When her beloved husband died, Mrs. Dignity did not seem to care and
went on day to day in her now rote fashion of living. It seemed impossible to
her children that this indifference to her life could be the product of "mental
illness," but they found it difficult to believe that a doctor would prescribe
medications that could have such catastrophic effects.

Mrs. Dignity's family tried to convince her to stop seeing the doctor. She
complained in retrospect that he rarely if ever spent more than a few minutes
at a time with her. He never involved her now-deceased husband or children
in the treatment process. And she didn't particularly like him. Yet, she refused
family pressure to change doctors.

Mrs. Dignity was in her early sixties. In the elderly—people over fifty-five
are considered elderly in this scientific literature—the rates of tardive dyskinesia after exposure to antipsychotic drugs are astronomically high. Controlled
clinical trials have repeatedly shown that the risk of developing permanent abnormal movements is at least 20 percent per year in older people. That huge
risk accumulates from year to year, so it's at least 40 percent after two years.[5]
Unlike in younger patients, tardive dyskinesia in the elderly commonly develops after only days or weeks of exposure. Older human beings should never be
put on these drugs.

Although drug companies and some doctors promote the newer antipsychotic drugs as less prone to causing tardive dyskinesia, this speculation remains
unproven.[6] The FDA continues to require the same class warning about tardive
dyskinesia for the entire group of drugs, including newer ones like Zyprexa,
Risperdal, Abilify, and Seroquel. Unfortunately, there are no effective treatments
for tardive dyskinesia. Sedative drugs can sometimes calm the movements temporarily by quieting the nervous system. When the movements are disfiguring
or disabling, sometimes Botox injections can temporarily paralyze the muscles,
providing some relief.

Mrs. Dignity was sitting next to her two daughters at Sunday church
when they noticed that she was making odd movements. Mrs. Dignity was
gasping as if having trouble breathing and her arms seemed to be moving out

of control. Despite how distressing the symptoms seemed, she didn't seem to notice or to care.

Spellbound by a combination of acute drug effects and by persistent drug-induced brain damage, most tardive dyskinesia (TD) patients fail to recognize their symptoms. As a result, even after stopping drugs, some patients remain unable to recognize their twitches and spasms. One of the pioneers in this arena, Michael Myslobodsky (1986), found that an astonishing 95 percent of tardive dyskinesia patients displayed "emotional indifference or frank anosognosia [not knowing]" toward their abnormal movements.[7] The rates have varied in subsequent studies but they are usually high.[8]

One of Mrs. Dignity's daughters made an appointment with their family physician. Although the doctor was unable to diagnose the specific disorder of tardive dyskinesia, he immediately recognized that Mrs. Dignity had a neurological problem that was probably being caused by her medications. He referred her to a neurologist who diagnosed tardive dyskinesia and the antipsychotics were stopped. Unfortunately, it was too late—the disorder had become irreversible.

Now the neurologist faced a daunting problem. Mrs. Dignity's abnormal movements had become so painful, exhausting, and disabling that something had to be done to control them. The only effective way to suppress the movements was to give her the same kind of drugs that had caused her disorder. As already described, the antipsychotic drugs mask or suppress the disease even as they cause it, until over time the tardive dyskinesia movements becomes so severe that they break through the masking effect.

The neurologist brought the family together with his patient to discuss the alternatives. Together they decided to resume antipsychotic drugs in order to provide Mrs. Dignity some relief. Giving her the offended agents sealed her fate. Mrs. Dignity's underlying disorder is not likely to improve and she may get worse, but in the meanwhile she will experience some relief.

Later when Mrs. Dignity and her family sought my medical opinion, I approved the decision and the manner in which it was made by involving the doctor, the patient, and the family. The medication dose was relatively low and did not suppress her mentally as much as her previous treatment that caused her disorder.

When I evaluated Mrs. Dignity in my office, she was continuing to take the medication that suppressed her abnormal movements; but despite the masking effect she was nonetheless unable to sit still. Every few seconds or minutes, her hands and feet moved uncontrollably. Her head continuously bobbed forward and her chest gave little heaving movements. She walked on her heels because her feet were stiff. When I flexed her elbow, it snapped back in spasm.

Mrs. Dignity's jaw spasms were among the worst of her symptoms, causing her constant pain and interfering with her swallowing. Eventually the jaw spasms will probably cause her teeth to come loose.

Her face was distorted by muscle spasms and her voice sounded badly distorted and sometimes unintelligible. Mrs. Dignity was so embarrassed by her appearance and the sound of her voice that she had become more reclusive.

Mrs. Dignity regretted that she had not responded years earlier to her family's urgent requests to change doctors. She came from a social background where people tend not to question authority and she could not believe that her doctor would do anything to harm her. But that does not fully account for why she would continue to take medications that were literally stupefying and disabling her. Nor does it account for why she would fail to respond emotionally to her husband's death. It especially does not explain why she failed to notice or care about the early but obvious signs of her now disabling abnormal movements. The real reason is that the drugs had spellbound Mrs. Dignity for many years.

Antipsychotic Dementia

Mrs. Dignity's mental capacities were significantly diminished at the time I saw her. She was functioning on a much lower intellectual level than required to raise a family, to socialize, or to earn a living as she had done so effectively in earlier years.

Although the medical profession often resists the tragic facts, there can be no doubt that patients taking antipsychotic drugs for many years not only tend to develop tardive dyskinesia, they also lose some of their cognitive abilities. Many develop frank dementia—a generalized loss of intellectual ability accompanied by mood instability—called tardive dementia.[9]

By the time I evaluated Mrs. Dignity after her years of antipsychotic drug exposure, she thought and spoke with the innocent simplicity of a child. She was unable to describe what medications she was taking or precisely why she needed them. While she sat back seemingly unconcerned, I had to review with family members issues surrounding her future treatment and prognosis. The drug-induced dementia rendered her unable to fully appreciate or to react emotionally to her dire circumstances.

Through it all, this remarkable woman maintained a sense of humor and expressed surprisingly little resentment. She is what many people would describe as a "good soul."

We can only hope that the medications will continue to partially mask Mrs. Dignity's abnormal movements without worsening them in the long run. As she grows older, the constant movements will also cause wear and tear on her muscles and joints. The aging process itself may compound the disorder. But I know this proud, good woman will do her best to keep up her spirits and the spirits of those she loves.

LITHIUM DOLDRUMS

MOOD STABILIZERS LIKE LITHIUM and Depakote have an impact on neurotransmitters different from the antipsychotic drugs, but they have similar if less intense effects. Because they cannot be used like the antipsychotic drugs to abruptly subdue the individual, they are reserved for the long-term control of so-called bipolar disorder. Nowadays they are given to many children and adults who have but the faintest signs of a maniclike problem, such as irritability and mild mood swings in adults or temper tantrums in children.

Lithium was the original mood stabilizer. It was discovered when it was accidentally found that injections of lithium into guinea pigs immediately made them inactive and even flaccid.[10] Numerous studies of normal volunteers have confirmed that lithium knocks people out of touch with their feelings, puts a dark glass between them and other people, and reduces their motivation to do anything. In the process it leaves many people with memory dysfunction and other cognitive deficits.[11]

The FDA has also approved a group of antiepileptic drugs specifically to treat "bipolar" disorder, especially the long-term suppression of mania. These include Equetro (carbamazepine), Depakote (divalproex sodium), and Lamictal (lamotrigine). A complete list is found in the appendix. These drugs were originally approved and used as antiseizure drugs. They tend to suppress the electrical activity of the brain. In sufficient doses, they cause sufficient sedation to slow down the brain and mind, and hence are used in psychiatry to control behavior. They disable the brain in a global fashion and there is nothing specific about their effects for any "mental illness."

Dotty Novick took lithium for almost six years. The drug virtually wiped out much of her fourth decade of life, emotionally clamping her into a deep, chronic depression. She might have been spellbound for the rest of her life, if the drug hadn't caused her kidneys to fail.

Coming from a difficult childhood and an ongoing conflicted relationship with her mother, Dotty had tough times but surmounted them. She graduated college at a precociously young age and later returned to graduate school to get a master's degree.

Before Dotty could finish her last class in the master's program, her father was diagnosed with cancer. Dotty had always felt closer to him than to her mother and didn't want him to go through his last weeks or months without her. She returned home, which also meant putting off the completion of her degree and returning to live under her mother's domination.

It took her father many months to die and during that time Dotty reestablished herself in her community with a good job. She often felt sad, especially after her dad's death, but she carried on.

Then good things started to happen. She fell in love, became engaged, and moved in with her fiancé. He was doing well professionally and they planned to move to another state after getting married, so she quit her job and began preparing for the wedding. Seemingly without warning, a few weeks before the wedding her fiancé abruptly ended the engagement and moved away.

Dotty was overwhelmed by her father's death and her fiancé's abandonment of her. She became fearful, suspicious, and paranoid, and was admitted to a mental hospital with a diagnosis of brief psychotic break. From my reading of the records, it was an abrupt onset stress reaction that can usually be treated by an experienced therapist in an outpatient office rather than by hospitalization or psychiatric drugs.

Dotty became panicked in the hospital. At the age of nineteen, a man with a knife had chased her through a park, almost catching her. Now she became terrified that she would be assaulted in the hospital. A mental hospital can be a humiliating and terrifying experience for anyone, especially a vulnerable, emotionally wounded woman. Dotty grew worse in the hospital, and she was numbed with injections of the antipsychotic Haldol.

The Haldol quickly subdued Dotty. Then, without giving her natural healing processes a chance, she was put on lithium. This is typical of modern psychiatric care. Unable or unwilling to relate to their patients in a healing manner—utterly lacking what I call a healing presence in *The Heart of Being Helpful*—my colleagues nowadays rely solely on drugs. A person coming out of a psychotic episode needs a clear head and patient, experienced guidance—not a brain full of toxins that will only complicate her ability to take charge of her emotional life.

As an HMO outpatient, Dotty now began almost six years of outpatient lithium treatment. The medical record confirms that the lithium made her feel slowed down and depressed. By interfering with the overall electrical processes in the brain, lithium gums up the brain and, hence, the mind.

As already mentioned, lithium is such a spellbinding drug that patients easily become severely intoxicated without realizing it, so patients on lithium are required to have blood tests to check the concentration of the drug in the bloodstream. Lithium is toxic not only to the brain but to many other organs in the body including the skin, thyroid, and kidneys. Patients on lithium need periodic thyroid and kidney function tests. The HMO doctors ordered kidney tests periodically over more than five years but failed to check on them or to compare them to each other—or they would have noticed that the results were gradually moving from the normal to the abnormal range, indicating that her kidney function was gradually deteriorating. Dotty never gave the tests any thought and assumed she would be informed if anything abnormal was showing up. By the time the test results were noticed, Dotty was already displaying symptoms of weakness and fatigue with excessive urination and thirst. She could barely take a walk without having to sip the bottled water that she carried with her everywhere.

Meanwhile, Dotty became so listless she was unable to work and had to live on disability. In her spellbound state, she had no idea what was happening to her. Without having the mental energy to come to any conclusions or to take any positive actions, Dotty blamed her condition on the death of her father, the stress of living with her mother, giving up her job when she thought she was getting married, and the betrayal by her ex-fiancé. She never guessed that there was something more physical crushing her vitality.

For a few weeks after starting lithium, Dotty saw a therapist. The social worker noted in the chart that Dotty "feels 'blah'" and had "decreased motivation," but did not recognize these symptoms as typical lithium effects. Too spellbound by lithium to benefit from therapy, Dotty stopped going. Meanwhile, the HMO made it hard for her to get any further help except for lithium.

By the time her lithium-induced kidney disease was finally diagnosed, Dotty was left with permanently impaired kidney function. Worst of all, her kidney specialist warned her that it was too risky for her to become pregnant any time in the foreseeable future—abruptly ending one of her most cherished dreams.

The HMO doctors switched her from lithium to Depakote. Recognizing that her HMO doctors had betrayed her, Dotty did what many other intelligent but injured patients finally do—she started reading on her own about drugs on the Internet and at the library. Dismayed at what she found, Dotty tapered herself off medication.

Dotty came to me for help in staying off psychiatric drugs and in getting her life together. She was already on the road to regaining her sense of self after almost six years in a drug stupor. She also wanted to consult with me about a lawsuit against the HMO and its doctors. I located an attorney who was willing to take her case and agreed to work on it as well. My list of medically negligent acts was extensive, including the failure to respond to her worsening kidney tests and the years of unnecessary, brain-clouding medication. My notes on her damages from the malpractice were also extensive, including more than five and one-half years of drug-induced depression, emotional dulling, and apathy; financial dependence; social isolation; complete disruption of her educational and career opportunities; and partially disabling kidney disease.

During the time the HMO doctors were treating her with lithium, they made Dotty feel hopeless about recovering. She had been misled into believing that she was chronically mentally ill, requiring lifelong drug treatment, and that she must settle for a stunted life when, in fact, she was spellbound by lithium.

Due to legal technicalities in suing the HMO, Dotty's lawyer encouraged her to settle for a mere one hundred thousand dollars. Pro-industry lobbying has given the misperception that patients frequently and successfully sue innocent doctors for malpractice. As mentioned earlier, in reality, it is very difficult and expensive to bring a malpractice suit, and the vast majority fail regardless of their merit.

Fortunately, Dotty was able to stay off all psychiatric drugs and to learn how to understand and deal with her drug-free emotions. That resulted in a big bonus: a return of her sense of self, her ability to feel, and her capacity to make use of therapy as an avenue for personal growth. Having lost so many years trapped within drug-induced oblivion, it was slow going, as if climbing out of a bottomless pit, but she continued to grow and regain control over her life.

A few years later Dotty Novick came back to see me again because of the abrupt onset of another, in her words, "paranoid" episode. She was extremely frightened and having trouble sleeping. She had a good, stable job in a relatively secure work environment, but she was certain her employer was conspiring against her with the government and equally certain that the CIA was spying on her.

Because I never start patients on psychiatric drugs, I have to make myself more available to them. I decided to see Dotty for an hour every day for three or four days in a row. In that brief time, the strength and safety of our relationship was able to reconnect her to reality.

Psychosis is a devastating loss of confidence and trust in other human beings. When social relationships become unendurably terrifying, and other people become objects of terror, the individual becomes lost in the nightmarish state called psychosis. People going through what psychiatrists diagnose as schizophrenia are enduring a horrific loss of relationship to other people, usually accompanied by overwhelming feelings of distrust, humiliation, and powerlessness.[12] If the patient's disturbed condition has not become cemented into place by years of toxic drugs, a caring, reality-oriented relationship with an experienced therapist can often quickly reverse the downward spiral.

Dotty returned to work in a few days—more quickly than I had advised—and showed no signs of paranoia or severe disturbance the following week. She has continued to do well without therapy over the following years.

Unfortunately, because of their total reliance on drugs and electroshock, modern psychiatrists are ill equipped to build trusting relationships with disturbed people. Having been actively discouraged from trying drug-free psychotherapy with disturbed patients, they have no inkling that acute psychotic breaks often quickly respond to skilled human intervention. Instead of building rapport with their patients, they reflexively resort to pressuring or forcing them into hospitals against their will, further humiliating and alienating them. A few hours or days of disturbed behavior are nowadays treated as a cause for a lifetime sentence to drug treatment when all that's really required is short-term, experienced help.

During their training, modern young psychiatrists hardly ever see a disturbed patient who is not already snowed under with drugs. When the patient initially appears in the emergency room, clinic, or private office, drugs are immediately begun without any attempt at psychotherapy. Psychiatrists who have been trained in the last few decades only get to see drug-free patients who have recently stopped their medication. Instead of recognizing that the patients are undergoing withdrawal, their flagrant symptoms are seen as a reason to immediately resume medication, by force if necessary.

DRUG-WITHDRAWAL MADNESS

THERE ARE TWO EXCEPTIONS to the rule that antipsychotic drugs crush spontaneity and enforce robotic docility. One exception is akathisia, an experience of inner torture with a compulsion to move, which we've seen as a result of exposure to SSRI antidepressants. The *DSM-IV* recognizes that neuroleptic-induced akathisia can produce suicidal and violent behavior, and a general worsening of the individual's condition. It estimates neuroleptic-induced akathisia to occur in 20 to 75 percent of patients.[13]

Withdrawal is the other exception in which neuroleptics can cause activation with anxiety and agitation rather than more stupefied reactions. During withdrawal, as described earlier, Regina experienced an intense lethargy and depression. More often, withdrawal reactions from antipsychotic drugs produce overexcitation, anxiety, and other intensely disturbing manifestations of emotional pain and suffering, including psychosis. Whenever the brain is subjected to drugs that suppress its function, the brain fights back. When the drug is stopped, abruptly lifting the lid off the suppressed brain, it can be as explosive as snatching the top off a pressure cooker.

Withdrawal from antipsychotic drugs can drive people into tardive psychosis—a state of madness worse than before the drugs were started. Guy Chouinard and Barry Jones, among the earliest to recognize tardive psychosis, estimated that it occurs in 30 to 40 percent of patients withdrawn from long-term treatment with antipsychotic drugs.[14] As Jones put it, "Some patients who seem to require lifelong neuroleptic therapy may actually do so because of this therapy." For the remainder of their lives, these unfortunate patients remain more disturbed than they were before the drugs were prescribed to them.

Severe emotional disturbances can occur during antipsychotic-drug withdrawal even in patients who have not been previously disturbed. A large percentage of children who are prescribed antipsychotic drugs to control their behavior in institutions undergo similar withdrawal reactions. After being withdrawn from the antipsychotic medications, their behavior frequently becomes more disturbed and uncontrollable than before they were placed on the medicines.[15]

On rare occasions when a patient stops taking antipsychotic drugs and commits a horrendously violent act, drug advocates and the media are quick to howl that patients must never stop taking their drugs. In reality, the occasional patient who goes berserk shortly after stopping antipsychotic drugs is almost certainly suffering from a drug-induced withdrawal psychosis. These already unstable persons have no idea what's happening to them as they descend further into madness.

In my clinical experience, few clinical challenges are more difficult and hazardous than removing a patient from antipsychotic drugs after years of exposure. The brain damage and dysfunction unmasked during withdrawal are often emotionally unendurable and the distressed behaviors are too often dangerous. The victim remains locked for their lifetime into taking these very uncomfortable, often agonizing, generally stupefying, potentially disabling, sometimes lethal, and very brain-damaging chemical agents. Because it is so difficult to stop taking long-term neuroleptics, I have urged my colleagues to view the drugs as "addictive" in their capacity to compel people to continue taking them.[16]

Similarly, patients who stop taking the "mood stabilizer" lithium will be exposed to a much higher risk of having a manic episode than they were before taking the drug.[17] In other words, they risk suffering from withdrawal mania. Instead of admitting that a patient is suffering from withdrawal mania, the doctor is likely to say, "See, I told you that you need to take lithium for the rest of your life." What the withdrawal victim really needs is a chance to get through the withdrawal period without being subjected to additional brain-disabling chemicals.

In the last few decades, psychiatry has tried to stake out a claim to being both therapeutic and scientific based on the results obtained from using antipsychotic drugs to treat "schizophrenia" and mood-stabilizing drugs to treat "bipolar disorder." In reality, these very toxic substances simply disable the brain, producing profound deactivation, and spellbinding. Instead of using physical restraints to control the patient, modern psychiatry disables the brain and mind, producing relative degrees of apathy and indifference. The intensity of this lobotomy-like effect depends upon the individual's sensitivity to the drug and the size of the dose, and has nothing to do with the individual's psychological problems or supposed mental illness. This is intoxication masquerading as therapy.

Chapter 17

Dilemmas and Difficulties in the Role of the Medical Expert

CAN MEDICAL EXPERTS LIKE me believe what we are told by people who claim that their bad behaviors were driven by drugs? Have they been spell-bound by medication or are they conning us with misleading stories? Can medical experts really determine whether or not individuals have control over their behavior or if, instead, they have been driven to act by drug intoxication and medication spellbinding?

Of the hundreds of people I have evaluated for medical-legal cases, only four or five have been caught lying, usually by withholding information about prior offenses. In a few other cases, patients in outrageously manic states have made up colossal lies that were patently and ridiculously false. Although these bizarre lies have hurt their cases in the eyes of juries, they are consistent with spellbinding—compulsive lying without appreciation of the consequences.

More commonly, my legal clients have been determined to tell their version of truth, even when it hurt their cases. In several cases in this book, drug spellbinding caused a level of naiveté and incompetence that drove the victims to tell "the truth" as they saw it—even when that truth was so absurd that it was bound to lead to their conviction.

ZERO RECIDIVISM

I AM AWARE OF only one of my cases in which a former legal client with a medication-related crime was arrested again for committing a crime. He had a

DUI a year or more after my involvement in his legal case, breaking probation, and leading to his reincarceration. Alcohol was a lifelong problem for this individual. However, his original crimes occurred solely under the influence of psychiatric drugs and did not involve alcohol.

It is remarkable that not one of my legal clients that I know of has become a repeat offender. However, I must add the caveat that I do not have systematic follow-ups on all of my legal cases. If a few do someday offend again, the record of so many others returning to crime-free lives is very confirmatory that their offenses were indeed related to medication intoxication and spellbinding, and that it was safe for them to return to society. A zero or near-zero recidivism rate is not characteristic of ordinary criminals and crimes.

Given the especially senseless, impulsive, and compulsive nature of many of the crimes described in this book, one would expect the likelihood of recidivism to be especially high in this group. That is, given how out of control these people behaved during their perpetrations, they would seem especially likely to become repeat offenders. As my research assistant Ian Goddard reminded me while editing this chapter, that these individuals returned to being law-abiding, responsible citizens—that none of them repeated bizarre crimes when free of psychiatric drugs—further confirms the drug-induced nature of their misdeeds. In addition, if they had been lying about their mental condition in order to avoid conviction or to lighten their sentences, some of them at least would have repeated their harmful behaviors after being released.

Similar observations can be made about individuals who became depressed and compulsively suicidal while taking psychiatric medications. Given the repetitive nature of suicide attempts in depressed people, we would have expected some of these individuals to make repeat suicide attempts after they became drug free. Furthermore, if the antidepressants had been helping them, as many of their doctors contended even after they attempted suicide while taking them, then the likelihood of suicide attempts would have been greatly increased, rather than reduced to zero, after removal from the drugs. The absence of any further suicide attempts in any of the cases in this book confirms that the original suicide attempts were medication-induced.

DISTORTED PERCEPTIONS OF REALITY

LYING IS NOT the biggest problem in determining the facts about what happened to the person who endured spellbinding drug intoxication. A more common problem is the tendency for all psychoactive substances to cause the brain and mind to distort reality.

Derealization—a feeling of remoteness from reality—often sets in at the time of the drug-induced incident or shortly afterward. People often say, "It was like a dream," or "Like watching a TV in the distance." Depersonalization—a feeling of remoteness from oneself—often goes along with derealization or remoteness from the events and the outside world. A man will report, "I looked down and saw this hand holding a gun pointed at this person but it wasn't my hand." Reports like this do not help in court—they carry a frank admission of perpetrating the crime, they are too common to justify an insanity defense, and they seem unbelievable—and, therefore, the individual has little reason to make them up.

My research assistant Ian Goddard pointed out to me that the continuum of depersonalization proceeds from being uninvolved to being overinvolved. At one extreme of depersonalization, individuals feel so remote from what was happening that they do not see themselves as actors in the drama. The unfolding events are experienced as "not about me." At the other extreme of the continuum, individuals feel as if "it's all about me." In a psychotic state, Melvin Worthy thought he was the center of an alien plot to take over the world and to exterminate all human beings. In this sense, being totally self-centered can be viewed as a form of depersonalization—another manifestation of distorting one's role in what is taking place.

Drug-induced depersonalization can make people feel as if they are going insane. A new patient arrived in my office after two weeks on Prozac 20 mg that had been prescribed for anxiety and mild depression. Within a day or two of starting the Prozac, in his own words, "I lost track of myself as a person. I didn't feel like a human being or like I fit in with other people. It was as if I got up each day and had to re-create myself from scratch. I was asking all the time, 'Who am I?' It sounds corny but I was scared to death."

Instead of realizing he was having a drug reaction, he was so spellbound at times by Prozac that he imagined he had reached the "essence of what life is really like" and that life was too horrible to endure. He told me, "I even thought, 'If this is all there is to life, I might as well die right now.'"

An artistic and intelligent nineteen-year-old college student, he had at times in the past felt alienated from other people, but this is not unusual among sensitive young people. More than most, he often wrestled with philosophical problems. But the Prozac had pushed him far over the edge into a state of utter existential dread and obliteration of identity, something he had never come close to experiencing ever before in his life. He was sinking deeper into despair and depression, horrified that he might be like this forever.

On my recommendation, he stopped the Prozac immediately. With much reassurance and frequent office visits, he gradually recovered over several drug-free weeks.

Derealization and depersonalization are found in response to almost any kind of severe psychological stress, including witnessing an accident, committing or enduring a violent act, or dealing with the unexpected death of a loved one. They are so common among children and adolescents that doctors often consider mild cases to be normal. Depersonalization and derealization cannot be considered unique to spellbinding but they can be especially severe when drug-induced. They complicate how to evaluate the observations made by people who are intoxicated by medications.

ARE MEDICATION MADNESS RECOLLECTIONS RELIABLE?

MEDICATION SPELLBOUND individuals often suffer from serious memory problems surrounding the period of acute intoxication. Memory loss, much like depersonalization or derealization, can be caused by psychological trauma as well as by brain dysfunction. However, when people forget events because they are too emotionally painful, they make little or no effort to recollect what happened to them. Instead, they recoil from recalling what happened, feel relieved rather than frustrated by the amnesia, and do not go to great lengths to fill in the blanks. If pressed, they will become distressed and actively resist the return of the painful recollections.

By contrast, when people lose their memory functions because of physical trauma—such as a blow on the head, electroshock treatment, or drug intoxication—they feel frustrated and resentful. They typically try hard to recapture their lost memories by asking friends about their prior shared experiences, by looking at picture albums, and even by studying police and medical records in the hope of reconstructing what happened.

Psychoactive drugs do not seem to disrupt immediate memories as much as they prevent the storing of these memories for long-term retrieval. As a result, medication spellbound memories are the clearest shortly after the episode of intoxication and then often fade with time. It is similar to awakening from a nightmare: the recollections are initially vivid, if fragmented, and then fade from memory within minutes or hours. Similarly, the person who "freaks out" on drugs may give vivid descriptions of his behaviors to the first policeman or

EMT who responds to the crisis. Then, within a few hours or days he may find it difficult or impossible to recall anything about the events. Typically, the prosecuting attorney in a trial will use this delayed memory loss to impugn the individual's honesty. The attorney will sarcastically observe, "You told the policeman all the details and now you're telling the jury you don't remember?" Rarely are these people covering up what they've done. Usually, they do not deny the accuracy of the reports, and they feel dismayed and horrified by their actions.

Psychoactive drugs can also disrupt the chronology of memories. As a typical effect of brain damage and dysfunction from any cause, some memories surrounding the trauma and its aftermath may remain intact but they may be jumbled. For example, the individual may feel convinced that something happened on a particular day when in fact it did not. Or the individual may be unable to put a series of events into proper order.

In summary, the stories told to me by survivors of medication spellbinding are often confused by memory dysfunction and derealization or depersonalization, and much more rarely by conscious deception. It bears repeating that to overcome these impediments to getting at the truth, I always try to reconstruct what happened based on other sources, such as medical records, pharmacy records, and police reports.

THE ROLE OF THE MEDICAL EXPERT

WHEN I EVALUATE a criminal case prior to a formal hearing or a trial, I am often the first person to take an in-depth look at what happened, including the details of the perpetration of the crime. As the first evaluator, I often establish the direction of the case, and in particular whether or not an involuntary drug-intoxication defense will be made. This puts enormous responsibility on me as a medical expert. The role requires that I take on the complex and subtle tasks of interpreting the medical and police records, reviewing collateral information from school or work records, and interviewing the defendant and numerous witnesses. I will usually have photographs of the crime scene or suicide. In some cases, I may be asked to evaluate the crime scene itself. Like a criminal investigator, I will try to reconstruct what actually transpired.

After trying to establish the facts of the case, I then evaluate the role of medication in influencing or causing the individual's behavior. I can easily spend twenty intensive hours on the initial stages of the case on behalf of the

accused before anyone from the prosecutor's office has evaluated it. I will often spend additional hours when a complicated report is required.

A medical expert carries a heavy burden of responsibility. If I decide that
there is insufficient evidence to make an involuntary intoxication defense, the
attorney and his client will probably drop that line of defense. If I determine
there is sufficient evidence that medication influenced the individual's behavior, then it becomes almost certain the defense will rely on this opinion.

Even after the case has begun, my expert report or testimony often influences the course and outcome of legal events. In some instances, charges have
been reduced and jail time has been avoided. In others, people have been ac-
quitted of crimes based on an involuntary intoxication defense.

Although not couched in terms of morals and ethics, the end product of
any expert's evaluation necessarily draws complex conclusions concerning
guilt and innocence, including the perpetrator's degree of moral responsibility
for his or her actions. These opinions usually affect the outcome of a case even
before there is a formal hearing in front of a judge and, even more commonly,
before there is a trial. For example, prosecutors commonly decide to plea bargain more leniently in cases where there is a convincing medical report.

Countless medical experts in criminal cases repeat the process I have described. However, the process has serious flaws. Most important, it places too
much responsibility on one individual—the medical expert—and to some extent undermines the basic adversarial checks and balances built into the criminal justice system. If I've been misled in my analysis, then everyone is misled.
If my judgment is flawed, then often there is little or no countervailing opinion to correct it unless the prosecution hires a competent medical expert of its
own or the case goes to trial.

Although I work hard to overcome the limitations of my role, medical experts are not properly equipped to determine all the facts. We are not criminal
investigators and we are not lawyers or judges. Nor are we a one-person jury
of peers. Yet, as psychiatrists in criminal cases, we end up to some degree playing the roles of criminal investigators, lawyers, judges, and even juries, especially early in the process.

I don't believe that a medical expert, however wise or well intentioned,
should play the role of criminal investigator, defense or prosecution attorney,
judge, and even jury, ultimately influencing outcomes before the case is argued
in court before a judge and jury. I don't believe medical experts on their own,
including myself, should have so much influence on a case prior to a factual
determination of guilt or innocence.

Consistent with reforms suggested by others in the legal arena, I believe that a determination of guilt or innocence should be made *before* psychiatric experts become involved. Put simply, the facts of what actually happened—objective guilt or innocence—should be determined separately from issues surrounding motivation, intention, and "sanity." When and if the accused is convicted of perpetrating the crime, then medical experts could be appropriately involved to testify before a judge or jury about mitigating circumstances such as involuntary intoxication that might reduce the sentence.

Under this system, a person could not be found "not guilty by reason of involuntary drug intoxication" or "not guilty by reason of insanity." Opinions concerning involuntary drug intoxication or insanity would be reserved for postconviction sentencing in regard to mitigating the sentence.

Medical experts do have a very important role to play—to offer testimony and to help in understanding how and why the individual acted in a particular fashion, including the possible role of medication intoxication and spellbinding. Medical experts could appropriately testify concerning whether a person's destructive behavior was in part the result of a head injury or Alzheimer's disease. But this testimony should be limited to the sentencing phase. After hearing medical testimony, in cases of involuntary drug intoxication the judge or jury could conclude, "Yes, he is guilty of committing the crime, but there are mitigating circumstances. He was intoxicated by prescribed drugs, had little or no moral responsibility for what happened, and is not likely to repeat the crime. Therefore, he can serve a relatively short sentence or be set free."

Compared to criminal cases, the role of the medical expert in malpractice and product-liability cases does not require substantial reform. Often, these cases have already gone through the criminal justice system to determine objective guilt or innocence, and the experts rarely duel over these issues. Instead, the experts focus on the role played by drugs in the commission of harmful acts, as well as the alleged negligence of the doctor or the drug company.

Overall, lying and reality distortions by patients play a relatively minor role in cases against drug companies. As the following chapter documents, drug-company distortions and deceptions are by far the biggest impediment to justice.

Chapter 18

Drug Companies on Trial

IF YOU ARE WONDERING if you can trust your doctors to tell you the truth about psychiatric drugs, the answer is, you can trust your doctors only to the degree that you can trust the drug companies who provide them with most of their drug information directly and indirectly.

THE DARK SIDE OF ELI LILLY AND PROZAC

DRUG COMPANIES go to great lengths to protect their products and in the process they keep doctors and the public in the dark about many of their adverse effects. Eli Lilly set the standard for the determined pursuit of self-interest in defending Prozac from any and all criticism. Despite the company's best efforts, by 1994, there were already so many lawsuits against Eli Lilly that a federal judge in Indianapolis combined an initial 160 cases into a consortium called the multidistrict litigation or MDL. This enabled one lead attorney to manage the overall investigation called discovery, including gathering documents and taking depositions from Eli Lilly. The lead attorney would also select a medical expert or experts to evaluate the underlying basic scientific issues and medical data about Prozac suicide and violence, and to help construct the negligence case based on that information. This information and its analysis would then be made available to the dozens of other attorneys in the combined MDL cases.

In addition to reviewing and mastering the scientific evidence, the medical expert would have to address numerous issues that would decide the merits of the initial cases. Did Prozac cause or contribute to the murder or suicide? Did negligence on the part of Eli Lilly in hiding information contribute to the murder or suicide?

The MDL lead attorney began looking for an expert to review the initial cases and, above all else, to provide a medical and scientific basis for claims that Prozac was causing mayhem, violence, and suicide. I was informed that many physicians and scientists were being interviewed for the role of medical expert for the seemingly endless number of cases. Ultimately, I was interviewed and selected.

At the time I had only limited experience in the courtroom but in other ways I was a natural candidate for this position. Ten years earlier, I had published a medical textbook on adverse drug effects, *Psychiatric Drugs: Hazards to the Brain* (1983). Then in 1991, in *Toxic Psychiatry,* I became the first expert to warn the public and the profession that Prozac could cause a constellation of stimulating cocainelike adverse effects resulting in violence, suicide, and mania. Based on my clinical experience, research, and documents obtained from the FDA through the Freedom of Information Act (FOIA), I warned in *Toxic Psychiatry* that Prozac was causing "murderous and suicidal behavior." I suggested that Prozac's stimulating effect could be one of the causes of this abnormal behavior: "Like amphetamine or cocaine, Prozac can produce the whole array of stimulant effects, such as sleeplessness, increased energy, jumpiness, anxiety, artificial highs, and mania."[1]

I was not the first doctor to notice the dangerously stimulating effects of Prozac. Credit for that goes to the FDA's Richard Kapit whose observations remained buried within voluminous other documents inside the FDA until I obtained them through the Freedom of Information Act and made them public. Kapit derived his conclusions from the drug company's own data. Eli Lilly knew and initially failed to disclose the fact that its drug was dangerously overstimulating many patients. In order to hide this danger, Eli Lilly secretly and against FDA rules prescribed tranquilizers to many of the patients who were taking Prozac in its clinical trials used to obtain FDA approval for the antidepressant.

Without informing the FDA, Eli Lilly's top scientist, Ray Fuller, signed an in-house memo—not copied to the FDA—modifying the rules for the clinical trials to permit the administration of tranquilizers along with Prozac in the clinical trials:[2]

Some patients have converted from severe depression to agitation within a few days. In one case the agitation was marked and the patient had to be taken off the drug. In future studies, the use of benzodiazepines [tranquilizers] to control agitation will be permitted.

Permitted by whom? Permitted by the company, and not by the FDA.

As illustrated in many of the cases in this book, turning patients with depression into patients with *agitated* depression is potentially very hazardous. Unlike most forms of depression, which tend to immobilize and subdue, agitated depression tends to energize the individual toward potential suicide or violence.

After Eli Lilly submitted all of its clinical trials to the FDA, the agency's evaluation showed Prozac to have little or no benefit, especially when the illegitimately tranquilized patients were removed from clinical trial data. Incredibly, the FDA did not exercise its authority to protect the consumer from dangerous and ineffective drugs. Instead of throwing out the bogus trials, negating any possibility of Prozac being approved, the accommodating federal agency allowed the tranquilized patients to be counted as if they were legitimate participants in the drug trials. Then, and only then, did the clinical trials demonstrate effectiveness for Prozac—and even that was marginal at best.[3] The public and the profession still do not realize that instead of approving Prozac for the treatment of depression, the FDA covertly approved the combination of Prozac with addictive tranquilizers, and even then the drug combination proved very hazardous and only marginally effective.[4]

THE INFAMOUS WESBECKER CASE

IN MY ROLE AS MEDICAL EXPERT for the combined Prozac cases, I interviewed FDA officials about how they approve new drugs and in particular about problems involved with Prozac during the approval process. I studied federal regulations governing the FDA, and took intensive seminars intended for drug company officials concerning the operations of the FDA and the procedures for obtaining drug approval. I located and then reviewed hundreds of published studies concerning Prozac, especially how it causes adverse effects. At the same time, I reviewed innumerable large storage boxes of sealed Eli Lilly memos, letters, and studies concerning the development and marketing of Prozac, some obtained on my own through FOIA and some obtained from the drug company by the consortium of lawyers.

The Wesbecker case[5] was scheduled to be the first one to go to trial from among the deluge of combined cases for which I was the scientific and medical expert. Joseph Wesbecker was a classic if horrific example of "going postal," except he was employed by a printing plant, not the U.S. post office. Unlike almost all the other cases in this book, Joe was predisposed to anger before he committed violence on a psychiatric drug. At one point he had been psychiatrically hospitalized and the medical record indicated that he had made threats to harm his coworkers long before starting Prozac. I testified that his preexisting feelings had been activated by the drug, pushing him toward violent actions.

Despite a past history of resentments, Joe was doing relatively well in 1989, when his psychiatrist added Prozac to his treatment regimen. On the follow-up visit one month later, his doctor found that Joe had become agitated and suffered a delusion that he was sexually abused by his boss in front of an assembly of employees at work. Joe had never before shown frank symptoms of psychosis and the doctor observed, "Patient seems to have deteriorated." According to the doctor's progress note, Joe was "weeping" and displayed an "increased level of agitation and anger."

Joe's doctor questioned whether Prozac was causing the deterioration, and he wisely stopped the medication. Three days after Joe stopped taking the Prozac, while most of it remained active in his body,[6] he took an arsenal to his former place of work and marched zombielike through the building shooting twenty people, killing eight, and then killing himself.

Despite his long-term, serious problems, including preexisting violent feelings toward his workplace, Joe had never before voiced delusions about his coworkers, and he had never acted violently until he was put on Prozac. I concluded that Prozac had complicated his condition and amplified it by making him agitated, paranoid, and psychotic, so that he could no longer control his preexisting aggressive impulses.

After reviewing the available records, I also concluded that Joe's psychiatrist had not committed malpractice. He had recognized the probable onset of Prozac toxicity and psychosis, and prudently stopped the drug. He had no way of knowing how dangerous it was to start the drug because Eli Lilly had withheld critical information from the FDA about the risk of Prozac-induced violence and suicide.

Joe's prescribing physician could not know, for example, that Prozac commonly causes akathisia, a disorder than can drive an already depressed patient into a dangerous state of agitation and depression. He had no way of knowing that Eli Lilly possessed data confirming very high rates of agitation and suicide attempts on Prozac. He had no way of knowing that Prozac caused mania in patients who had never before undergone mania. Eli Lilly had hidden all of this data from the public and the profession, and some of it from the FDA as well.[7]

Despite Eli Lilly's conduct, the case against the company had problems, especially the glaring fact that Joseph Wesbecker had threatened to harm his coworkers long before starting on Prozac. I concluded that I could *not* state within a reasonable degree of medical certainty that Prozac was the sole cause of his murderous impulses. But I *could* say that the drug had tipped him over—pushed him over the edge—into perpetrating outright violence for the first time in his life.

In contrast to the other cases in this book, Joe Wesbecker's predisposition to paranoid feelings and anger made the case against Prozac and Eli Lilly comparatively weak. How then did the Wesbecker case get to be the first and, therefore, most influential case brought against Lilly by the MDL consortium? Knowledgeable lawyers have told me that Eli Lilly maneuvered the case calendar to make sure it had a strong chance of winning its first trial. But the company wasn't going to leave anything about the trial to chance.

The Legal Arena of Smoke and Mirrors

After I started to work on the Prozac cases, I disagreed with the approach of the lead attorney who was initially in charge of the consortium. After much soul-searching, I made what seemed like a momentous decision. I withdrew as the medical expert for the combined Prozac cases, leaving behind one of the most potentially worthwhile projects of my career. Soon after I quit, this attorney was replaced and in 1993 I was rehired by his replacement, the esteemed Chicago lawyer Leonard Ring. Unfortunately, Leonard Ring died that same year and was replaced by Paul Smith, a Dallas attorney. Smith took over as the attorney in charge of research for all of the combined MDL cases as well as the attorney for the Wesbecker case. He became the point man for the entire legal assault on Eli Lilly and I continued as his medical expert for all of the cases, starting with the first one to go to trial in the fall of 1994.

Things did not seem right from the start with Paul Smith, but I was slow to accept the painfully disillusioning truth. Unlike every other attorney who has ever hired me in any case of any significance, attorney Smith spent almost no time going over the case with me. He made few communications to me while I examined the materials that I already had in my possession and he sent me little or nothing new. What I did not know—and was then too inexperienced to realize—was that Smith had gathered a roomful of additional documentation that he was not sharing with me, including medical records, a history of Wesbecker's childhood, and about twenty depositions taken by Eli Lilly, including people who knew Wesbecker before the rampage. Although I didn't realize it, he was keeping me in the dark about the great majority of discovery materials gathered for the case itself. Nothing like this has happened to me before or since.

When I arrived in Louisville, Kentucky, for the trial, I was dismayed to find out that Smith had sequestered me in a hotel that was miles away from where his team of other experts and attorneys was staying. In every other case I've ever participated in, attorneys have always put me in the same hotel with them to facilitate working together. I became more suspicious when Smith refused to discuss and to practice my upcoming testimony. In the Wesbecker case, the issues were enormously complex, requiring great coordination between the attorney and the expert, but he wanted me to get on the witness stand without any preparation or practice, and then to respond "spontaneously" to whatever questions he asked me.

I thought that Smith was either emotionally overwhelmed or incompetent— but he was neither.

In the few days remaining before I went on the stand, I spent hours alone in Smith's temporary office in a Louisville law firm while he conducted the ongoing trial. I now discovered that he had never sent me or told me about voluminous documents, including a color-coded detailed chart documenting the details of Joseph Wesbecker's childhood. The chart had been created by Eli Lilly based on reports from its investigators and many depositions of people who knew Wesbecker. It contained many facts, some damaging to the case, about Wesbecker's troubled childhood. It was exactly the sort of information that I needed in order to prepare my testimony and to handle cross-examination.

When I demanded my own copy of the biographical chart, Smith refused, making excuses like his assistants were too busy to copy it. He gave in only after I took possession of the original and refused to give it back. Needless to say, it was a confusing and demoralizing conflict. Until I stepped onto the witness stand, I had no idea just how crucial this document was.

Meanwhile, Smith persisted in refusing to discuss my testimony with me. An expert's testimony on the witness stand cannot be spontaneous; courtroom procedures require that the witness answer specific questions from the attorney. So I laboriously wrote out questions for him to ask me in the form of several dozen hand-printed note cards. After another confrontation with Smith at a dinner with the assembled legal team for the case, he agreed to ask me some of my prepared questions when I took the stand. By now, we were openly arguing with each other.

From my viewpoint, my testimony went surprisingly well. Rereading it years later, I can see where I'm actually asking and answering my own questions, orchestrating the testimony. Thinking that I was dealing with incompetence rather than a strategem, I tried to salvage my testimony as best as I could.

Smith asked me some of the prearranged questions. He must have feared that I would become suspicious if he refused to ask me any of the pertinent questions that I'd worked so hard to press on him. I testified that the company knew that Prozac was overstimulating the patients and, to cover up the effect, had broken the rules by putting patients on sedatives to calm them down in the clinical trials. I analyzed data showing that the placebo-controlled clinical trials demonstrated an increased rate of suicide attempts among Prozac patients compared to patients taking placebo or older antidepressants.

Before I got on the stand, Smith had told me in a shouting match not to dare to bring up one particular smoking gun. From my FOIA inquiries to the FDA, I had found that initial drafts of the Prozac label had listed "depression" and "abnormal thoughts" as two of the three most commonly reported adverse reactions to the drug. In these drafts, the company in effect admitted that its own principal investigators—the scientists conducting the clinical trials—were reporting that their patients frequently became more depressed on Prozac. Combined with an increase in "abnormal thoughts," this indicated that the drug was making many people worse and even potentially dangerous. I then discovered that shortly before the label was made official, "abnormal thoughts" was dropped from the list of top three adverse effects and replaced with the more innocuous "abnormal dreams." Then, on the last day before the label was officially approved, an FDA official scratched out "depression" from its prominent place in the label. Depression as a serious adverse effect of Prozac went from being "frequent" to being nonexistent. The company, in combination with the FDA, had expurgated some of the most damning information from the label shortly before its publication. Attorney Smith outright refused to let me testify about this.

When Eli Lilly's attorney cross-examined me, he spent no time trying to undermine my scientific testimony. He simply ignored all of my testimony about the drug company conduct. The only detailed factual cross-examination by the drug company focused on predisposing factors in Wesbecker's troubled childhood—the very information that attorney Paul Smith had tried to keep from me.

The chronology of Wesbecker's early life turned out to be a blueprint for cross-examining me on the witness stand. I happened to have the document in my hand during the cross-examination; otherwise I would have seemed totally uninformed about Wesbecker's early years. It would have been embarrassing to me and very damaging to the case.

At the conclusion of my testimony and cross-examination, one attorney who had been listening among spectators said that I had conducted the best handling of a cross-examination he'd ever seen. Considering the circumstances, I thought I had done well on the stand but not that well. I had been too handicapped by my own side. Meanwhile, attorney Smith was enraged at me when my testimony was over. When I asked him why, he denied he was angry and would not discuss it. In retrospect, I concluded that I may have partially undermined his agreement with Lilly to present a weak case against the company.

The jury came back with a verdict in favor of Eli Lilly. Despite my watered-down testimony, however, the jury was nearly hung. The company won by a vote of nine to three. Under Kentucky law, one more vote against Eli Lilly would have hung the jury and created a public-relations nightmare for Prozac.

I still had no idea what had really transpired at the trial. That the trial had been a sham still eluded me but I was exhausted and disillusioned. It took more than a year for the truth to begin to unfold in public. Soon after the trial, presiding judge John W. Potter concluded that Eli Lilly had secretly manipulated the trial. Lilly had promised a huge sum of money in a secret settlement in return for which Smith had presented a weakened case to the jury.[8]

Judge Potter concluded that in return for a promised payment the trial had been covertly settled toward the end. But from my direct, first-hand experience a deal was in the works from the beginning. Otherwise attorney Smith would have sent me significant discovery materials, prepared me for trial in advance, and not tried to undermine my testimony on the stand.

Judge Potter confirmed that attorney Smith had flimflammed the entire MDL consortium of attorneys with Prozac cases who were depending on his collection of discovery materials. Instead of giving the discovery materials to the other lawyers to use in their own cases as originally agreed and required by law, he sent them back to Eli Lilly and Company where they disappeared into the usual places that telltale documents go—deep within the recesses of drug-company storage. Two years after the trial, this would lead the trial judge, John Potter, to ask, "Was Smith's agreement to secretly return documents to Lilly a failure to adequately represent the MDL [the combined Prozac cases] plaintiffs?"[9] I am not aware that Judge Potter ever gave a formal answer to the question, but the question itself confirmed this aspect of the secret agreement.

Judge Potter, meanwhile, was especially outraged because he believed both Eli Lilly and Smith had lied to him or at least mislead him. While the trial was still ongoing, the judge had become suspicious and called both sides into his chambers to ask if they had made a secret settlement. Both Eli Lilly and Smith had denied it.[10] Judge Potter specifically recalled being reassured that money had not secretly changed hands during the trial.[11] After concealing the truth from the judge, Smith and Eli Lilly went ahead with perpetrating the fake trial.

Eli Lilly, of course, attacked me during its summation to the jury. But attorney Smith said nothing to defend me in his summation. In his summation, Smith also failed to bring up the scientific data I had presented in order to demonstrate the company's negligence.

After reviewing the evidence, Judge Potter decided to change the verdict of the trial. He threw out the jury verdict and changed it to settlement with prejudice by Eli Lilly. Although the fake verdict in favor of Eli Lilly received widespread news coverage, this dramatic turn of events with such enormous importance to medicine and public health was almost entirely ignored by the major media. There were no headlines in *Time, Newsweek,* or *The New York Times* declaring, "Drug Company Fakes Trial: Data Reveals that Prozac Causes Suicide and Violence."

If either the media or the FDA had examined the data I generated for the MDL consortium, followed by the fake trial, it might not have taken twelve more years for the FDA to acknowledge that antidepressants cause suicidality, and by now the agency might also have recognized that they cause violence as well. Many lives continue to come to tragic ends because of these delays.

It was several months or more before I heard anything about the trial being a sham and that information came to me entirely by chance. I was in New Jersey for a case when an attorney told me that the state law journal had published an article in March 2005, entitled "Kentucky Fried Verdict Up for Grabs."[12]

The trial ended in 1994, but the Kentucky Supreme Court did not empower Judge Potter to investigate the case until May 30, 1996. By the time the truth about the secret settlement came out, Eli Lilly had negotiated settlements favorable to itself with most of the remaining hundred or more cases. Even after that, the overturning of the verdict and its implications never became widely known, even in the legal community. As far as most lawyers knew, the drug company had won the big test case fair and square, and was invincible.

In 1997, three years after the trial, a small Bloomberg News report published in *The Indianapolis Star* in Eli Lilly's hometown summed up succinctly:[13]

> Survivors and heirs of the dead sued Lilly, claiming it wrongly suppressed information about the risks of Prozac patients becoming violent. The jury decided Eli Lilly wasn't liable. Lilly said then that "the verdict represents a reaffirmation of Prozac's well-established safety." Later, however, [Judge] Potter learned that Lilly had promised money to the plaintiffs, who agreed not to introduce evidence that could hurt Lilly's defense.

After the judge threw out the verdict and declared the case a settlement, Eli Lilly appealed the judge's decision up to the Kentucky Supreme Court, which concluded that Eli Lilly had "manipulated" the judicial system and further opined that the drug company might even have committed "fraud":[14]

> A careful and thoughtful examination of the entire record in this case indicates that some sort of settlement was reached before the case was submitted to the jury. . . .
>
> In this case, there was a serious lack of candor with the trial court and there may have been deception, bad faith conduct, abuse of the judicial process, or perhaps even fraud.

The Supreme Court authorized Judge Potter to go forward with a full hearing to determine the specifics of the secret deal. The hearing would likely have made public the amount of money that had been paid to the plaintiffs in settlement. Numerous plaintiffs were involved in the Wesbecker case including those who had been injured and their surviving families. Lawyers who were later involved in divorces among the plaintiffs were startled by the large sums that had been paid out by the company. Unfortunately, as Jeff Swiatek reported in 2000 in *The Indianapolis Star,* the anticipated hearing never occurred.

> Faced with fully disclosing the deal, Lilly officials had a change of heart. They agreed in 1997 that Potter could change the official judgment in the case to dismissed "as settled." That made the hearing unnecessary and ended the dispute, ruled Kentucky Judge Edwin Schroering, who replaced Potter when he stepped aside. Schroering's January 1998 ruling said Lilly and other parties to the secret deal did "nothing improper." By then, losing the dispute over wording may hardly have mattered for Lilly. The drugmaker already

had squeezed most of the public relations value out of the 1994 jury verdict, and Prozac lawsuits were on the wane.

According to Swiatek, one Eli Lilly executive credited the company's overall defense strategy in the Prozac suits with defusing a "deadly serious" threat to the company and its star drug. Swiatek's report also cited outrage aimed at Paul Smith by other attorneys involved in litigation against Eli Lilly, including one lawsuit that labeled Smith as "Lilly's puppet." As a part of this ruse, there was an agreement between Lilly and Smith that the attorney "had to pretend he had lost the trial and won no settlement," Swiatek said.

Swiatek sums up the collaboration between Smith and Lilly as a "deal to essentially buy off the plaintiffs with a huge cash payment, secretly negotiated even as the trial went on." As someone who could not be bought, and as the main expert against the drug company, I was inevitably the object of attack from both Paul Smith, the attorney who hired me, and Eli Lilly, both of whom wanted to undermine my testimony and my credibility as an expert.

Swiatek reported that interviews with four jurors after the trial indicated that, despite the secret agreement in the Wesbecker case, Eli Lilly almost lost. The final jury vote, as already mentioned, was nine to three in favor of the drug company. In my opinion, even the combined efforts of Smith and Eli Lilly could not fully hide the evidence against the drug company. My testimony, most of it delivered against Paul Smith's active resistance, may have influenced some of the jurors to believe that Eli Lilly had been negligent. It is no wonder that Smith was so angered at my determination to present my complete analysis of Eli Lilly's conduct.

After the trial, Smith refused to cooperate with the other attorneys in the combined suits, and he unceremoniously quit his role as keeper of the documents. He was supposed to turn over his all-important discovery documents to the other attorneys who had cases against the drug company, but instead he returned them to the drug company.

Events surrounding the Wesbecker trial left me exhausted and extraordinarily disillusioned. For a few months, I thought I would quit being a medical expert. Eventually, with urging from others, I recovered my morale and resumed acting as a medical expert in many legal cases, including numerous ones against Prozac and Eli Lilly. Because of my knowledge about the background documents showing how the company had hid the drug's dangerous effects, most of my subsequent cases against Lilly have been settled satisfactorily for the plaintiffs without admission of fault by the company and none has gone to trial.

Why has Eli Lilly and Company gone to such extreme lengths to defend Prozac, even undermining and defying the American court system in the process? For many years the economic survival of Eli Lilly depended on that one single drug. In the mid-1990s, Prozac was generating over two billion dollars per year in revenues, accounting for nearly half of the company's total income. This lopsided dependency on one drug undoubtedly motivated the company to go to extremes in defending the drug and attacking its critics.

By contrast, most other major drug companies have a much more diversified portfolio of products. Now Lilly has developed a similar dependence on Zyprexa, and as I've already documented, it continues its pattern of failing to disclose important information about the potentially dangerous effects of its drugs.

In retrospect, it is much clearer to me now why attorney Paul Smith and Eli Lilly would want to try to discredit me at the trial by undermining my testimony. At that time I was the only psychiatrist in the world who had the inside scoop—the details of the sealed data concerning Eli Lilly's negligence in the developing and marketing of Prozac. I was also the only psychiatrist at that time who was willing to stand up to the company in court and in the media, as well as in the scientific community.[15] I was literally the biggest threat to the company's most important source of revenue, Prozac.

Over the ensuing years, I have tried my best to communicate what I know about Prozac and Eli Lilly's cover-ups, for example in 1994 in *Talking Back to Prozac,* and then in 1997 in the original edition of *Brain-Disabling Treatments in Psychiatry,* and with an updated edition in 2008. Unfortunately, following the 1994 fixed trial Lilly was indeed invincible, and my attempts to tell the truth went largely unnoticed.

To this day, most psychiatrists have no idea about the fake trial and tend to believe that Prozac has been exonerated in court. Most of the cases in this book took place long after the Wesbecker trial. If Eli Lilly had not perpetrated this sham trial, many product-liability cases might have been won in trial or the settlements might have been financially crippling to the company. Professional and public attitudes would have become much more skeptical toward Prozac, and toward all the newer antidepressants that were subsequently marketed. Many lives would have been saved from ruination or death. Eli Lilly's manipulation of the court in the Wesbecker case continues to cast a shadow over the truth about the dangerous effects of these drugs.

BLOWING THE WHISTLE ON THE "MISSING" ELI LILLY DOCUMENTS

After the Wesbecker trial Paul Smith broke with the consortium of attorneys and returned all of the critical discovery materials to the drug company. There were twenty-eight large legal storage boxes.

In late 2005, an anonymous source sent some of the most eye-opening Eli Lilly documents to reporter Jeanne Lenzer at the *British Medical Journal* (*BMJ*). Since I knew these documents most intimately, she asked me about their genuineness and also reviewed their contents in detail with me. On January 1, 2005, Lenzer published a report on the documents in the medical journal. Simultaneously, the *BMJ* forwarded the documents to other authorities, including New York congressman Maurice Hinchey and the FDA.

Congressman Hinchey distributed the documents to other individuals and organizations, including me. The drug company never asked for the return of the documents, instead arguing that they contributed nothing new.[16]

The first key document is a July 1985, in-house analysis by Eli Lilly that found a statistically significant increase in suicide attempts for patients taking Prozac during their placebo-controlled clinical trials. Twelve suicide attempts were found in the Prozac group and only one each in the control group and the comparison drug, a tricyclic antidepressant. Even after the company's hired consultants threw out six of the suicide attempts—an action that scientific veracity did not permit—the remaining 6:1 ratio was alarming.[17]

This bombshell—proof that Prozac caused suicide attempts—was never released to any drug-monitoring agency, including the FDA. After the *BMJ* made it known, Eli Lilly ignored this smoking gun while defending itself on more irrelevant issues in advertisements and to the media.

Another group of key documents included two in-house Eli Lilly memoranda written by Eli Lilly employee Claude Bouchy in November 1990. Bouchy wrote from Germany to Leigh Thompson, a high-ranking Eli Lilly official in the United States. Bouchy complained in the memos how the company was purposely hiding Prozac-induced suicidal ideation and acts under misleading categories, effectively keeping them from inquisitive eyes.

In one memo Bouchy expressed dismay at how his company was hiding data on suicide:

Finally, on a very simple and nonscientific basis, I personally wonder whether we are really helping the credibility of an excellent ADE [adverse drug event] system by calling overdose what a physician reports as suicide attempt and by calling depression what a physician is reporting as suicide ideation . . . Of course by the end of the day we will do what we are told to do but Hans and I felt that we had to bring these to attention.

In the other memo, Bouchy displayed profound personal shame over participating in the deceptive hiding of suicide data under misleading categories.

I do not think I could explain to the BGA [Germany regulatory agency], to a judge, to a reporter or even to my family why we would do this especially on the sensitive issue of suicide and suicide ideation.

Another set of key documents involves a 1991 study conducted by the FDA concerning the disproportionate number of reports of "hostility" and "intentional injury" that were spontaneously sent to the agency concerning Prozac. Compared to another less-stimulating antidepressant, trazodone (Desyrel), hostility and intentional injury reports were twenty times more frequent for Prozac. This massive increase took into account the greater numbers of prescriptions for Prozac. The initial spike in Prozac reports occurred even before there was any public controversy surrounding the drug as a potential cause of violence.

Before and after the Wesbecker trial, I repeatedly attempted to obtain the FDA study through the FOIA requests. The FDA finally wrote me that the documents were "lost." This group of documents also included graphs showing a forty-fold relative increase in reports of suicide attempts, overdose, and psychotic depression on Prozac compared to trazodone.

The last key document was an in-house Eli Lilly study of "Activation and Sedation in Fluoxetine [Prozac] Clinical Trials" dated November 8, 1988. It found that 38 percent of Prozac-treated clinical trial patients developed symptoms of stimulation as compared to 19 percent taking placebo. It did not mention that many of the Prozac-treated patients showed these symptoms despite being sedated in the clinical trials by tranquilizers that were supposed to be excluded from the study. In addition, the criteria for stimulation were relatively narrow. From my investigations as the scientific expert for the original Prozac suits, I found out that this study was requested by the German drug regulatory agency but as far as I have been able to determine Eli Lilly never turned it over in full to the Germans or to the FDA. After these documents were released by the *BMJ,* in order to show that it had not hidden the data, Eli Lilly pointed to an obscure source where a passing reference had been made to a significant percentage of activated patients, but the observation was buried in a larger article and the all-important study of activation had apparently never been released in its entirety.

Lilly Defends Itself

Deeply stung by the revelations, Eli Lilly took out full-page ads in newspapers around the world claiming that it had withheld nothing and that the documents contained nothing new. Very cleverly, the company did not challenge the authenticity of the documents, their contents, or their implications. Any attention given to the actual documents would have highlighted the contents and proven the accusations, including that Eli Lilly had known for decades that Prozac increased the suicide attempt rate in its controlled clinical trials.

Meanwhile, the company threatened the *BMJ* and successfully intimidated the medical journal. During the legal assault by Eli Lilly, I spoke by phone with *BMJ* lawyers. They were clearly frightened about the possibility of a financially crushing lawsuit from a multibillion dollar corporation and they were looking for an easy escape route.

Eli Lilly did not claim that the documents should have remained sealed or secret and they never asked for them to be returned. They did not express outrage at the *BMJ* or "anonymous" for releasing them. The company had a more distracting tactic. It wanted to force an apology out of the medical journal—any kind of apology! The press would then pick up the apology without looking at whether or not it undermined the validity or meaning of the documents.

On January 29, 2005, the *BMJ* issued a very short "Correction and apology." It had two parts, one about this writer. In regard to me, the *BMJ*'s apology declared:

> The same article described Dr. Peter Breggin as "the medical witness in the Wesbecker case." He was, in fact, the expert witness for the plaintiffs.

As if anyone would have mistakenly thought that I was testifying on behalf of the drug company.

The other part of the apology said, "At the end of the trial, all the documents were preserved by Court Order or were disclosed by Eli Lilly to the plaintiff's lawyers in related Prozac claims." Therefore, the *BMJ* apologized, saying, "These documents did not go missing." It was a fine point, turning on the word "missing." Since they were sealed, the documents were certainly missing from the public domain, and unavailable to physicians and researchers. The most significant in-house reports about increased suicidality on Prozac had never been revealed to the FDA. Neither had the in-house memoranda displaying guilt and shame over Lilly reclassifying suicide reports so that they disappeared from view.

Eli Lilly's strategy worked. The worldwide press quickly picked up on the *BMJ* apology as if it undermined the documents themselves. Although the apology withdrew none of the most significant accusations against the company, the press from then on dodged the controversy, and it disappeared from public view. Once again Eli Lilly managed a brilliant public relationship coup at the expense of the truth.

So, the *BMJ* backed down and said the documents never went missing. In my opinion, even that very limited apology went too far because the documents did in fact go missing. On one occasion, armed with an order from a judge in yet another product-liability suit against Eli Lilly, I went into the supposedly complete Prozac files at the company headquarters, and looked for the many cartons of missing documents. Because I knew how they were numbered for indexing, they should have been easy to find—but none of the relevant boxes could be located. If I hadn't been knowledgeable about the Wesbecker trial documents, I would not have observed their absence.

During the *BMJ* controversy, one of the lawyers who had been deprived of these documents, Jerrold Parker,[18] declared that as an attorney in the combined Prozac cases, he never saw or knew about the missing documents. In *USA Today* on January 6, 2005, psychiatrist Martin Teicher was quoted as confirming that he never saw the documents, even though Eli Lilly had supposedly cooperated with him in revealing its internal data on suicide. Furthermore, Dr. Teicher says that Eli Lilly specifically told him that there was no data confirming his own studies of Prozac-induced suicidality. Lilly has always said that no such data existed—misleading the FDA, the profession, and the public.

Finally, Richard Kapit, the psychiatrist at the FDA in charge of reviewing the adverse effects of Prozac before its approval, told the *BMJ* that these were important documents and that he had never before seen them.[19]

The Continuing Master of Manipulation

Eli Lilly remains a master of manipulating the legal system. On June 15, 2005, the company settled a multicase product-liability suit for 690 million dollars involving life-threatening diabetes associated with its relatively new antipsychotic drug Zyprexa. Because the drug is directly toxic to the insulin-producing cells, some patients are dying in hours from the acute or sudden onset of diabetes and pancreatitis. Other patients endure a more gradually developing and chronic insulin-dependent diabetes.

I was an expert hired by Hersh and Hersh, a California law firm involved in that multisuit, multistate legal action. In that capacity I evaluated chronic and sometimes lethal cases of diabetes and pancreatitis caused by Zyprexa.[20] Cases continue to come forward and a recent estimate placed total potential "payouts" or settlements by the company at 1.2 billion dollars![21]

Eli Lilly continues to deny any wrongdoing in the Zyprexa diabetes cases. Imagine paying more than a *billion* dollars just to get the lawyers to drop false charges? As a part of the settlement, all of the most revealing documents remained sealed. Although I announced the initial settlement on my Web site, relatively few people heard about it or the sealed documents.

Instead of encouraging the kind of transparency that a democracy should require of its corporations, Eli Lilly fights for its right to hide itself beneath the dark mud of corporate secrecy. The company is not protecting trade secrets; it is protecting information about potentially lethal adverse effects, including diabetes.

Unlike earlier Lilly public relations successes, in the case of Zyprexa the truth came out with a big bang.[22] Alaskan lawyer and heroic psychiatric reformer Jim Gottstein obtained the sealed documents. Jim founded and is president of the Law Project for Psychiatric Rights (www.PsychRights.org), whose mission is to mount a strategic litigation campaign around the United States against forced psychiatric drugging and electroshock.[23]

Jim released the documents to the public, including evidence that Eli Lilly pushed the drug for off-label (unapproved) uses and hid the risk of Zyprexa causing pathological weight gain and diabetes—accusations that the drug company has denied.[24] The secret documents were featured in a series of *New York Times* articles.[25] In a remarkable editorial on December 19, 2006, *The New York Times* reviewed some of Lilly's documents and called for "Congressional hearings that should focus on how well the industry complies with existing laws and how effectively the FDA regulates the industry's marketing materials."[26]

Lilly stormed into the public relations disaster with its usual overwhelming force, obtaining court orders that forced Jim to return the documents. But the *New York Times* articles had been published and the actual documents were already circulating on the Internet.

As much and probably more than any other drug company that I've encountered, Eli Lilly has perfected the art of dodging any boomeranging bullets that it fires at unsuspecting patients. Eli Lilly is probably the main reason that the public remains unaware that millions of persons may have been hurt and may even have been killed by newer antidepressants like Prozac and newer antipsychotics like Zyprexa. By so vigorously and successfully protecting itself from criticism, the company has helped to raise an almost impenetrable shield around the entire pharmaceutical industry, especially in regard to psychiatric drugs.

THE DARK SIDE OF PAXIL AND GLAXOSMITHKLINE

PROBABLY BECAUSE PAXIL IS among the most toxic of the SSRI antidepressants, in recent years I have been deluged with inquiries about cases of Paxil-induced mayhem, murder, and suicide. Most of my inside information concerning Paxil was accumulated in late 1999. At that time I was asked by California attorney Don Farber to be the medical expert in a product-liability case that was brought by the family of Reynaldo Lacuzong (his real name) in California against the Paxil manufacturer, GlaxoSmithKline (GSK).

The Lacuzong Case

On the third day of taking Paxil 10 mg, the smallest available dose, Reynaldo drowned himself and his two small children in a bathtub. Before his death, Reynaldo received excellent evaluations as an employee at a high-tech firm. He had no prior history of mental problems, psychiatric treatment, or counseling. He was never violent or suicidal. For a number of years he had been accustomed to enjoying one or two drinks in the evening at home and infrequently he had gotten tipsy at weekend parties. To avoid embarrassing himself at occasional parties, he had stopped drinking. The Paxil may have been prescribed in order to relieve tensions that he felt when abstaining from his customary one or two evening drinks.

Almost immediately after starting the antidepressant, Reynaldo developed akathisia—the painful inner agitation accompanied by a compulsive hyperactivity—as well as maniclike signs of irritability and anxiety. As already documented in this book, antidepressant-induced akathisia is known to be associated with violence, suicide, psychosis, and an overall mental deterioration.[27] In my clinical experience, patients who are already anxious are prime victims for developing antidepressant-induced mania, depression, violence, and suicidality. The drug aggravates the preexisting anxiety or agitation, causing an escalating deterioration.

As the medical expert in Reynaldo's case, I was empowered by the court to examine hundreds of cartons of sealed drug company files concerning Paxil that were contained in GSK's record room. Attorney Farber and I, with the help of my assistant Ian Goddard, spent three days going through the materials that included FDA correspondence and the company's worldwide clinical trials and adverse drug reports for Paxil.

Don Farber was new to this complex business of evaluating product negligence documents and part of my duty was to educate him. He was a quick learner and has gone on to participate in many additional suits against the company.

On July 21, 2001, my expert report in the Lacuzong case was sent to the court. It was very lengthy and detailed in its charges of negligent behavior on the part of GSK. It addressed the drug company's practices in the development and marketing of Paxil, and, in particular, its alleged withholding or manipulation of information about the drug's dangerousness in regard to producing violence and suicide. Drawing on GSK's proprietary files that to this day have never been made public, my report examined many issues including the actual rates of Paxil-induced suicidality in the company's adult clinical studies.

The case against GSK was eventually "resolved" to the satisfaction of the Lacuzong family. GSK denied and continues to deny all of the allegations of negligence in developing and marketing Paxil. Although the amount was not disclosed, my impression is that a substantial amount of money was involved in the resolution of the case. Attorney Farber went from working out of his home to working in a private office, and has become one of a handful of highly experienced attorneys in the arena of antidepressant litigation.

GSK refused to unseal its records for public use or to allow me to make public my findings, regardless of their potential public health significance. The FDA, the medical profession, and the public would remain unaware of what I had discovered. Both Don and I found this appalling, and he went to court to try to force the company to allow me to publish my report with its revelatory data and my critique of GSK negligence. Unfortunately, the judge supported the company's right to withhold its proprietary information, including my analysis of it, regardless of any public health consequences.

A few years after the Lacuzong case was resolved, I was hired as a medical expert in another case in which Paxil was implicated in a suicide and I urged the new attorney to bring in Mr. Farber as a consultant. My report for the case was hampered by the fact that everything I had learned in the earlier Lacuzong case was sealed, apparently including my original report. Then, GSK asked the judge to dismiss the suicide case on the grounds that my new report provided insufficient evidence to justify the case continuing in the court. Attorney Farber countered the company's argument about lack of evidence by producing my extremely detailed Lacuzong report as a demonstration of how much information was already available concerning GSK's negligence in developing and marketing Paxil. The judge sided with Mr. Farber and the plaintiffs, rejecting the drug company's attempt to reject my testimony and to stop the case from going forward.

Although I did not realize it at the time, submitting my Lacuzong report to the new court turned it into a public document. When I discovered that this legal miracle had occurred, I asked attorney Derek Braslow to obtain a copy of my report from the court and then I placed it on my Web site (www.breggin. com). I also wrote a series of three articles in 2006 for *Ethical Human Psychology and Psychiatry,* analyzing and replicating large portions of it.[28]

In 2006, the FDA had demanded that the antidepressant manufacturers review the data from their controlled clinical trials in order to reevaluate the risk of antidepressant-induced suicide in adults. In 2004 to 2005, the FDA had previously concluded that these drugs do indeed cause a suicide risk in children.

In May 2006, before the last of my three reports was published, GSK published to the world the results of its new FDA-mandated reevaluation of its clinical trials. The reevaluation showed that Paxil increased suicidal behavior in adults. This was nearly five years after I had tried and failed to get the company to allow me to release my findings demonstrating that Paxil increased suicidal behavior.

My evaluation of GSK's internal secret documents confirmed that the company had hidden the true rate of suicidality by failing to report all suicide attempts on Paxil and by artificially inflating the number of suicides for patients taking placebo. Indeed, when the company received many of its suicide reports, it didn't list them as such. Instead, it listed the suicides under the relatively benign category of "emotional lability" (emotional instability). No one on the face of the earth looks for suicide data under the category of emotional lability. As a result, anyone scanning the company's database would be unable to discover all the suicide attempts on Paxil.

My report in the Lacuzong case, based on sealed company data, also showed that the company systematically avoided reporting cases of akathisia, and that some of the suicide cases were related to that anguish-inducing drug reaction. It also showed that the company systematically disguised the stimulating effects of Paxil by, among other things, making up many different subcategories for overstimulation, such as nervousness, anxiety, hyperactivity, and agitation, and not adding them up to show the high overall rates of stimulation.

In addition, my searches into the company files disclosed correspondence from the FDA warning the drug company that its advertising and marketing practices were promoting an unfairly positive picture of the drug in comparison to other antidepressants, and ordering the company to stop.

One of the key issues in the Lacuzong case was Reynaldo's abrupt deterioration into murder and suicide after a few small doses of Paxil 10 mg. Did the drug company have information confirming that two or three daily doses cause severe adverse drug reactions, including abnormal behavior? I spent hours inside GSK combing through the case reports of adverse reactions to determine if they were being reported after very short exposures. It turned out that the first few days are the greatest time of risk. Perhaps in the same way that the first few sips of alcohol or puffs of a cigarette have such strong effects on the previously uninitiated drinker or smoker, so, too, the first few doses of an antidepressant in the uninitiated can have the most overwhelmingly harmful impact. Unfortunately, many healthcare practitioners remain unaware that the first few doses, or dose changes, present the greatest risk of causing severe adverse psychiatric reactions.

All of these findings from my investigation of GSK's files are documented in the series of three articles[29] and the report on my Web site.

The Spooner Case

The case through which the Lacuzong report was made public involved a man I will call Elliot Spooner.

Elliot was prescribed Paxil 20 mg by his family doctor who wrote that his patient suffered from "marital problems . . . some depression over the last six months or so. There is some associated anxiety, mood swings, irritability, and anger. . . . He has had some thoughts of suicide, but he is not really making any plans and does not think that will be any problem." He diagnosed Elliot with depression, anxiety, and family problems.

The doctor had no way of knowing that Paxil can worsen all of the symptoms that his patient was displaying. The FDA had not yet forced the antidepressant manufacturers to add the warning about "Clinical Worsening and Suicide Risk" described in chapter 5.[30] Elliot was already suffering from several of the symptoms that Paxil causes or exacerbates—anxiety, agitation, insomnia, irritability, hostility, aggressiveness, and impulsivity—so that Paxil became a prescription for disaster.

When asked under oath in deposition what kind of warnings he gave to his patient, Elliot's doctor explained, "I don't recall the specific conversation, but typically it would have probably been headache, nausea, and some sexual dysfunction." GSK advertising and promotion had created an environment in which many doctors believed that Paxil was a relatively harmless drug with no potential to cause madness.

A psychologist saw Elliot three or four days after he began Paxil and emphasized his patient's increasing anger and irritability. The psychologist also noted poor appetite, trouble sleeping, and depressed mood. He did not recognize this as a pattern of Paxil-induced overstimulation with the risk of drug-induced suicide.

On Elliot's last visit to his doctor, his prescription for Paxil was renewed and he was described as improving. The diagnosis remained depression and anxiety. Elliot may have reported feeling better due to the drug's stimulating effects. The artificially induced euphoria can feel like an improvement. That's why people abuse methamphetamine and cocaine. Paxil can also produce an emotional flattening or anesthesia that temporarily feels like an improvement. Probably more than most antidepressants, Paxil is a powerful spellbinder, making people think they are doing better when in fact they are doing worse.

Not quite two months after starting Paxil, Elliot committed suicide by hanging himself in a closet. It would be almost exactly four more years before GSK would issue its "Dear Healthcare Professional" letter in May 2006, admitting that Paxil causes suicidal behavior in depressed adult patients. GSK settled Elliot's case without acknowledging fault for an undisclosed amount of money. Similar cases have been settled for at least one million dollars.

Paxil is not substantially different from Prozac, Zoloft, Luvox, Celexa, Effexor, Wellbutrin, or any other of the newer antidepressants in its capacity to cause overstimulation and a variety of other dangerous adverse mental reactions. If Paxil causes suicide in adults, so do the other antidepressants. As already described, the FDA has mandated clear warnings that are identical for the drugs. But because it is so short-acting and potent, Paxil probably poses a more frequent and more severe risk than some of the other antidepressants.

I have spent years documenting drug company influence in what the medical profession learns and fails to learn, but you no longer have to only rely on what I say. Physicians from the heart of establishment medicine have recently begun writing books with titles like *The Truth About the Drug Companies,*[31] *Overdosed America,*[32] and *Medicines Out of Control?,*[33] and also in journal articles like "Medical Journals Are an Extension of the Marketing Arm of Pharmaceutical Companies."[34] In her brilliant new book, *The Myth of the Chemical Cure: A Critique of Psychiatric Drug Treatment* (2008), British psychiatrist Joanna Moncrieff has subjected the basic assumptions of biological psychiatry to scientific scrutiny in an easily readable style. These books and articles confirm the unholy, corrupting influence of pharmaceutical money on research and practice in the healing professions.

At the end of the day, you cannot trust what your doctor tells you because you cannot trust the information your doctor is getting from drug companies. In my clinical experience, the best approach is to avoid taking so-called "antidepressant" drugs. As documented in chapter 2, antidepressants lack effectiveness and cause many serious hazards to the body and mind. They can also produce painful and even dangerous emotional reactions during withdrawal. Depression can be treated by psychotherapy and family therapy without resorting to drugs, as well as by many other positive alternatives from exercise to religion.[35]

Chapter 19

Marketing Myths and the Truth About Psychiatric Medication

MODERN PEOPLE SWIM IN A SEA of psychopharmacological advertising and promotion amounting to an all-pervasive propaganda campaign designed to shape the way we think about our lives and ourselves. We take for granted pronouncements like, "You have a biochemical imbalance," and "Mental disorders are like diabetes," and can easily feel shocked when someone challenges their factual basis. In reality, these are not scientific observations—they are promotional slogans, so adamantly repeated in the media and by individual psychiatrists that people assume them to be true. The psychopharmaceutical complex fosters these falsehoods in order to promote the widespread use of their products.

MARKETING MYTH: PSYCHIATRIC DRUGS CORRECT BIOCHEMICAL IMBALANCES

THIS IS THE THEORETICAL EDIFICE that psychiatrists stand on when instructing their patients to take drugs: "You have a biochemical imbalance." Reluctant patients, by the millions, are pushed into taking drugs by doctors who tell them with no uncertainty that they need medication.

Causing Biochemical Imbalances

If you have a biochemical imbalance in your brain, the odds are overwhelming that your doctor put it there with a psychiatric drug. In fact, these are the only *known* biochemical imbalances in the brains of psychiatric patients—the biochemical imbalances caused by drug treatments and electroshock.

Psychiatric drugs don't correct biochemical imbalances—they cause them. Even the American Psychiatric Publishing's adamantly pro-drug *Textbook of Psychiatry* admits that antidepressant-induced biochemical imbalances may be the cause of the increased suicidality produced by these drugs.[1]

Psychiatric drugs are developed precisely with the aim of causing biochemical imbalances in the *normal* brain. The first step is to find a chemical agent, such as Prozac, that induces some kind of biochemical malfunction in the brain of an experimental animal, usually a rat. Prozac, for example, blocks the *normal* removal of serotonin from its active place in the synapse or cleft between brain cells. This floods the area with excess serotonin, creating a decidedly abnormal biochemical imbalance. Eli Lilly, the manufacturer of Prozac, screened many drugs before it found one that would cause this imbalance in the brain.

Probably, drug manufacturers would rather discover and market drugs that do correct biochemical imbalances but this cannot be done because no biochemical imbalances have been identified in the brains of patients with diagnoses such as anxiety disorders, depressive disorders, bipolar disorder, or schizophrenia. Therefore, the drug companies are limited to giving toxins to rats until they find ones that disrupt the rat's normally functioning brain, causing biochemical imbalances. Then they try to argue that this particular intervention has beneficial effects.

In the mid-1980s, when Prozac was still in the experimental stage, Lilly researchers discovered that the brain fights against the abnormal accumulation of serotonin by shutting down its production of serotonin for a period of time.[2] This compensatory reaction produces additional, unpredictable imbalances, and may account for why so many cases of antidepressant madness occur shortly after starting the drug or changing doses.

The brain also takes long-term measures to fight the effects of any accumulating extra serotonin, for example, by reducing the number of receptors to which the serotonin molecules can attach, a process called down-regulation. Sixty percent of the serotonin receptors can disappear and the effect can last long after treatment has ended.[3] This persistent loss of serotonergic function may cause or contribute to the apathy that antidepressant-treated patients can develop over years of treatment.[4]

Drug companies do not want you to know about these lasting antidepressant-induced biochemical imbalances and anatomical changes in your brain. In a product-liability suit against the company, Lilly's head of research,

Ray Fuller, was asked under oath in deposition if his company had ever conducted studies to determine the potential permanency of Prozac-induced serotonin receptor loss in the brain. Dr. Fuller replied that the company had not conducted any such tests. When asked if it might be important to know if Prozac permanently changes the brain, Fuller replied, "I don't see that that would be of any value to know. . . ."[5]

Correcting Biochemical Imbalances

Given that psychiatric drugs can cause biochemical imbalances, can they also correct them, thereby producing beneficial outcomes? There's little or no chance that a drug will beneficially alter a human experience as varied and complicated as depression, anxiety, or psychosis. Drugs are gross intrusions into an infinitely complex and largely unexplored biological system called the brain, so that any given drug "treatment" is bound to impair normal functioning. Depression, anxiety, and other so-called psychiatric disorders are the result of that enormously complex psychological phenomenon called the mind, itself the product of the brain, environmental influences including childhood and culture, as well as the subjective judgments and decisions made by the individual as he or she deals with life.

Meanwhile, we know much too little about the brain for neuroscience to contribute anything to our understanding of an individual's problems or how to ameliorate them. Furthermore, it will almost certainly prove impossible in the long run to reduce the mental states of distressed or disturbed people to their brain biochemistry. In my clinical experience, childhood plays a powerful role in how we think and feel, after which we continue to grow and to develop through our adult experiences, modified by our individual values, our courage, and our choices. Mental or emotional phenomena like depression, anxiety, and "schizophrenia" can only be understood by using all the intellectual tools available to us for understanding an individual's psychological and spiritual life in the context of family, culture, and society.

I first began shredding the biochemical theory of depression in 1991 in *Toxic Psychiatry*. I pointed out the absurdity of attributing a complex human phenomenon like depression to any specific or even several neurotransmitters when there are two hundred or more interacting with one another and with myriad other brain mechanisms—some known and most undiscovered—that facilitate chemical and electrical communication inside the brain.

Once again, psychiatry has just barely begun to catch up with scientific reality. Again, turning to the American Psychiatric Publishing's *Textbook of*

Psychiatry as our illustrative source of conventional wisdom in psychiatry, after much hemming and hawing, the textbook has been compelled by science to admit that all the hocus-pocus about biochemical imbalances remains entirely unproven. In other words, the chemical imbalance theory is dead.[6]

The next time you think, "I have a biochemical imbalance," let it go. There are much better psychological and spiritual ways to understand, manage and learn from your emotions. I have tried to express my own broader approach to life in *Beyond Conflict* (1994) and *The Heart of Being Helpful* (1997), and I suggest seventeen principles of living in the concluding chapter of this book. However, no one person and no one therapeutic approach can have "the answers." Solutions to personal distress and suffering lie in all the accumulated wisdom of humankind as well as within the realms of individual, subjective values, and choice.

People who are depressed or anxious often suffer from a variety of physical discomforts and emotional reactions that seem like they are rooted in physical illness. They often worry about being physically ill. If you suspect that something physical is causing you to feel depressed, you should begin by seeing an appropriate medical specialist, not a psychiatrist, to check for the many genuine physical ailments that can contribute to feeling depressed or anxious, such as hypothyroidism, diabetes, Lyme disease, and any physical disorder that's debilitating or causes fatigue. However, beware of your family doctor's response if you mention feeling depressed, sad, or even tired. Your general practitioner may be enamored with mythical biochemical imbalances and is likely to urge you to take a psychiatric drug.

If you do turn out to suffer from one of the genuine physical disorders that can cause depression, anxiety, and other psychiatric symptoms, or even if you suffer from some as yet unknown and unidentified biochemical imbalance, taking a psychiatric drug will only add additional imbalances to your already malfunctioning brain

But the Drug Made Me Feel Better

The fact that a drug sometimes makes us feel better does not mean that it's correcting a biochemical imbalance. Recreational drugs such as alcohol and marijuana are used by hundreds of millions of people to "relax," but few if any scientists believe that these chemicals are correcting imbalances in the brain. Instead, everyone recognizes that they impair brain function. No psychiatric drug is known to correct anything in the brain.

Lessons of Drug-Withdrawal Symptoms

Drug-withdrawal reactions confirm that psychiatric drugs throw the brain into severe biochemical imbalances and malfunctions, so much so that the individual goes through painful, dangerous reactions when the drug is removed. In one of my legal cases, nineteen-year-old Virgil Ackerman skipped a dose or two of Paxil and assaulted a close friend while she was sleeping. They were platonic friends taking a nap in separate seats of a van but when he awoke in the seat behind her, he happened to see a heavy object on the floor, and bludgeoned her into unconsciousness. Then he touched her sexually. The behavior was totally out of character for the young man and most probably resulted from drug withdrawal.

The judge dropped the physical assault charge but the charges growing from the sexual touching of the unconscious young woman were not legally subject to mitigation. The young man's sentence was reduced in regard to the charge of physical assault and the woman fortunately made a full physical recovery, although she undoubtedly will carry the emotional scars indefinitely.

Charles Medawar and Anita Hardon (2004) have documented how GlaxoSmithKline, Eli Lilly, and other companies have fought recognizing the severity of withdrawal problems from Paxil, Prozac, and other SSRI antidepressants. A few years ago I was a consultant in a California suit to force the manufacturer of Paxil to increase its warnings concerning withdrawal. Don Farber, with whom I also worked in the Lacuzong case, was the attorney.[7] GlaxoSmithKline (GSK) "resolved the case"—without admitting wrongdoing. At about the same time, GSK—simultaneously under pressure from the FDA—agreed to upgrade the warning on its label concerning Paxil withdrawal.

Under a bold black heading, "Discontinuation of Treatment with PAXIL," the label now summarizes reports that it has received concerning withdrawal reactions:[8]

> Dysphoric [painful] mood, irritability, agitation, dizziness, sensory disturbances (e.g., parethesias such as electric shock sensations), anxiety, confusion, headache, lethargy, emotional lability, insomnia, and hypomania. While these events are generally self-limiting, there have been reports of serious discontinuation symptoms.

The label goes on to note that these symptoms can become "intolerable." It recommends slow withdrawal with resumption of the previous dose if the suffering becomes intolerable. The slow taper hopefully gives the brain time to correct the imbalances caused by the drug. Psychiatric drugs do not improve bio-chemical imbalances, they cause them, and withdrawal reactions are one result.

MARKETING MYTH: PSYCHIATRIC DRUGS DON'T PERMANENTLY HARM THE BRAIN

THINK OF PSYCHIATRIC DRUGS as pollutants. The brain is wrapped in thin protective membranes and defensive chemical reactions that try to pre-vent the entrance of pollutants. The protective system is called the blood brain barrier. All psychoactive substances including psychiatric drugs pierce these defenses. Once inside they wreak havoc with the brain's biochemical ac-tivities.

We now know that atmospheric pollutants in minute concentrations can inadvertently pose hazards to the life on Earth. Compared to most atmos-pheric pollutants, psychiatrically induced brain pollutants are highly concen-trated and they are specifically tailored to disrupt normal functions.

Mounting laboratory evidence—reviewed in more detail in my medical book, *Brain-Disabling Treatments in Psychiatry* (2008)—indicates that psychiatric drugs can cause permanent brain dysfunction and damage. The antipsychotic drugs cause obviously observable brain damage in the form of tardive dyskine-sia and a variety of studies show that they kill or maim brain cells.[9] Similarly, there's growing evidence that the stimulants we give to children can perma-nently change the function of the brain.[10] Here, I will focus on a particularly ominous body of literature confirming that the SSRI antidepressants can per-manently damage the physical structure of the brain, including various parts of brain cells (neurons). This scientific literature is becoming extensive.[11]

When researchers do admit that antidepressants cause persisting brain dys-function and damage, they typically spin the results by claiming that the abnor-malities represent an improvement. For example, one group of researchers found that antidepressants given to children produced an abnormal shrinkage in a part of the brain that governs many life functions—the thalamus—but then claimed that these children probably had too much thalamus to begin with.[12] Another group of researchers claimed that the opposite effect—an antidepressant-induced abnormal increase in brain-cell growth—was "protective" of the brain.[13] The two studies illustrate that no matter how the antidepressant harms the brain—by causing overgrowth or by causing shrinkage—researchers will ignore the obvi-ous pathological implications while touting the highly speculative and even ab-surd benefits.

On December 19, 2005, a headline in a promotional bulletin called *Johns Hopkins Medicine* made an astonishing claim:[14]

Popular Antidepressants Boost Brain Growth, Hopkins Scientists Report

The university's Office of Corporate Communications distributed this Johns Hopkins Public Relations Release. It touted a recently published study by medical center researchers showing that antidepressants increased the density of nerve trunks in many regions of the brain including the frontal lobe and limbic system. These are the highest evolutionary centers that regulate the individual's overall mental and emotional life—everything having to do with intelligence, reason, and emotion. A drug-induced over-growth in nerve connections in this region represents a serious abnormality with unpredictable mental and emotional consequences.

Principal investigator Vassilis Koliatsos, MD made drug-promotional lemonade out of these medical lemons, declaring "It appears that SSRI antidepressants rewire areas of the brain that are important for thinking and feeling, as well as operating the autonomic nervous system." It required a mere four weeks for Prozac to accomplish this "rewiring." By comparison, an older tricyclic antidepressant had no such effect, confirming the greater toxicity of the newer antidepressants.

If you are a patient taking antidepressants, do you want your mental and emotional centers rewired? Every doctor should ask himself or herself, "Do I want to rewire the frontal lobes of my patients?" Of course, it is not a rational rewiring but rather a haphazard overgrowth produced by the brain's abnormal reactions to a toxic substance.

Dr. Koliatsos argues that patients should welcome this abnormal growth of brain cells as "more tangible evidence of a real effect in the brain." Yes, antidepressants do have a "real effect" on the brain—the production of gross, widespread, physical abnormalities, including areas of abnormal growth.

The hypocrisy behind this spin on brain damage is apparent if we look at how the same medical center, Johns Hopkins, treated brain changes caused by recreational drugs, that is, drugs without corporate sponsors. In late 2002, another Johns Hopkins public-relations bulletin displayed this alarming headline:[15]

Recreational Use of Ecstasy Causes New Brain Damage

Both of these press releases—the one spun in favor of antidepressants and the other more rationally critical of Ecstasy—were picked up by news agencies around the world. They had a great deal of influence on how people view the prescribed medication versus the illegal recreational drug.

Why do Johns Hopkins public relations officials and researchers report honestly on the harmful effects of Ecstasy but rationalize the harmful effects of the widely used antidepressants? The answer involves influences such as money, prestige, power, professional standing, and the control exerted over research by the psychopharmaceutical complex.[16] Most research in psychopharmacology is supported by the pharmaceutical industry and most careers related to psychiatric drugs eventually involve receiving money from the companies.

The Brain Is Vulnerable to Injury

Meanwhile, it should be no surprise that the brain is not well suited to receive drugs. It lives in a delicate harmony with itself, an organ with complexity far beyond our current understanding and imagination that provides the biological basis of our humanity. It contains approximately one hundred billion neurons—nerve cells that send the chemical messages that run our brains and influence our bodies. There are more neurons in our brain than there are stars in the universe. Some of these individual neurons make ten thousand or more individual connections with other neurons. These neurons and their connections are ignited by a couple of hundred different neurotransmitters, such as serotonin and dopamine. The neurotransmitters we know best we nonetheless know little about; most of the others we know nothing about and haven't even as yet identified.

Beyond the neurotransmitters, our brain functions are affected by assorted other kinds of support cells, many chemicals such as sodium and potassium, and various hormones. The overall brain activity generates electrical fields that reflect and influence brain function in ways no one can yet grasp. We don't even understand the operating system of the brain—how it organizes and runs itself.

Each brain is more complex than the entire physical universe of stars, galaxies, black holes, gravity, and electromagnetic fields. That is the nature of life and especially of the mammalian brain—it is complex far beyond our current understanding and far beyond anything in the inanimate physical universe.

So the next time some "expert" tries to explain a subtle manifestation of human behavior in terms of brain function—or tries to convince you that a biochemical imbalance is at the root of your problems—you should wonder about his pecuniary motives. You should suspect that it's in the expert's interest to convince you that you're a much simpler biological organism than you are.

A principle to remember: Tampering with the human brain to influence human emotions and actions is not a good idea.

MARKETING MYTH: PSYCHIATRIC DRUGS IN SMALL DOSES ARE RELATIVELY HARMLESS

THE PREVIOUS CHAPTER described the case of Reynaldo Lacuzong who drowned himself and his two children in a bathtub after taking only two or three doses of the smallest available dose of Paxil (10 mg). Despite how often doctors tell their patients, "Don't worry, it's a small dose," many people have serious adverse effects from one or two doses of a drug, often in relatively small amounts. Here is a simple rule: If a drug dose is large enough to affect your brain and mind, then it is also large enough to cause serious dysfunction in your brain and mind, including compulsive violence and suicide.

Of course, toxicity is to some degree dose-dependent. The frequency and intensity of most adverse drug reactions will increase with the dose. But there are always exceptions, like the occasional drinker who gets "tipsy" on a few sips of wine and the person who becomes manic on small doses of antidepressants, stimulants, or the tranquilizer Xanax. People who are ill or elderly are more susceptible to adverse drug reactions. Impaired liver and kidney function can increase the impact of drugs by raising their blood levels and slowing their deactivation or removal from the body.

Up to 10 percent of the population have a genetic lack of liver enzymes necessary for the effective breakdown of many medications, including the newer antidepressant drugs such as Prozac.[17] These people are called "poor metabolizers." They are more likely to suffer adverse drug reactions because the drug concentration builds up in the bloodstream when it cannot be destroyed or eliminated efficiently. If medicine were conducted on a more rational basis, all patients would be tested when possible in advance of taking psychiatric drugs—or any drugs—where there is a risk of abnormal liver metabolism affecting the treatment result.

The drug companies have been reluctant to recognize this problem or to make laboratories available to perform tests for these liver enzymes. In many of my legal cases, the attorneys have been reluctant to test their clients for a genetic defect in liver function for fear that the results might be confusing to a judge or jury. They felt that it was sufficient to show that even in the presence of normal liver function the drug was known to cause abnormal emotional and behavioral reactions. In the few cases where liver enzyme tests were conducted, no deficiencies were found.

Since each group of liver enzymes metabolizes many different drugs, when two or more drugs are overloading the same enzyme system it can lead to severe toxicity. Dangerous drug combinations can usually be identified in sections labeled "Drug Interactions" in pharmacology handbooks and in the annual *Physicians' Desk Reference* or *Drug Facts and Comparisons*.

Doctors very often fail to take into account that the recommended dose of a drug is based entirely on the premise that the patient is taking no other drugs. When combined with other drugs, a small dose can become a large one, and a large dose can become a mammoth one.

Drug trials used to determine appropriate dose ranges for a drug never combine similar drugs, and they usually exclude all other psychiatric drugs. Physicians often fail to realize that they can easily overdose a patient by prescribing combinations of several psychoactive drugs, even though each one is prescribed within the suggested dose range.

Clever advertising can confuse physicians about the potential for dangerous drug combinations. For example, Eli Lilly marketed Strattera as "the nonstimulant" treatment for ADHD. However, it is a very stimulating drug that causes all the usual stimulant adverse effects from insomnia and agitation to mania. As mentioned earlier, if you look in the *Physicians' Desk Reference*'s table of contents, Strattera is listed under stimulants. A physician who swallowed the Eli Lilly marketing slogan would not recognize the risk involved in combining Strattera with another stimulating drug.

Strattera is the only nonaddictive stimulant used to treat ADHD. By calling Strattera a nonstimulant, Eli Lilly was probably trying to avoid the stigma associated with dependence and abuse. The company did not call Strattera the nonaddictive stimulant, perhaps because it wanted to avoid informing physicians that the drug can cause overstimulation of the brain that can become clinically dangerous.

SSRI antidepressants such as Prozac, Paxil, and Zoloft are said to be "selective" because they mainly affect the neurotransmitter called serotonin. Selectivity, in this case, is a misleading concept. The serotonin system is the single most extensive neuronal network in the brain. It originates deep within the confines of the midbrain and then spreads out, reaching into the nooks and crannies from the memory centers in the temporal lobe to the emotional and intellectual centers of the limbic system and frontal lobes. In addition, when the serotonin system is disrupted by antidepressants, other neurotransmitters go into imbalance as well, including dopamine, the main nerve route between the basal ganglia deep in the brain, and the limbic system and frontal lobes.

It has often been observed that the dose determines whether a medication is therapeutic or poisonous. For example, a small dose of a cardiac toxin may slow the reactivity of the heart muscle but ultimately improve heart function by stopping a dangerous arrhythmia. This observation has been used to justify psychiatric drugs that slow down or otherwise impair brain function.

A simple analogy may help explain the difference between impairing cardiac function and impairing brain function: A heart transplant and a brain transplant have very different implications: the one replaces a pump, the other replaces the person. Drugs that impair the higher centers of the brain will inevitable impair the function of the mind and dampen or distort what we call the human identity and spirit—much as we have seen in the cases in this book.

MARKETING MYTH: PSYCHIATRIC DRUGS ARE NECESSARY TO PREVENT SUICIDE AND VIOLENCE

THE CASES AND SCIENTIFIC EVIDENCE presented in this book should convincingly demonstrate that antidepressants cause suicide. Given that psychiatric drugs can cause suicide, is there evidence that any of them actually reduce suicide? The answer is no. Particularly in the case of the antidepressants, drug companies and their paid researchers have tried for years to show that these drugs reduce the suicide rate, but no compelling evidence has been forthcoming. The opposite has been proven—that they cause suicidal behavior. As a result, no drugs are FDA-approved for treating suicidal feelings or behavior.

The cases and evidence in this book also demonstrate that psychiatric drugs can cause violence. Do any of them prevent violence? Again the answer is no. Psychiatric drugs stop violence only to the extent that they temporarily immobilize the individual. Certainly, a shot of Haldol in the emergency room frequently renders people so mentally numb and physically stiff—a virtual mental and physical straitjacket—that they are temporarily rendered unable to commit violent acts. But the effect is hardly therapeutic—no more than a blow on the head or physical restraint. It is a simple matter of temporarily knocking the person out of commission.

When I worked in emergency rooms and acute treatment hospitals, approaching the most disturbed patients in a peaceful and reassuring manner almost always worked. Few of my colleagues felt they had enough time for it, when in reality they lacked the interest, skill, and patience for relating to very disturbed people in a caring manner. It would not have dawned on them to behave like my friend who helped his hospitalized, sleeping-walking father by gently interpreting his dream content so that he felt comfortable returning to bed. Most of my psychiatric colleagues would have behaved much more like the doctors who initially responded to my friend's sleepwalking father by calling security, holding him down, and forcing Haldol into his body.

MARKETING MYTH: PSYCHIATRIC DISORDERS ARE DISEASES LIKE DIABETES

COMPARING "MENTAL DISORDERS" like anxiety, depression, and mania to diabetes, as is often done, is false and misleading. Diabetes has all of the hallmarks of a real disease, including many biological markers, such as an elevated fasting blood sugar. It has known biological causes, such as reduced insulin production and reduced cellular capacity to utilize insulin. Finally, it has several specific, rational physical treatments, such as dietary control and medication, including insulin replacement. Psychiatric disorders meet none of these criteria. They have no biological markers, no known physical causes, and no rational physical treatments.

Ironically, doctors who treat diabetes show much more concern for the feelings, attitudes, and self-determination of their patients than psychiatrists who treat mental problems. Without exception, experts in diabetes emphasize changing lifestyle as central to the treatment. Books and educational pamphlets given to patients focus on how the patient must take responsibility for diet, exercise, and even stress reduction. They point out that everything should be done to control the disorder without resort to medication.

In contrast to doctors who treat diabetes, psychiatrists almost never talk about lifestyle changes or stress reduction. Mostly, they push drugs. It is strange that doctors who treat diabetes place more emphasis on the patient's responsibility for lifestyle changes than psychiatrists who are in fact treating lifestyle problems. It is bitterly ironic that doctors treat diabetics with much more personal attention, respect, and care—that is, much more like real people—than doctors treat patients with emotional problems.

To counter the criticism that people with mental problems do not have "real diseases," extreme claims have also been made that psychiatric problems can be visualized with brain scans. In several of my books, I have systematically debunked this concept. More recently, psychiatrist Grace Jackson (2006) reviewed these studies and concluded, "Contrary to reports that have been emphasized by the major news outlets, there is no evidence at this time to justify the claim that brain scans discern the presence of psychiatric disease, based upon anatomic or physiological abnormalities in the brain." No ethical physician will make believe he or she can use a brain scan to diagnose a psychiatric problem.

While psychiatrists are eager to make believe they are treating real diseases, they rarely admit that they are causing them. Medication madness is a real neurologic disease—one that my medical and psychiatric colleagues are far too eager to ignore.

MARKETING MYTH: "THE DRUG ONLY UNMASKED YOUR UNDERLYING PSYCHIATRIC DISORDER"

DRUG ADVOCATES often claim that that drugs can only "unmask" preexisting psychiatric disturbances rather than cause them. When a child loses touch with reality while taking a stimulant like Ritalin, Adderall, or Strattera—when he fears the world is conspiring against him, sees little creatures crawling out of the walls, and becomes violent toward his parents—the parents are almost surely to be told that the drug merely "brought out" the child's underlying bipolar disorder. When a woman's moods become wildly unstable while taking an antidepressant like Prozac, Zoloft, Paxil, or Effexor, when she wastes her family fortune, starts having multiple affairs, and is found running naked in the streets—in almost all cases the prescribing doctor will inform the patient and her family that the medication merely "unmasked" her "bipolar disorder."

With this twisting of the truth, every adverse drug reaction becomes the patient's fault and is used to justify prescribing even more drugs. Meanwhile, the medication-spellbound patient usually lacks the confidence or certainty to reply, "Well, maybe I was harboring mania for twenty years but I harbored it pretty damn well until you started writing prescriptions for me."

Common sense and a variety of scientific studies confirm that sometimes there are predisposing factors for adverse drug reactions. For example, if a person has been diagnosed with a manic episode in the past, then an antidepressant is more likely to cause mania again. But as we've seen in our cases and confirmed in the literature, people with no apparent manic tendency can also be driven into mania by the drugs. In either case, stopping the offending agent is the primary treatment, and prescribing additional psychiatric drugs is likely to do more harm than good.

It is worth repeating that, with only very few exceptions, the stories of medication madness in this book describe people with no discernable predisposition toward madness prior to taking the drugs. After going through medical records, school reports, personnel reports from work, and interviews with family and friends, I found no evidence of a predisposition to act in the way that they did when under the influence of psychiatric medications. As a group they seemed especially law-abiding, most had led exemplary lives, and many seemed more self-controlled and responsible than average.

MARKETING MYTH: "YOU WILL HAVE TO TAKE THEM FOR THE REST OF YOUR LIFE"

WHEN A PSYCHIATRIST TELLS YOU, "You will have to take medication for the rest of your life," he's making a pernicious speculation that's bound to do you much more harm than good. To begin with, we don't have any rest-of-your-life clinical studies.

In fact, the typical psychiatric-drug study lasts only four weeks, maybe six at the most. Why? One reason is that psychiatric drugs are so ineffective and cause so many adverse effects that many, if not most, patients drop out before the study can last four to six weeks! It is a constant lament in psychiatry that most patients stop taking their drugs after a few weeks or months, and then drop off the psychiatric radar screen.

There is no science to back up claims that long-term dosing with psychiatric drugs does any good, even in regard to the antipsychotic drugs that are forced on people for a lifetime.[18] On the other hand, there is mounting evidence about permanent harmful effects from long-term exposure to these drugs. For example, most patients given antipsychotic drugs for many years will endure permanent brain damage in the form of tardive dyskinesia and tardive dementia.[19] We've also seen that antidepressants and stimulants can produce persistent and probably permanent abnormalities in the brain. These risks afflict children as well as adults. For example, although there are fewer studies of children, they probably share the same astronomically high rates for TD as studies have found in adults.[20] I have evaluated dozens of children afflicted with tardive dyskinesia by the newer antipsychotic drugs such as Risperdal and Zyprexa.

MARKETING MYTH: YOUR PSYCHIATRIST IS A BRAIN EXPERT

AS AVIDLY AS THEY push drugs, physicians tend to know very little about them. What about finding a specialist, for example a psychiatrist like me who has a subspecialty in clinical psychopharmacolgy—a psychiatrist who knows more than most about drugs? Almost without exception, doctors who specialize in knowing about psychiatric drugs are the worst possible sources of unbiased scientific information about drugs. They are listening to drug company salespersons. They are listening to drug-company advertising. They are listening to paid drug-company consultants giving presentations at medical meetings and sponsored dinners. And if they are really respected in their field, they are listening to all the money they are getting from the drug companies to put their name on drug-company-authored papers, to give seminars, and generally to lend their name to company products and profits. Who aren't these "experts" listening to? Their patients.

Even if your doctor kept up with the latest scientific research, there is simply too little known about how your brain works, how your mind works, and the risks that psychoactive substances pose to both. There is no comparison, for example, between the knowledge of computer hardware and software possessed by a competent computer expert and the knowledge of your brain and mind possessed by any neurologist or psychiatrist. The computer specialist knows pretty well what he is doing and is unlikely to harm your machine's hardware; your psychiatrist is feeling around in the dark with rough hands and is very likely to harm your delicate brain.

Computers are man-made. They come with blueprints. The programs we put into them are man-made as well. Therefore, it's usually possible to find people who know something about how computers work and how they can be repaired. No one brings a computer back to the same specialist week after week for years in the hope that constant tinkering might finally pay off.

Compared to a computer specialist's well-defined knowledge of his machine's hardware and software, the psychiatrist's knowledge is a pitiful, fuzzy collection of drug-company-sponsored "theories" about the brain and the mind. You would think our comparative ignorance as psychiatrists would lead us to treat your brain with at least as much care as your computer expert treats your computer. Not so. Although it would make sense to treat our delicate, complex, largely mysterious living brain and our almost unknowable mind with greater care than we treat a man-made machine, psychiatrists and other physicians treat the human brain and mind in ways so cavalier, uninformed, and destructive that the same approaches would *never* be inflicted on a computer or its software.

If your computer technician poured liquid junk into the back of your computer the way your psychiatrist pours junk into your brain, you would be justifiably outraged. If, in desperation, the computer expert suggested putting electrodes onto the motherboard of your computer to shock it, you would realize that you had already purchased a surge protector specifically to prevent excessive jolts of electricity from disrupting your computer's function. Hopefully, you would grab your computer and run for the hills. Well, when a psychiatrist wants to pour junk into your brain or to shock it, you might want to do the same thing—grab your brain and run for your life.

Many books have been written in an effort to fathom why psychiatry has such a long and dreadful history of abusing its patients and their brains.[21] There are innumerable approaches to explaining this phenomenon but in many ways I think it comes down to this: When people treat other people as objects rather than as treasured beings, they end up abusing them. Put another way, if we do not openly love and treasure the people we try to help, we will end up hating and abusing them. Modern psychiatry persists in taking the pseudoscientific position that people are biochemical devices to be corrected with toxic chemicals and jolts of electricity. Because they are despairing and sometimes even depressed and self-hating, many people who seek psychiatric help find it difficult to resist or to argue against these assaults on their brain.

MARKETING MYTH: YOUR DOCTOR KNOWS WHAT'S BEST FOR YOU

ALTHOUGH PEOPLE are less likely to accept medical authority as meekly as they did in earlier generations, most psychiatrists remain devoted to the view that they know what's best for their patients. As a result, organized psychiatry fully supports involuntary psychiatric treatment.

As psychiatrist Thomas Szasz first pointed out decades ago, involuntary treatment is not treatment at all. Despite the argument that it is "for their own good," locking up people for psychiatric reasons is arbitrary and wrong in principle. It also takes place without the careful legal protections provided to accused criminals and is, therefore, subject to constant abuse.

Locking up people against their will should not be called therapy.[22] Despite centuries of implementation, there are no scientific studies to show that anyone benefits from involuntary "treatment." In my experience, this kind of coercion makes people resentful, fearful, and uncooperative toward those who are supposed to be helping them. Fear of being locked up involuntarily also keeps people from seeking help. When they find themselves unexpectedly detained against their will, many understandably become much more emotionally distressed and angry.

Involuntary treatment provides the public with little protection from violence because these patients tend to be released once their insurance coverage runs out or when the state facility feels compelled to lower its census to save money. Many violent people are able to play to the overconfidence of psychiatrists and con them into thinking they can "cure" dangerous people. It would be far safer, as well as more consistent with constitutional rights, to rely on the criminal justice system to determine how long dangerous individuals should remain incarcerated and how they should be monitored after release.

My own patients have told me that they feel more able to talk with me about their painful and "crazy" feelings because I will never lock them up. In the meanwhile, in forty years of private practice, none of my patients has committed suicide or seriously harmed another person during treatment with me. Some of that is luck; any psychiatrist or therapist can have patients who harm themselves or others. But the relative lack of these bad outcomes in my decades of clinical practice confirms the safety and effectiveness of treating people without ever forcing them into mental hospitals and without treating them with psychiatric drugs.

As I describe in *The Heart of Being Helpful* (1997), good therapy begins with a caring, empathic relationship offered by a therapist with the capacity to create a healing presence. While I practice a combination of relationship and insight therapy, there are many varieties of therapy that work because of the human capacity of the therapist to connect with patients in a meaningful, encouraging way. In helping relationships, there is no place for authoritarianism or fake biological theories and drugs.

Opposition to involuntary treatment is a cornerstone of "the survivor movement"—an international effort led by victims of psychiatry.[23] I count many of my oldest friends among this group of former psychiatric patients and inmates, including David Oaks and Leonard Roy Frank, men who suffered abuse at the hands of psychiatry and who then went on to live enormously productive lives as leaders in the psychiatric-reform movement.

David Oaks is the executive director of MindFreedom, the leading survivor organization in the world fighting for psychiatric patient rights and resisting psychiatric abuses. He edits the group's magazine, organizes protests against psychiatric abuses like electroshock treatment, and in general inspires reform-minded professionals and victims alike. David and I like to joke that we have a lot in common: we both went to Harvard. I then volunteered in the local state mental hospital[24] while he was forced into a private one in Boston. Both experiences led us to become reformers.

After Leonard Roy Frank was subjected to forced electroshock and even more damaging insulin-coma shock as a young man, he helped found the psychiatric reform movement in the early 1970s. We worked together closely in those years opposing lobotomy and shock treatment. At that time, Leonard also began to collect quotations in order to exercise his shock-battered mental functions and to replace his obliterated college education. He is now the author of a series of brilliant books of quotations published by Gramercy Books, including his most recent, *Freedom: More than 600 Quotes Celebrating Independence, Liberty, and Justice* (2007). Leonard has also written a book and a carefully researched scientific publication on the damage wrought by shock treatment.[25]

For those of you who have been injured by psychiatric treatment, it's worth knowing that many others have transcended that abuse and gone on to live marvelous, inspired, and inspiring lives.

Chapter 20

Spellbound by Drug-Withdrawal Reactions

IMAGINE THIS SCENE UNFOLDING in front of you on the checkout line at the grocery store. The woman ahead of you in line looks to be in her late forties. She is well groomed, dressed for professional work, and seems very pleasant as she smiles back at you. Then the checkout clerk asks her, "Have you counted your items? This line is for fourteen items or less."

The previously congenial lady shouts at the top of her voice, "Count them? You want me to count them? All right, I'll count them." She picks up the first item, a can of food, shouts "One!" and slams it down onto the counter, shocking you and the checkout lady and startling customers within a fifty-foot radius.

Now she picks up the second item, shouts "Two!" and slams it down as well. You and the checkout girl stand mesmerized by the scene as the woman slams down fourteen items one by one and concludes at the top of her voice, "I've got two items too many. I must be in the wrong line!" The fuming woman throws the items back into her cart, whirls around—nearly hitting you in the process—brushes by a stand of sundries that shakes, nearly topples over, and pushes her cart away toward the regular checkout.

You wonder to yourself, "What in the world is going on with that person?" Well, I can tell you, because she was my patient at the time that she blew up.

Christine Zeltner was a fifty-year-old social worker and mother who had lost her husband after a long and difficult illness several years earlier. Christine was stressed by having to work while tending to her chronically ill husband and raising her infant daughter. So she went to a psychiatrist for help in perking up, especially explaining to him that she wanted to take better take care of her child. Without offering any counseling, the psychiatrist began prescribing a series of antidepressants and mood stabilizers. For the next ten years, through her husband's painful death and then raising her daughter into her early teens, Christine remained on combinations of mood stabilizers and antidepressants.

Christine began to suspect that the drugs were putting her into an emotional fog. Rather than helping her to be a better mother, they rendered her emotionally remote and aloof. Her daughter was doing well by almost any standards but Christine felt unable to fully connect emotionally with her daughter.

Christine began to taper herself off the medications and then came to me for help in the final stages of withdrawal. She was already down to taking only one-half of a 10 mg tablet of Celexa each day. Together Christine and I decided to slowly taper the last of the Celexa. Her life at the time was very stable, including a convenient part-time job and a nurturing boyfriend.

In the process of weaning Christine, I reminded her on each visit about the risks associated with antidepressant withdrawal including crashing into depression and suicidality, or becoming irritable and overreactive to ordinary frustrations. Because Christine had already cut back on the drug before seeing me and because she seemed to be doing well, we took only one month to remove her altogether from the Celexa.

Three days after completely stopping the Celexa, Christine came to me for a scheduled follow-up visit. She looked good, perhaps a little too good in the way she began by joking and kidding around with me. Withdrawal seemed to bring out a slight touch of elevated mood. Abruptly she said, "I don't think I can go on like this."

I quickly became concerned. Was she talking about feeling suicidal? No, she was afraid she was losing control of her behavior. I asked for examples. She explained that on the previous day she became extremely annoyed at coworkers for not performing more expeditiously. They were discussing how to proceed on a project and then discussed it "over and over again" before getting down to work. She now realized that her anger over this had been "silly," and she was afraid she had offended a good friend by vociferously complaining about all the talking.

I asked her for another example and it was similar. Christine explained that she had become irritated with her boyfriend over nothing of any great importance. Finally, with enormous embarrassment and remorse, she told me the story about her wild display of outrage at the grocery store. As she recounted what happened, she felt embarrassed and wanted to apologize to the store clerk but she also saw the events as comical. The withdrawal reaction was causing both irritability and a heightened mood that fell just short of euphoria or mild mania.

I reassured Christine that she was going through a classic case of "irritability" in response to withdrawing from one of the new antidepressants, in this case Celexa. I reminded her that we had talked about this possibility during each of our several visits. She now remembered our conversations but somehow when the reactions occurred, she had failed to identify them as drug-withdrawal symptoms. Spellbound for ten years while antidepressants made her emotionally remote, she was still spellbound by Celexa during withdrawal. As an educated professional social worker, Christine had some experience with medications but she had nonetheless been dumbfounded by the drugs and been driven into a potentially dangerous state of aggression.

I reviewed once again with Christine that these were temporary symptoms of withdrawal, that they would not go on forever, and that we could quickly abort them by resuming a small dose of Celexa. I reminded her about staying in touch with her daughter, her boyfriend, and me, so that we could help her assess what was going on. I also suggested she take sick leave for the next day of work and coddle herself over the weekend.

Christine felt relieved and decided she could handle remaining off the Celexa in anticipation of the irritability subsiding. Unfortunately, in the following weeks she continued to feel so emotionally unstable and irritable that she decided she needed to return to taking small doses of the drug. Typical of withdrawal reactions, she immediately felt somewhat better.

For some months, Christine remained unable to completely taper off the newer antidepressants. She continued to grow in her understanding of herself, increasing her ability to feel and to express her feelings, and to manage her irritability and anger. Eventually, she succeeded in becoming drug-free.

A MORE TRAGIC OUTCOME

SEVENTY-THREE-YEAR-OLD CRAIG KINGMAN and his wife had been married for more than fifty years. Craig may have been struggling with aging but in addition he had lost his son to a chronic illness three years earlier. His daughter had gone through a period of personal problems but was now doing much better. Craig ran a family business where his wife and daughter worked with him.

For a few months, Craig seemed to his wife to be getting anxious, as well as fidgety, short-tempered, and stubborn. His wife urged him to get some help and he went to his general practitioner. The doctor made no notes on the first visit, in retrospect claiming that he had only a few minutes to chat with Craig in the hallway of the hospital. He did prescribe Paxil 10 mg for his patient.

Three weeks after starting the medication, Craig went unannounced to the doctor again. Without realizing it, the doctor described a possible delusion when he wrote, "Complains of being depressed facing potential financial doom." There was no apparent explanation or exploration of this ominous and apparently unfounded fear. The doctor also described a potential state of activation or incipient mania: "Having a hard time focusing, stopping his mind from running." The fact that Craig made a walk-in appearance was in itself reason for concern. Despite these warning signs, the doctor continued the Paxil and did not refer his patient to a mental-health specialist.

At about this time, shortly before he would have finished the bottle of thirty tablets, Craig told his daughter that the medicine made him "feel bad" and that he had tried to stop but that withdrawal made him feel even worse. His daughter had heard bad things about Paxil and was dead set against Dad taking it. Unfortunately, her father trusted the doctor and was already feeling "hooked" on the medication.

One week later, now a month after starting Paxil, Craig once again returned to see the doctor who wrote that the Paxil was working well during the day but that his patient needed more toward nighttime. The doctor listed depression and anxiety as current problems. He increased the morning dose to 15 mg of Paxil CR (long-acting) with a note in his record to consider an extra Paxil in the evening if necessary. Taking two Paxil CR 15 mg would have tripled the original 10 mg dose.

Craig told his wife about the dose increase and explained to her that he had expressed a desire to stop the Paxil but the doctor had insisted it was safe and that he hadn't been taking it long enough. Craig explained to his wife that the doctor had told him that the drug was so safe he would give it to his own family.

After the increased dose, Mrs. Kingman watched her husband deteriorate:

I noticed it right away. His whole behavior was different. He got a little handheld tape recorder, and started going around taping things. He had temper outbursts. He was pacing the floor. He didn't sleep. He went into the computer room and closed the door. He never did that before. This went on the entire weekend, and I became extremely worried.

Craig was experiencing symptoms of stimulation or activation including akathisia, that potentially deadly combination of drug-induced agitation with hyperactivity.

Four days after her husband restarted the medication at the increased dose, Mrs. Kingman called the medical office to warn the doctor that her husband was becoming much more "moody and depressed." The nurse told her to have her husband double the dose but Mrs. Kingman considered it such a bad idea that she did not pass the recommendation on to her husband. Those who knew Craig confirmed Mrs. Kingman's observations that he was becoming erratic and unpredictable in his moods.

Craig told family members and his friend and employee Danny that the medication was making him feel funny, moody, or weird. According to Danny, he said, "They're going to have to get me on something else, because this medication isn't cutting it."

Now five weeks after his first dose of Paxil, Craig was at the office of the family business when he called his daughter, saying he "needed her." It was an odd call and she hurried to see him. When she arrived, her dad was leaning against his pickup truck, swaying back and forth, and holding something long propped up in a blanket. Her mom and Danny were trying to talk with him.

His wife asked, "Craig, what's wrong?"

Her husband replied, "I'm going crazy."

She reassured him, "You're not crazy."

He replied, "The voices tell me I have to do it, and that if I don't I'm a coward." Craig pulled a shotgun from beneath the blanket and pointed it at his wife and friend.

As best as his wife can recall these terrifying events, her husband said with grim determination, "I'm going to have to take you with me."

She replied, "Craig, why do you hate me so?"

He responded, "I don't hate you; I love you, and that's why I have to take you with me, because there'll be nobody to take care of you after I'm gone."

She told her husband that everything would be fine, that he needed to go to the hospital, and that the family would take him right away. Craig refused, protesting that they would lock him up, that he would get visitors only a few times a week, and that he didn't want to live like that. His wife pleaded with him not to abandon his grandchildren whom he loved beyond description. He responded that he didn't want them to see him locked up like that.

Craig rambled on irrationally about the business, saying that their inventory was gone, a natural consequence of good sales at that time of year. He had a "crazed look" in his eye and was pacing "like a caged animal."

Meanwhile, Danny dialed 911 on his cell phone. After what seemed like an eternity—twenty minutes during which Craig brandished his shotgun, rambled, and issued warnings—the sheriff finally arrived. SWAT team members positioned themselves on the perimeter of the yard of the business where the little group was gathered around Craig and his truck. A helicopter began to circle overhead.

Craig told his wife, "Well you're safe; the police have arrived."

Gun still in hand, Craig ran around the corner of their office building. When his daughter tried to run after him, Craig motioned vigorously to her not to follow and then disappeared from view.

A loud shot rang out and Craig was found dead from a shotgun wound.

In a note to his sister that Craig had typed on his computer, he had written, "Sis, I'm on Paxil and it focuses my attention on doing away with myself." He then stated, "The rest of the Catch-22 is if I stop taking the Paxil I become so paranoid and panic stricken, and depressed, I can't stand it." Craig's case is unusual in so graphically illustrating how a man can recognize that he is suffering from medication madness while being unable to stop taking the drug due to the horrible feelings associated with withdrawal.

All psychiatric drugs can cause withdrawal symptoms. If you've been on any psychoactive drug for a month or more, it is safest to assume that the drug should not be stopped abruptly. Meanwhile, there is no guaranteed safe way to taper off or to withdraw from psychiatric drugs but the next chapter will offer some useful safety guidelines.

Chapter 21

Making Drug Withdrawal as Safe as Possible

REMEMBER THAT IT IS NOT only dangerous to start taking psychiatric drugs, it is also dangerous to stop them. Experienced clinical supervision during drug withdrawal can be lifesaving, especially if you have been taking medications for many months, or if you're taking multiple medications, or if you have serious emotional problems.

A few types of drugs pose life-threatening physical risks during withdrawal, such as seizures and blood-pressure spikes. These physical risks can usually be avoided by taking at least ten days to withdraw. However, the feelings of physical and emotional discomfort associated with drug withdrawal can become overwhelming, sometimes necessitating many weeks or months to complete the taper. As a very rough gauge, it's not uncommon to require a month of withdrawal for every year of drug exposure, so that if you've been on a medication for five years, you might need five months to withdraw from it.

In addition to seeking experienced clinical guidance, during withdrawal from psychiatric medications it is important to take your time to slowly taper the drug. Don't let yourself be talked into a rapid withdrawal without good reason and do not push yourself beyond your emotional limits! Insist on maintaining a cooperative effort with any professional who is helping you and do not be shy about expressing your opinions about how the taper is progressing.

BEFORE STARTING TO TAPER YOUR DRUG

BEFORE TRYING TO WITHDRAW from psychiatric drugs, you should take four basic steps:

1. Inform Yourself about the Drug, Including Withdrawal Risks.

Keep in mind that medical books and establishment Web sites or publications, while worth reading, tend to minimize adverse effects, especially withdrawal problems. Although you will have to sort through junk, it would be good to search the Internet, including consumer Web sites. Because these sites' quality may vary in the future, I cannot recommend specific ones, but there is a great deal of information available. Even if your professional guide seems well informed, I strongly advocate taking the necessary steps to educate yourself as much as possible about medications and how to withdraw from them.

2. Ask a Health Professional with Experience in Drug Withdrawal to Monitor Your Progress.

In too many cases, healthcare providers who advocate psychiatric medication resist and even resent being asked by their patients for help in withdrawing from them. In an ideal world, your psychiatrist would be eager to help you learn to live without toxic substances in your brain, but in the real world most psychiatrists try to keep their patients on medications indefinitely.

Whether you are working with your original prescribing physician or with another professional, do not hold back from sharing with the professional everything you have learned on your own, and don't hesitate to bring along a friend or family member. Unfortunately, you are likely to have difficulty finding an informed professional willing or able to handle drug withdrawal. In that case, you can ask your family doctor to evaluate you, to write your prescriptions, and to help monitor your condition. If you think it would be helpful, share this book chapter with him. Especially if you've been taking the drugs for a long time or have emotional problems, find a caring therapist (such as a psychologist, social worker, counselor, or family therapist) to see on a regular basis to help you with the emotional aspects of withdrawal. You and your professional helper may also find it useful to read the recent edition of my book with David Cohen entitled, *Your Drug May Be Your Problem: How and Why to Stop Taking Psychiatric Medications* (2007).

3. Inform Friends or Family that You Are Withdrawing from Medication and Ask Them to Keep a Daily Eye on You.

Tell someone you trust to be on the lookout for any odd, unstable, or danger-ous behavior on your part. Your best protection during withdrawal is an in-formed family or social network. Drug withdrawal can be spellbinding and you may be the last to realize that you're losing control over your emotions or behavior.

4. Seek Advice and Counsel but Rely on Your Own Judgment about Withdrawing from Medication.

Doctors who prescribe medication too often feel slighted or disrespected when patients ask to stop taking their drugs. Don't accept one physician's opinion, especially the original prescribing doctor, about whether or not you should spend "the rest of your life" on a drug. Get second opinions. Research the drugs for yourself. Ultimately, make up your own mind.

THE WITHDRAWAL PROCESS

UNLESS FACED WITH AN EMERGENCY SITUATION where you must abruptly withdraw from medication under a physician's supervision, remember that a slow taper is usually safest.

One Drug at a Time

By tapering, I mean a gradual reduction of the dose over a period of time. It is almost always better to taper one drug at a time. Otherwise, you put excessive stress on your brain and your body. Also, if you develop withdrawal symptoms while stopping more than one drug, you won't know which drug is causing the problem. If you or your child is taking multiple psychiatric drugs, very thorough medical monitoring becomes especially important during with-drawal. It has sometimes taken more than a year to withdraw patients from a mixture of four or five drugs.

If one of the drugs is posing a special risk, such as an antipsychotic drug causing abnormal movements or a tranquilizer making you feel "drunk," taper that drug first.

If you have recently started a drug and do not believe it is having much effect on you, that's probably a good one to start initially tapering because your risk of severe withdrawal problems is reduced by your short time of exposure.

If you are concerned about getting enough sleep at night, do not taper or stop the evening sleeping pill until last. It is very helpful to get enough sleep during the withdrawal process. If you're taking a tranquilizer or any other se-dating drug several times a day, remove the evening dose last in order to stave off insomnia.

If the medications are causing you to feel too sedated, sleepy, or "drunk" during the day, then you may want to begin by tapering one of the morning sedative doses. It is important to feel alert during the day when you're tapering off drugs. Also, if your medication is jazzing you up too much during the day, begin by tapering the morning dose before the evening dose. In general, how-ever, the sleeping medication should be the last to be stopped, especially if you have been taking it for several months or more.

If you've had a tendency to get manic or unrealistically "high" in the past, you may want to remove your mood stabilizers toward the end of the with-drawal process. You will also want to be carefully monitored.

These observations are common sense but your physician may not take the time to think through the withdrawal process. When stopping multiple drugs, be sure you talk it through carefully with your doctor and also be sure to say what you think. When I take patients off medication, it's a highly collaborative venture that often includes not only the patient but also other family members.

Your Feelings Are the Most Important Signal During Drug Tapering

How you feel during the drug-withdrawal process is the single most impor-tant signal for how well you are doing. Unless it's an emergency and you are being very closely supervised, do not withdraw faster than you feel comfort-able. Unfortunately, there is always a risk that spellbinding will mislead you into thinking you're doing better than you are during withdrawal, making adequate monitoring by a professional and by friends or family especially im-portant.

If you begin to feel too physically or emotionally uncomfortable, you can usually solve the problem by returning to the previous dose. For example, if you become depressed or fatigued within a few days of reducing your Paxil from 20 mg to 15 mg, you can immediately return to your 20 mg dose, and that should solve the problem if it's due to withdrawal. Similarly, if you feel more anxious and are unable to sleep after reducing your Xanax dose from 1 mg to 0.5 mg at night, then you can return to the 1 mg dose.

Special Risks and the Length of Withdrawal

Check to see if your drug has been FDA-approved to control high blood pressure (some antihypertensive drugs used in psychiatry are listed in appendix A). Sudden withdrawal from antihypertension drugs can cause a dangerous rebound rise in blood pressure.

Also check to see if your drug has been FDA-approved to treat seizures (some antiseizure drugs used in psychiatry are listed in the appendix) because sudden withdrawal can cause rebound seizures. Similarly, if you've been taking a tranquilizer/sleeping pill (see appendix A), assume that it can cause seizures if you stop too quickly.

Most of the physical risks of withdrawal, such as blood pressure spikes or seizures (convulsions), are vastly diminished if ten days are taken to gradually withdraw. In drug labels that can be found in the *Physicians' Desk Reference,* manufacturers often stipulate the amount of time required to withdraw from their particular drug in order to avoid a dangerous physical adverse effect, such as seizures or blood-pressure spikes. The suggested withdrawal time may be no longer than a few days or a week.

Beyond the warning to take at least ten days for gradually tapering drugs that pose life-threatening physical risks during withdrawal, there are no formulas to tell you how long to take when withdrawing from a drug. However, as mentioned earlier, I sometimes suggest to patients that they consider taking a month or more for every year they have been on the drug or similar drugs from the same category such as antidepressants, neuroleptics and mood stabilizers, stimulants, and tranquilizer/sleeping pills. The main point is to emphasize caution.

When determining how long you've been exposed to a drug, be sure to take into account drugs that are in the same category, such as tranquilizers or stimulants. Thus, if you've been on Valium for six months and Ativan for another six months, you have been taking benzodiazepine tranquilizers for a year and will probably require a month at least for withdrawal. Similarly, if you took Ritalin for four months and Adderall for five months, you've been exposed to addictive stimulants for nine months. If you have been taking many different kinds of antipsychotic drugs over a ten-year period, your total exposure to antipsychotic drugs is ten years. Overall, if you've been taking almost any psychiatric drug or class of psychiatric drugs for twelve months, you might need at least a month to withdraw comfortably—and that may not be sufficient!

The following sections address unique aspects of withdrawing from the individual categories of psychiatric drug.

Antidepressants

Both the newer and the old antidepressants are listed in appendix A. All of them can cause withdrawal problems, including emotional reactions that can become manic or depressive in quality with a heightened risk of aggression or suicidality. All of the newer antidepressants such as Prozac, Paxil, Lexapro, Zoloft, Celexa, and Effexor can be extremely difficult to withdraw from. If you have been taking these drugs for several months or years, you probably need counseling as well as drug-monitoring with an understanding, informed professional.

Some doctors will switch patients from the short-acting Paxil to the longer-acting Prozac in the hope of attenuating the withdrawal reaction. To avoid adding complexity by switching drugs, I have preferred to keep patients on Paxil while weaning down to very small doses. In tough withdrawal cases, I may end up prescribing Paxil Oral Suspension (the fluid form) administered by means of an eyedropper for the last tiny doses. In these cases, I make sure that the pharmacist and my patient communicate about exactly how to use the eyedropper.

Antidepressant-withdrawal symptoms include not only the whole range of emotional reactions from anxiety to depression and mania, but also physical ones such as ringing in the ears, dizziness, and feelings of instability, or a variety of horrible sensations often compared to shocks or electricity in the head, body, or skin. Here's a summary of relatively common antidepressant-withdrawal symptoms:[1]

- Psychiatric—mood swings; anxiety and severe panic; depression, mania; suicidal feelings, irritability and excessive anger, insomnia, vivid dreams
- Abnormal neurological sensations—dizziness, spinning, or feelings of instability; abnormal skin sensations; abnormal sounds and noise hypersensitivity; shocklike feelings especially in the head
- Abnormal movements—tremor; muscle spasms; impaired balance and drunklike walking
- Gastrointestinal—anorexia; nausea; vomiting; diarrhea
- Whole body—weakness; extreme tiredness and fatigue; muscle pain; chills; sweating
- Others—visual problems; hair standing on end; flushing (persistent blushing)

These symptoms are physical, not psychological, in origin. If a pregnant mother takes antidepressants, then the infant will go through toxicity in the uterus and then undergo withdrawal symptoms after it is born. These drugs also enter into breast milk, causing toxicity and withdrawal symptoms in the nursing infant.

Although it seems counterintuitive, antidepressants can cause depression, anxiety, and mania while they are being taken as well as while they are being tapered and stopped. This is true for many withdrawal symptoms: they can occur while an individual is taking the drug and also during withdrawal. Keep in mind that if you develop depressive, anxious, irritable, or manic feelings within days or a few weeks of starting to taper an antidepressant, it is most likely a withdrawal reaction rather than the return of your original emotional problems. Recognizing that the emotional changes are induced by withdrawal and probably short-lived can help you to weather them.

Antidepressant withdrawal much more commonly causes depression and anxiety compared to mania, but mania can be an especially disastrous if unusual withdrawal reaction. Mania is so spellbinding that you are likely to be the last person to realize what's happening to you. Be alert, and ask your family, friends, and doctor to watch for any signs that you're getting "high," euphoric, impulsive, or otherwise unrealistically exuberant about yourself and your life.

Do not stop antidepressants secretly. It is too dangerous to be alone and isolated during the process. Try to find a sympathetic, experienced professional and be sure to enlist family members or a friend in the process of keeping an eye on you.

In my experience, many patients notice that their antidepressant-withdrawal symptoms begin to abate after a few days or one week, and finally disappear entirely over a few weeks. For some unfortunate people, they persist for many months and sometimes seem to become permanent. Recently, one of my patients decided to resume taking Celexa 10 mg per day because, over a drug-free period of several months, feelings of dizziness and instability had not gone away. She experienced some relief of these distressing symptoms within three days of restarting Celexa, but has not returned to normal. She had been taking antidepressants for many years, during which time she became progressively emotionally dulled, and in order to avoid that happening again, she plans to attempt withdrawal once again in the future.

Stimulants

All stimulants—they are listed in appendix A—pose the potential for causing withdrawal reactions. The most common withdrawal reaction is "crashing" with fatigue, depression, lengthy periods of sleep, and overeating. It's the opposite of being stimulated. The biggest risk is suicide. Much like the antidepressants, these drugs are a suicide risk while being taken and while being stopped. If your child has been taking stimulants continuously for several months or more, withdrawal should require at least several weeks with careful parental and professional monitoring.

If your child has routinely come off stimulants with no signs of difficulty on weekends and school holidays, then there is probably not much risk involved in simply stopping the drug. After all, you've already stopped the drugs many times before without anything going wrong. Nonetheless, I always prefer to taper stimulants for a few weeks just to be on the safe side.

While your child is coming off a psychiatric drug such as Ritalin, you should check with his or her teachers to see if any unusual behavior has been observed, but you may not want to tell the teachers what you are doing. Too many teachers have become ardent promoters of drugs to control their classrooms. When one of their students misses a drug dose and shows signs of withdrawal, they mistakenly believe that the student "needs" the medication, when in reality the child needs a chance to experience a tapered withdrawal. In most cases, keep your child's teacher in the dark but stay in touch with the school to see how your boy or girl is doing.

Parents often find it best to taper their child off medications during vacations, especially the long summer break. That way the children aren't simultaneously going through the stresses of school while stopping their medication.

Here is advice that cannot go wrong: While your child's medication is being tapered, be sure to keep in touch whenever your child is alone during the day, and also in the morning before going to school, in the afternoon on arriving home, at dinner, and before bed. If you make it a habit to smile at your child and to look for the gleam in his or her eye whenever you meet, and if you check on how he or she is feeling a few times a day, you might find that you want to keep up this loving, rewarding routine long after the drug is no longer an issue.

Keep in mind that children who take stimulants have an increased risk in young adulthood of abusing street drugs such as cocaine. You may even want to warn your children about it. They may think they want to experiment with drugs, but for them it's too risky. Their brains have adapted to these drugs, making them vulnerable to seeking drugs in the future and making them more sensitive to addictive drug effects when exposed at a later date.

I have actively campaigned to stop prescribing stimulant drugs to our children. As I describe in *Talking Back to Ritalin* (2001) and *The Ritalin Fact Book* (2002), there are always better alternatives. In addition to my books, the shelves of any large bookstore are lined with manuals about how to teach and to raise children without diagnosing and drugging them. Rather than suggesting my own favorites, I urge you to page through a number of them until you find one or two that appeal to you. Many parents also find parenting classes very useful and they are often offered free or at little charge by city or county family programs.

Tranquilizer/Sleeping Pills

Tranquilizers (antianxiety drugs) and sleeping medications are listed in appendix A. Although all are potentially very hazardous to withdraw from, Xanax and Halcion are among the worst. I have also seen people have grave difficulty withdrawing from Ativan and Klonopin. All of the drugs in this group can cause seizures and catastrophic levels of anxiety and insomnia during withdrawal. High levels of anxiety and loss of sleep can lead to agitation and depression, and ultimately to destructive behaviors. Nausea, vomiting, weight loss, hypersensitivity, muscle twitches, and painful muscular spasms are common during withdrawal after prolonged exposure to these chemicals. Delirium, confusion, paranoia, hallucinations, and delusions can occur in severe withdrawal cases.

If you've been on these drugs for several days or more, anticipate difficulties coming off, particularly insomnia and anxiety. Patients taking Xanax for panic disorder for only several weeks often had grave difficulties withdrawing from the drug, and a significant number are unable to stop. You can find these dreadful facts buried in the label for Xanax in the *Physicians' Desk Reference.*

If you've been taking tranquilizing drugs or sleeping pills for several months or years, be especially prepared for a tough time: enlist all the help you can get, and go slowly. Expect some of your withdrawal symptoms to persist for several weeks or more, although in all likelihood they will eventually disappear. Unfortunately, I have worked with a few patients who for months after withdrawing have experienced continuing memory and concentration problems, and various physical discomforts, such as abnormal feelings in the skin, leg cramps, or inflammationlike pain in the nerves to the feet.

The long-term prescription of tranquilizers and sleeping pills is a very bad idea. If you've been taking these drugs for more than a few weeks, consider tapering off them as soon as possible, while keeping in mind that withdrawal can be dangerous and difficult.

Antipsychotic Drugs

Although prescribing physicians often seem oblivious to this clinical fact, withdrawing from antipsychotic drugs can be extremely difficult and sometimes impossible. As already described, children or adults who have taken these drugs for months or years often become more psychotic than ever when they try to withdraw. The phenomenon is called tardive psychosis. They may also undergo frightening and sometimes painful withdrawal dyskinesia—abnormal movements that hopefully will disappear with time but may turn into permanent tardive dyskinesia. Patients may also become nauseated and have trouble eating during withdrawal. Some become anorexic. In addition, these drugs can be very damaging to the mental processes over years of exposure, and stopping them can make more apparent the degree of cognitive impairment.

Withdrawing from antipsychotic drugs is so potentially difficult that a strong social network is imperative. Many people taking these drugs are impaired by their own emotional difficulties as well as by the drug, and to succeed in withdrawing they may need close monitoring, a day treatment program, and a family network. Without a supportive social network, it can be hazardous to help people come off long-term antipsychotic drug exposure. Yet, many of these people are relatively isolated from society, making it difficult or impossible to safely taper their medications.

On the other hand, there is always reason to hope that previously disturbed patients will do very well when removed from long-term antipsychotic treatment. Especially when very disturbed patients have been alerted and mobilized by signs of tardive dyskinesia, I have seen them rise to the necessity of living drug free. For example, recently I was chatting on the phone with a Canadian attorney about a tardive dyskinesia malpractice case that I am currently working on concerning a woman who at the age of thirty developed drug-induced mouth movements (puckering); facial grimacing; turning movements of her head and twisting movements of her neck; severe arching of the back; jerking, twisting, flailing, and other abnormal movements of her arms and shoulders; tremors of her arms and hands; and increased tone of her limbs. Although not all of these symptoms afflicted her at the same time, she was always severely impaired.

This tardive dyskinesia victim had been taking antipsychotic drugs for at least five years before she eventually developed this florid, disabling case while taking Risperdal for the final few months. The attorney remarked to me with considerable surprise that despite her continued severe abnormal movements, she was doing very well emotionally and much better than when she was taking her prescribed drugs. I explained to him that this was common in my experience.

Many tardive dyskinesia patients I have treated have felt fortunate that their neurological symptoms led to the discontinuation of their mind-blunting drugs. After stopping the drugs, their quality of life—except for the tardive dyskinesia—has improved. When the tardive dyskinesia has turned out to be mild or when on occasion it has gone into remission, these patients find themselves living far better than when they were on the drugs.

The lesson from this? Antipsychotic drugs do make patients and inmates more compliant and numb in the short term, thereby easing management problems, but they end up doing much more harm than good. If long-term patients can go through the potentially tormenting withdrawal process, most will end up much better off without these toxic, mind-bending agents that also pose life-threatening risks such as neuroleptic malignant syndrome, liver disease, stroke, diabetes, pancreatitis, obesity, and elevated cholesterol levels.

Mood Stabilizers

Some mood stabilizers were originally FDA-approved to treat epilepsy. With these drugs, there is a risk of undergoing a seizure during abrupt withdrawal. Other drugs sometimes used as mood stabilizers have only been approved to treat hypertension, and there is a risk of a dangerous blood-pressure spike if these drugs are not tapered. These medications are listed in appendix A.

Stopping lithium has been shown to cause mania or maniclike withdrawal symptoms, as well as a general rebound worsening, including depression.[2] This risk must be communicated to anyone withdrawing from lithium, as well as to family members. After withdrawal is complete, there is increased risk of suffering a manic episode in the next few weeks or months. Since mania is especially spellbinding, it's critical for people other than the patient to be involved in a supervisory capacity.

It is not known whether tapering helps to prevent withdrawal mania, but stopping any mood-stabilizing drug slowly is usually a good idea. Although there's not much data on drugs other than lithium, be on the safe side and assume that stopping any mood stabilizer may increase the risk of emotional instability, including mania.

SPECIFIC TREATMENTS FOR WITHDRAWAL

There are at present no specific medications that help with drug withdrawal, other than tapering the offending agent or similar drugs. I do not know of any supplements with proven value for drug withdrawal but you can certainly find many suggestions in books and on the Internet. In general, remember that anything you take that "works," even if it is "natural," is adding to the load of chemicals that your brain must contend with.

Moderate exercise is healthy for all of us and can be very valuable when withdrawing from drugs. Eating healthy and getting plenty of sleep is also important. Spending time doing things you really enjoy is a great help in withdrawing, and in life in general. Spending time with people you like is also a good idea. Caring social contacts help keep us in touch with reality and provide some monitoring for how we are doing during withdrawal. *In short, when withdrawing from drugs, do all those emotionally and physically healthy things you know you should already be doing—and then keep on doing them for the rest of your life.*

GETTING PROFESSIONAL HELP

IF THE WITHDRAWAL IS DIFFICULT, counseling can be supportive and reassuring, and even lifesaving. If you've been taking drugs because of serious personal difficulties and emotional distress, then you need to find help during and after the withdrawal process. Do not delay getting help for the problems that led you to start drugs in first place.

Individual, couples, and family therapy can be very helpful during drug withdrawal. However, keep in mind that a therapy is no better than the therapist's personal ability; that therapies vary enormously from one to another in approach; that the cornerstone of therapy is the caring and trusting relationship with the therapist; and that you may have to shop around to find the right therapist for you. In my own practice, I always make drug withdrawal contingent on the individual being in therapy with me or with someone else whom we both trust. As an alternative to a psychiatrist, most of whom resist helping patients taper off their medications, find a family doctor who is willing to monitor your withdrawal while you find a helpful counselor or psychotherapist who is trained in talking therapy rather than in dispensing drugs.

Whenever possible, involve someone in your family in the withdrawal process, especially your husband or your wife. Couples therapy provides more than individual help—it can teach individuals to help each other. Many people also find it very helpful to become involved in church, Alcoholics Anonymous meetings, or other support groups. The more actively you are contributing to the lives of other people, the more successful you will be in your own life.

Don't make any big decisions while you are in the process of withdrawing from drugs. Wait until you feel clearheaded and on an even keel before deciding anything life-changing.

HOW LONG WILL WITHDRAWAL SYMPTOMS LAST?

UNFORTUNATELY, it is hard to come up with precise answers. In general, if the withdrawal symptoms start to subside in a few days, you're probably going to be symptom free in a relatively short time, perhaps in days or in weeks. If the symptoms do not subside quickly, there is no way to know with certainty how long they will last. Contrary to what most physicians tell their patients, some people experience lasting residual difficulties after they stop any class of psychiatric drug. Memory and concentration problems are especially common, as well as unstable moods and irritability, weakness, and fatigue.

Even if you have lasting mental difficulties that can be attributed to taking psychiatric drugs, do not let this prevent you from living a good life. My experience with patients, and with survivors of psychiatric treatment with whom I've worked in the psychiatric reform movement, has taught me that the human spirit can triumph over persistent impairments in mental function, such as memory problems or difficulty concentrating caused by exposure to drugs or to shock treatment. It is as if we have so much brain power in reserve that a determined spirit can overcome a great deal of drug-induced residual malfunction. In the psychiatric survivor movement especially, I have gotten to know people who have overcome the damage done by lengthy exposures to many devastating drugs and even electroshock. Although they remain aware of residual effects, so great is their courage and their spiritual strength that they have triumphed over these deficits to live satisfying, productive, and happy lives.

MEDICAL EMERGENCIES THAT MAY REQUIRE RAPID DRUG WITHDRAWAL

WHEN CONFRONTING DRUG-INDUCED EMERGENCIES of a *physical* nature, every effort must be made to stop the drug immediately or as soon as possible. For example, the development of abnormal movements while taking any antipsychotic drug such as Zyprexa or Risperdal, or any newer antidepressant such as Prozac or Paxil, should be cause for immediate concern. The abnormal movements could signal the start of tardive dyskinesia, the potentially irreversible drug-induced neurological disorder that afflicted several of our cases.

Antipsychotic drugs can cause a potentially lethal neuroleptic malignant syndrome and antidepressants can cause a potentially lethal serotonin syndrome. In varying combinations in these two disorders the symptoms can include fever, flulike aches and pains, rigidity or abnormal movements, unstable blood pressure or heart rate, and impaired consciousness. If these reactions are suspected, the medications must be stopped.

Any sign of diabetes or pancreatitis while taking the newer antipsychotic drugs requires the immediate withdrawal of the drugs. A new heart arrhythmia or other heart problem while taking almost any psychiatric drug, including stimulants, can be life threatening and requires immediate intervention. A seizure, serious rash, headache, gastrointestinal problem, liver disorder, joint or muscle pain, abnormal bleeding, or treatment-resistant infection while taking almost any psychiatric drug is another signal for an immediate evaluation and may require cessation of the medication. Loss of consciousness, faintness on sitting or standing up, dizziness and falling are wake-up calls for an immediate reevaluation of medications. Cognitive changes such as memory difficulties and confusion signal an immediate need to evaluate the medication regimen.

Because psychiatric drugs can impair the body's control centers in the brain, it is impossible to categorize all of the potential physical disasters that they can cause. Virtually every organ in the body is put at risk by one or another drug. *Any change for the worse in your physical condition should alert you to the potential need to stop your psychiatric drugs.*

Similarly, in severe drug-induced emergency of an *emotional* or psychiatric nature, immediate consideration should be given to stopping psychiatric medication. All categories of psychiatric drugs—antipsychotic, antidepressant, mood stabilizing, stimulant, and tranquilizing/sleeping medications—can cause serious emotional instability, including depression and anxiety with suicidality, agitation with aggression, and occasionally psychosis. Antidepressants, stimulants, and tranquilizers can cause mania, depression, and high-risk disinhibition. In all of these instances, professional help is needed to deal with the potential emergency and to determine how to stop the drugs as quickly and as safely as possible under the circumstances.

As already mentioned, any changes in memory and thinking should also be considered a warning sign about adverse drug effects. Many psychiatric drugs can cause confusion and delirium. *Any change for the worse in your mental or emotional condition, like any change in your physical condition, should immediately make you suspect a possible adverse reaction to your psychiatric medication and the potential necessity of weaning off as quickly and safely as possible.*

ADDITIONAL SOURCES OF INFORMATION

IN PHYSICAL AND EMOTIONAL DRUG-INDUCED emergencies, immediate consultation with a physician may be necessary. But keep in mind that your doctor may not recognize or know about the adverse drug affect that is afflicting you. Especially in regard to emotional or psychological adverse drug effects, he or she may not know as much as you have learned from reading this book. If you've spent a few intensive hours on the Internet looking up the potentially harmful effects of the particular drugs you are taking, you are likely to be better informed about it than the vast majority of physicians who simply do not have the time to keep up with every drug. If your physician says, "No, never, your drug could not possibly do that," he or she could easily be wrong.

You can also find many general sources of information on the Web such as www.WebMD.com but they offer conventional summaries that tend to advocate drug company viewpoints and cannot always be trusted. In your library or bookstore you can obtain the *Physicians' Desk Reference* or, even better, *Drug Facts and Comparisons* to find detailed up-to-date FDA-approved kinds of information such as your doctor probably relies on—but establishment information outlets must be supplemented with an Internet search for adverse effects that the medical profession or FDA refuses or neglects to acknowledge. You can also look up actual research studies on www.PubMed.gov.

You can find additional information on drug withdrawal in my books that focus on specific groups of medications, such as *The Antidepressant Fact Book* (2001) and *The Ritalin Fact Book* (2002), as well as the more comprehensive *Your Drug May Be Your Problem: How and Why to Stop Taking Psychiatric Medications* (with David Cohen, updated in 2007). For an overall understanding of the harmful effects of psychiatric drugs on the brain and mind, my 2008 edition of *Brain-Disabling Treatments in Psychiatry* is the most comprehensive text available.

DO WITHDRAWAL SYMPTOMS CAUSE PERMANENT DAMAGE?

SOMETIMES WHEN PATIENTS STOP their antipsychotic drugs, abruptly unmasking their underlying abnormal movements, ignorant or unscrupulous doctors will tell the patients that they "caused" their own symptoms by stopping too quickly. On the contrary, the drug was already causing the underlying disorder. The abrupt withdrawal merely brought out what was already happening and helped to prevent further deterioration caused by continued drug exposure.

There is no scientific reason to believe that the physical symptoms and pain suffered during withdrawal will cause further damage. Instead, they are signs of preexisting dysfunction or damage that hopefully will clear up with time when the offending agent is stopped.

A SUCCESSFUL WITHDRAWAL

AFTER WORKING without much enjoyment or progress at routine jobs through her mid-twenties, Emma Vitello decided to pursue her original love for music by returning to graduate school for a master's degree. She wanted to play and to compose.

Emma found grad school much more stressful than anticipated. Her teachers seemed more interested in putting their students through a grim academic hazing than in nurturing their sensitivity and creativity. For Emma, music came from the heart; it was spiritual. For her teachers, it seemed to come more from the mind, as if produced by a computer. Their music and their teaching felt mechanical to her. Several even made fun of Emma for her spontaneity.

Unfortunately, Emma didn't trust her own judgment and she was also unwilling to quit school. She went to the university clinic where she was prescribed Paxil 20 mg per day to get her through her anxiety.

Sometimes, Paxil exacerbates anxiety; sometimes, it blunts it. In Emma's case, the Paxil may have flattened her anxiety and enabled her to compete more compulsively, but her creativity declined. Emma got down to work and earned outstanding grades but along the way she lost interest in writing and playing music. By graduation she felt she had "nothing left."

Had Emma's teachers squelched her confidence and hence her spontaneous creativity and spirituality? Had the Paxil put a clamp on her more sensitive self? Or was it a combination? Emma was unsure what had happened. Sadly, she concluded that probably she was not really a creative person after all. She decided she would have to find something less artistic to do after graduation.

After graduation Emma continued on Paxil, now prescribed by her general practitioner, and she took a disappointing job as a music teacher. It was a default choice resulting from her loss of zest for writing and playing, and her subsequent loss of confidence in her abilities. She was now happily married but continued to languish in regard to her creativity. After nearly a year, she grew intolerably frustrated and unhappy, and decided to seek help. She came to me for therapy and for a reevaluation of her medication.

After a few sessions of horror stories about graduate school, it was clear that taking the master's degree had crushed Emma like a flower pressed inside a heavy academic tome. But why was she so unable to blossom once again? Was it the continuing Paxil?

Under my direction, Emma began slowly withdrawing from Paxil. She suffered bouts of anxiety and moodiness along the way but continued with the process. Eventually, she was able to do well while breaking her 5 mg tablets in half, and within a couple of more weeks she felt comfortable stopping altogether.

Everything went fine until two days after her last 5 mg dose of Paxil. Then, on day three over a weekend, the withdrawal hit: dizziness, a violently throbbing headache, and outbursts of sobbing. I had given Emma my home number and was glad when she overcame her usual diffidence and called me. She explained she could handle the mood swings. Her husband had been warned that she was going through withdrawal and he was supportive. He would keep her close by his side until she felt better. She also believed she could bear the headaches. But there was something terrifying about the bizarre sensations of imbalance, not so much a spinning but a feeling that she was so unstable she could topple over. The sensation became especially distressing when she moved her neck, causing her to sit still for long periods of time while holding herself rigid.

It took a while on the phone to figure out what was really scaring Emma. She could handle the immediate distress. But she was afraid the symptoms of imbalance were causing more damage that would end up permanently harming her. She asked if she should restart the Paxil to avoid doing permanent damage by allowing the dreadful imbalance sensations to continue.

I reassured her that the withdrawal symptoms could not in themselves physically harm her. The symptoms were distressing but not physically damaging. Because the symptoms indicated that Paxil had already been having a harmful effect, they confirmed the importance of attempting to complete the withdrawal process if she could weather the discomfort. I also reminded her that she could always stop the withdrawal symptoms by resuming the Paxil at the level of her last dose, and then we could reconsider the final withdraw steps later on when she felt stronger. After my reassurance that the symptoms in themselves were not harmful, Emma decided to remain drug free until our next session the coming week.

I phoned Emma again over the weekend to check on her. I left a message on her answering machine to remind her that I was concerned and available.

When I saw her in my office three days later, she was feeling much better and was confident about getting through the withdrawal period.

The bouts of sobbing lasted a week or ten days before abating and the sensation of imbalance lasted an additional week before completely disappearing. Soon after the headaches stopped as well.

Within a month of stopping the Paxil, Emma no longer suffered from obvious withdrawal effects and, much to her relief and gratification, she began rediscovering her love of music. She started to play music by herself with more energy. Then, for the first time since beginning Paxil four years earlier, Emma felt spontaneous impulses to jot down notes for possible musical pieces that were coming alive inside her. Within a couple months, she was once again active and earning a living as a writer and musician.

Once again, I want to emphasize that psychiatric drugs, one and all, reduce or cloud the highest human functions, including love, creativity, and spirituality—but many spellbound victims will not realize that this is happening to them. They will continue taking their drugs, oblivious to how much of themselves they have lost. Even young artists like Emma Vitello who are devoted to their creativity can end up rationalizing their diminished ability and interest, lapsing into relatively lackluster lives. Many people have no idea what they've been missing until they stop taking their psychiatric medications.

Chapter 22

The Tough Question of Personal Responsibility

"THE DRUG MADE ME DO IT!" No one likes the sound of that. Most of my patients and legal clients do not like it, either. After committing horrendous acts while taking psychiatric drugs, the people I have evaluated have almost always been horrified and at a loss to explain how they could have behaved so badly. Usually, they have approached the explanation of drug-induced madness with skepticism, often hearing about it for the first time from friends or relatives who have searched the Internet. After all, they had no idea that prescribed medications could have such drastic effects or they wouldn't have taken them in the first place. Even after they begin to realize that spellbinding and medication madness have afflicted them, they remain reluctant to embrace the full implications. Unless they have lost all sense of worth and efficacy, people want to believe in personal responsibility.

To what degree should society hold people responsible for succumbing to medication madness? The answer hinges in part on whether we think that these people were biologically driven or psychologically motivated—whether they were victims of brain dysfunction or guilty of bad decision-making.

Throughout this book, we have found irrefutable evidence that spellbinding—and its extreme of medication madness—is physical or biological in origin. At the risk of oversimplifying the many case studies and scientific points made in this book, here's a summary of reasons why we know that medication madness is biological:[1]

- If we place children or adults in controlled clinical trials, where some receive a psychiatric drug and others receive a sugar pill, those receiving the psychiatric drug are far more likely to develop a wide range of adverse mental reactions, including depression, mania, and suicidality. This has been proven time and again in clinical trials involving every kind of psychoactive drug. Psychoactive drugs cause madness.

- If we study children and adults in clinics and hospitals who are being treated with medications such as antidepressants and stimulants, the treated patients will develop many more severe mental reactions than those who do not receive the drugs.

- The FDA-approved labels for drugs often cite the risk of patients developing drug-induced mental aberrations from agitation, anxiety, hostility, suicidality, and depression through hallucinations, delusions, and psychosis. This is true for all psychiatric drugs and also for many nonpsychiatric drugs as well, even some antibiotics that affect the brain and mind.

- Many recreational drugs, including hallucinogens and alcohol, provide a familiar model for drug-induced spellbinding and madness.

- Episodes of medication madness can often be traced to starting the drug or to changing its dose, and the madness usually abates once the drug is stopped. In clinical studies involving challenge, dechallenge, and rechallenge we have seen patients develop obsessive suicidality while taking an antidepressant, lose it when the drug is stopped, and reexperience it when the drug is restarted. Similarly, few of our cases displayed any bizarre or criminal acts before taking the medications and *none* displayed them after recovering from them.

- Spellbinding often (but not always) is associated with obvious biological symptoms such as tremor or sweating, as well as cognitive dysfunctions such as memory impairment and confusion, which are consistent with brain dysfunction.

- Physically traumatic events such as head injury, electroshock, and lobotomy can also cause spellbinding, and can result in bizarre, potentially destructive, and out-of-character behavior.

Because most of the adverse drug reactions in this book manifest themselves as mental or emotional aberrations, it remains tempting to think that they are psychological in origin. Because they can occur in the absence of grosser bodily dysfunctions, such as a paralysis or tremors, there is a tendency to conclude that there is "nothing physically wrong" with the person. This is because the brain is the most sensitive organ in the body, and when damaged, the first signs are often mental or emotional. Furthermore, psychiatric drugs are selected for their capacity to impair brain function without obviously interfering with bodily functions.

The biological basis of spellbinding does not rule out the possibility that individual cases may be psychologically driven or that psychology may influence the direction or quality of the actions. That is why criteria have been developed for determining if a particular extreme behavior is most probably drug induced. As described in chapter 1, these criteria include:

- A recent change (up or down) in the dose of the medication;
- A relatively sudden onset and rapid escalation;
- Escalating symptoms of drug toxicity, such as insomnia, agitation, memory dysfunction, hallucinations, or other abnormal behaviors leading up to the event;
- An unusually violent, irrational, bizarre, or self-defeating quality to the behavior;
- An obsessive, compelling, and unrelenting quality to the behavior;
- A prior history indicating that the abnormal behaviors were uncharacteristic and unprecedented before exposure to the drug;
- The individual's subjective feeling that the feelings and actions are alien, inexplicable, and ethically repugnant;
- Gradual disappearance of the abnormal mental state after stopping the medication (although some residual effects may last much longer).

OVERWHELMED BY SEROTONIN

WHEN PATIENTS SUFFER from extreme drug toxicity, medication madness can occur along with gross and even life-threatening bodily dysfunction. For example, serotonin syndrome is a potentially lethal adverse reaction to the SSRI antidepressants and to other drugs such as Effexor that disrupt serotonin functions in the brain and body. In early stages, the syndrome causes hallucinations and confusion and in later stages it can be fatal. For some time, it has been known that the antidepressants can cause this reaction—I wrote about it in *Talking Back to Prozac* (1994)—but the drug companies have been slow to give sufficient recognition to it in their antidepressant labels.

In July 2006, the FDA at last forced the antidepressant manufacturers to put a warning in their labels describing the signs and symptoms of serotonin syndrome, including "restlessness, diarrhea, hallucinations, coma, loss of coordination, nausea, fast heartbeat, vomiting, increased body temperature, fast changes in blood pressure, [and] overactive reflexes."[2]

The FDA warning did not come in time to save a twelve-year-old girl whose story outraged and saddened me as much as any of my legal cases. Zoloft had been prescribed to this slip of a girl for several months when, two weeks before the catastrophe, her dose was increased to 25 mg per day and 25 mg at night when needed. (The use of "as needed" antidepressants is substandard and dangerous in part because the brain cannot adapt to the irregular dosing.)

A very good student and basically happy child, the young girl had been experiencing some anxiety, especially around schoolwork. One night she felt especially anxious about returning to school after winter vacation, and she asked her parents if she could take her elective evening dose of Zoloft. Her mother was in the shower at the time and thought that it would be okay for her daughter, for the first time, to take the pill unsupervised. By mistake, the child took her father's 50 mg dose, giving her a total of 75 mg—still well below the commonly used maximum dose for children and adolescents. Shortly after, she became severely agitated and displayed hallucinations. She was taken to the hospital where she displayed almost every one of the symptoms of serotonin syndrome described by the FDA, including hallucinations, except she did not lapse into coma.

The hospital doctors acted stupidly beyond belief, at one time ordering more Zoloft for her—even after diagnosing a Zoloft-induced serotonergic syndrome. It is unclear how much of the drug was actually administered to her, but the hospital bill charged for three doses of Zoloft 50 mg on the last two days in the hospital—even more than she had been previously prescribed before coming to the hospital. In another colossal misjudgment, the hospital then discharged her after only three and one-half days, before she had fully recovered. To make matters worse, the hospital staff issued conflicting orders to restart her Zoloft on discharge or to have her doctor restart it at the first visit.

Her private psychiatrist saw the child two days later—six days after the start of the severe adverse reaction to Zoloft—and he was smart enough not to resume the agent that had already intoxicated his patient. However, the drug was not through taking its deadly toll. Two days later, the lovely little girl hanged herself to death.

On autopsy, she still had Zoloft in her system, confirming that she was probably heavily dosed in the hospital, so that some remained in her body two days afterward. The association between physical and psychological symptoms in serotonin syndrome confirms the biological origin of the psychological symptoms.

CONVINCING THE LEGISLATORS

I WAS TESTIFYING before a committee of the Colorado State Legislature concerning why I thought the legislators should oppose the widespread drugging of schoolchildren. As a part of my presentation, I pointed out that medicating children causes some of them to become violent and others to become suicidal. The legislators had a close-to-home example of both in Eric Harris, who was taking Luvox at the time he slaughtered his classmates at Columbine High School and then committed suicide.

In response to my remarks, an earnest and sincere legislator challenged me about "making excuses" for violence. He pointed out that drunkenness is no excuse for bad behavior in the eyes of the law and that it shouldn't be.

I responded, first, by reminding him that we were talking about children. What if a small child were given alcohol by an adult and then behaved badly? Would the legislator hold the child to such a hard line of personal responsibility—or would he blame the alcohol and the person who gave it to the child? Similarly, both child and adult patients given psychiatric drugs are rarely forewarned about the potential for medication madness and have no expectation that their drugs could drive them to lose self-control. This lack of prior information increases the risk of becoming spellbound and establishes a potential criminal defense of involuntary intoxication.

MORALITY IN MOLECULES

I DON'T BLAME PEOPLE for resisting the moral implications of these stories. Many of my observations in this book fly in the face of everything I once believed about free will. Thirty years ago, as a young psychiatrist, I would have been outraged by the claim that drugs can influence human nature and human choice-making to such a degree. At that time, I rejected the idea that a drug could make any of us do anything we genuinely did not want to do.

Then in the early 1980s, I began researching more thoroughly into the adverse effects of psychiatric drugs and wrote *Psychiatric Drugs: Hazards to the Brain* (1983). The result? My growing clinical experience and the vast body of the scientific literature that I studied began to change my opinion about how much drugs can and do modify our behavior. The scientific data became overwhelming—psychoactive agents, including psychiatric drugs, frequently drive people to commit violence and suicide.

Philosophy drove my original conclusions; science refuted them. Desiring that people have free will and self-determination—wanting above all else for people to take personal responsibility for their actions—I had not looked in sufficient depth and detail at the data. Eventually, I would become one of the world's experts on that kind of data—but at the time I was relying mostly on idealistic philosophy with a dash of science thrown in from my basic medical and psychiatric training.

THE CRUX OF THE MATTER

THROUGHOUT THIS BOOK we have found that research studies and especially clinical trials demonstrate surprisingly high rates of medication madness. As I've previously emphasized, prescribe an effective dose of any psychiatric drug to one hundred people, and in the same experiment give an equal number of similar people a sugar pill, and you will invariably get the same result: Many more people on the psychiatric drug will develop psychological or psychiatric aberrations than those on the sugar pill, and the especially severe reactions will be limited almost entirely to those taking the drug.

This simple experiment—it's called a placebo-controlled clinical trial—has been repeated innumerable times with innumerable psychiatric drugs, always with the same result. To the degree that the drug has any psychoactive effect, all individuals will be changed in the way they think and feel, and some will develop reactions that noticeably impair them and lead to behaviors that they would otherwise not have undertaken. The drug reaction can range from slightly dulled emotions or increased irritability to a severely manic or psychotic episode.

As examples previously mentioned, studies of Luvox[3] and Prozac[4] in children found that those children receiving the drugs had very high rates of manic behavior (4 and 6 percent, respectively) while those receiving placebo had none. Rates for antidepressant-induced mania in adults in clinical practice are even higher (see chapter 6). Evidence like this leaves no room to doubt whether or not psychiatric drugs, and psychoactive substances in general, can make people behave in ways that are out of the ordinary for them, very disturbed and potentially dangerous.

Not everyone who takes Prozac becomes overstimulated and manic. Not everyone who takes Paxil becomes obsessively suicidal. The vast majority of people don't become dangerous to themselves or to others as a result of taking antidepressants, stimulants, or benzodiazepines. But there is a greatly increased likelihood of a worsening mental condition for those who take the drugs.

As far back as I can remember I have wanted to hold myself responsible for my actions. I realized that it was not only ethical but also effective to be in charge of myself. In my psychiatric practice to this very day I approach people with the aim of helping them become more able to take charge of their own lives. Responsibility for our personal lives, along with the promotion of liberty and of love, lies at the center of my philosophy and psychology. Even when people are suffering from drug intoxication during drug withdrawal, I encourage them to take more responsibility for themselves—but I do so while recognizing that the drug-induced impairments are making it more difficult for them.

THE IMPORTANCE OF VALUES

I HAVE NOT CHANGED my underlying philosophy about how people should conduct their lives. In every aspect of my life and work, I encourage people to take full responsibility for every action and to take overall charge of their lives. Even when I work with brain-damaged patients, I encourage them to muster all of their self-determination and to live by the best possible values in order to improve their lives and the lives of everyone they touch. In this regard, I place much more emphasis on principled living than the average psychiatrist who thinks he is treating a physical disorder. But clinical experience and scientific studies have given me a new respect for how badly drugs can disrupt our emotional stability and ethical capacity.

WHAT DO OTHER PSYCHIATRISTS HAVE TO SAY?

OVER MANY YEARS I have found that almost none of my psychiatric colleagues will dare to discuss or to debate the kinds of issues raised in this book, including medication madness and the brain-disabling effects of psychiatric drugs. The evidence is simply too strong in favor of what I am saying. Every decade or so, however, a ranking British psychiatrist agrees to debate me on his home turf.

For example, in April 2006, at a packed forum held in the *Guardian* news-paper building in London, I debated a respected British colleague on the question, "Do psychiatric drugs do more harm than good?" I argued for the proposition that psychiatric medications cause an enormous amount of harm and do very little, if any, good. In this formal debate, I was seconded by British psychiatrist Joanna Moncrieff and the opposing psychiatrist was seconded by a high-ranking official in a British psychiatric association. The debate was sponsored by my friend and colleague Bob Johnson, a courageous British psychiatrist.

As a physician and psychiatrist, and as a scientist, I focused my debate presentation on data similar to the studies I have reviewed throughout this book and even in more detail in my medical books and scientific publications. The opposition had little familiarity with this scientific literature and even if they knew the literature, it would not have supported their viewpoint. As a result, they had little to offer in rebuttal. At the end of the *Guardian* debate, the audience voted on the question of whose presentation was more convincing. The vote was 85 to 3 in favor of my proposition that psychiatric drugs do more harm than good. There were eight abstentions.[5]

Ten years earlier, in a one-on-one debate with the president of a large British psychiatric academy that was conducted in his own hometown, the result was almost identical. It has been even longer since a major American psychiatric figurehead has been willing to debate me on the subject of the risks and benefits of medication. The last time was 1987, on *The Oprah Winfrey Show*, when I debated Paul Fink, then the elected president of the American Psychiatric Association, on the merits of psychiatric drugs. He vociferously attacked me, claiming that I misrepresented the facts when I cited the high rates of serious adverse effects from antipsychotic drugs. But I had been quoting from a thoroughly documented American Psychiatric Association report on the subject, which I promptly retrieved from beneath my seat and read aloud to the audience of millions.[6]

Psychiatry cannot contest the facts presented in this book and it will not risk debating the opinions.

MILLIONS OF SPIRITUAL DEATHS

STORIES OF GROSS DRUG-INDUCED madness grab attention but hopefully they can also make us more alert to the underlying patterns that may manifest more subtly in less severe cases. Psychiatric drugs have worsened the lives of innumerable adults and children without anyone realizing what has happened to them. Such is the spellbinding power of these agents. There are millions of daily drug-induced tragedies—barely discernable spiritual deaths—that go unnoticed. Children live their lives dampened down or outright suppressed by stimulant drugs. Children and adults taking antidepressants never know how out of touch they have become with their real feelings and hence their real selves. Antipsychotic drugs and mood stabilizers produce a continuum of emotional flattening that ranges from barely perceptible to cataclysmic, depending on the dose and individual sensitivity to drugs.

Millions of individuals are kept on mind-numbing drug combinations, often including cocktails of antipsychotics, antidepressants, mood stabilizers, stimulants, and benzodiazepine tranquilizers. It is often apparent that the drugs are grossly impairing the overall function of these people. Yet, they keep taking the drugs. It is a worldwide demonstration of spellbinding—not the kind that leads to violence and suicide but the kind that leads to a slow spiritual decline under the crushing weight of drug-induced brain dysfunction and damage. The central aspect of spellbinding—the capacity of psychoactive drugs to block recognition of drug-induced mental and emotional impairment—is at work in all these cases.

Often the signs are subtle: A woman loses her former interest in art and becomes a drone with no interests outside work; a man forgets that he once felt passionately toward his wife and attributes his diminished feeling to aging; a young man has felt depressed for years and thinks it is his fate in life; or a young woman is glad to no longer feel "oversensitive" without realizing that she has lost the subtleties of her emotional life. None of these people recognize that he or she is suffering chronic toxic effects of prescribed psychiatric medication.

More than any other class of drugs routinely prescribed in private practice, the antidepressants change people's lives for the worse while enforcing the illusion that everything's better. A man feels his marriage has become more tolerable. He can manage it now. But his wife feels that he has drifted so far apart from her that it has become worse than being separated. His body is in the house and even in the bed but his spirit has departed. He blows her off when she tries to talk about the changes she sees in him. He was "really depressed" before he started his Celexa.

A single young woman tells her family doctor that she can no longer have orgasms since starting her Paxil but that it doesn't matter since she's not dating anyone. She's devoting all her energy to her career. What she doesn't tell him—because she does not realize it—is that the drug has taken the passion out of her life. Even at work she has been reduced to a zestless, indifferent kind of performance.

A forty-year-old man leaves the woman he has loved for twenty years, dissipates his meager financial resources by renting a luxury apartment and buying a sports car, and ends up neglecting his children's needs. A midlife crisis? That's what he jokingly calls it. He thinks his Effexor is "great" and swears by his doctor.

The myriad ways in which psychiatric drugs flatten and disrupt feelings, and render people disconnected from their inner selves, is rarely if ever mentioned in scientific publications. Most doctors do not stop to think about it when prescribing antidepressants or carrying out their occasional medication checkups. Meanwhile, millions of people have the zest, spark, or spirit rubbed out of their lives without appreciating what is happening to them. In a kind of emotional anesthesia, they have been lulled into believing that they are doing better because of medication. At the same time, they may undergo episodes of disinhibition, making fools of themselves or hurting the feelings of loved ones, without appreciating the nature or consequences of their actions.

THE ULTIMATE CHOICE

ON THE BASIS OF STATISTICAL ANALYSES of clinical trials and epidemiology data, it is easy to prove that psychiatric drugs can drive people crazy. But it's much harder to draw conclusions about drug effects in individual cases. We can weigh various factors, as I've done many times in this book, and conclude whether or not a drug probably caused or contributed to a reaction; but certainty is hard to achieve. We are hampered not only by our inability to know what went on inside the individual's brain and mind, we are also hampered by the inability of the victims to know or to describe what has happened to them.

On a more philosophical level, we can study but never resolve the ultimate question of the power of choice or free will in fending off adverse drug reactions. We can, of course, say unequivocally that individuals can make a choice to avoid taking psychoactive substances, including psychiatric drugs, that can compromise their mental faculties; but we can never know for sure the role of choice and predisposition in how they respond to the biological impact of the drugs.

To repeat, psychiatric drugs do more harm than good. They impair the function of the brain and mind, spellbinding individuals into believing they are doing better when they are often doing worse. They have no "curative" power and instead blunt the emotions, cause indifference, or produce artificial euphoria, creating an illusion of improvement in a life that's not going to improve without taking more rational control. Beyond that, reliance on drugs undermines the ultimate purpose of human life—learning to know and to guide our own mental processes and emotions in order to live as ethically and fully as possible.

Each person needs to make an informed choice about risking exposure to the negative effects of psychiatric drugs. If you are already taking them, remember that stopping psychiatric drugs can also be dangerous and needs to be done carefully and with as much experienced clinical supervision as possible.

It is wisest to avoid any exposure to these toxic chemicals. The best decision, I believe, is not to start taking psychiatric drugs. I have conducted my psychiatric practice since its inception in 1968, without starting anyone on psychiatric drugs, although I often have to prescribe these medications in the process of helping people withdraw from them. I have found that a deep commitment to helping people through psychotherapy—often with the cooperation of family and community resources—is far more effective and much less hazardous than inflicting toxic agents on the brain.

At best, psychoactive drugs paint a shiny mildly spellbinding veneer over our lives; at worst they spellbind us so profoundly that we no longer have any idea what we think and feel, and who we really are. The best measure for preventing medication madness is not to start taking psychiatric drugs; if you decide to take them, then take as few as possible at the smallest possible dose, and stop taking them as soon as you can.

To help prevent spellbinding and medication madness, physicians, other healthcare professionals, patients, and their families need to become much more aware of how psychiatric drugs impact on the mind, including their capacity to blind the individual to their adverse mental and emotional effects. They also need to be able to recognize the telltale signs of spellbinding such as the early symptoms of mania and depression that appear repeatedly throughout our cases. Especially when a psychiatric drug is started or the dose is changed, any changes in personality and behavior should sound alarms. Signs of stimulation such as insomnia, agitation, anxiety, hyperactivity, irritability, and hostility should immediately alert professionals, patients, and families to a probable adverse drug reaction with potentially serious consequences. Similarly, signs of depression and apathy, gloominess, withdrawal, or self-destructiveness should be taken as a warning that the individual may be suffering from adverse drug effects. Health professionals and prescribers far too often blame these symptoms on the patient's "mental illness" and end up raising the dose or adding additional drugs, instead of tapering or stopping the offending agent.

The array of adverse psychiatric-drug reactions is too vast and varied to be reduced to a formal list. Psychiatric drugs can cause the whole array of emotions and thoughts that lead to self-defeating and destructive actions. One reason for telling so many stories in this book is to familiarize the reader with the vast range of potentially harmful reactions caused by these medications. When you or someone else you know is taking a psychiatric drug, consider that almost any negative mental, emotional, or behavioral reaction can be the result of drug toxicity.

We must also take into account the harm done to cultural values and to society by the widespread use of psychiatric drugs. Instead of encouraging children and adults to take responsibility for their lives and to learn to manage their emotions in productive ways, we are creating generations of drug consumers who have no idea how to live with a clear brain and mind, and how to improve their lives through self-understanding, personal responsibility, principled living, and higher ideals.

From mass murders to domestic violence, medication madness takes a dreadful toll on others. It is difficult to show that psychiatric drugs offer even short-term help, and impossible to show they do any long-term good. By contrast, it is clear that psychiatric drugs impair the physical and mental well-being of millions of people, sometimes resulting in mayhem, murder, and suicide.

Chapter 23

Choose Your Last Resort Wisely

RELINQUISHING OUR RELIANCE on psychiatric drugs may seem at first like a giant leap off a cliff. Where would we be without our pills? The answer is simple but not easy—we would be where we always have been in this difficult existence on Earth. We would be required to take personal responsibility for learning how to live as ethically, as enthusiastically, and as courageously as possible in the face of life's difficulties.

From individual health and happiness to society's security and progress, medication spellbinding and medication madness impact adversely on every aspect of life. As a psychiatrist, I tend to focus on the tragic consequences for individuals and their families, but we must not forget that the cost to society is incalculable. Regardless of how much society decides to hold spellbound individuals responsible for their behavior, we also need to take into account the suffering these individuals inflict upon others and upon society while intoxicated by psychiatric drugs.

As documented in this book, not only has medication madness contributed to tragedies like the mass murders perpetrated by Eric Harris and Joseph Wesbecker, it has caused innumerable acts of violence inside of families. Sally Grimm and Reynaldo Lacuzong murdered their children and Melvin Worthy nearly killed his wife. Innocent bystanders can be injured as well. Only chance prevented Harry Henderson from committing homicide when he drove his automobile into a policeman.

Advocates of psychiatric drugs are forever claiming that these psychoactive chemicals save society untold millions of dollars by successfully treating psychiatric disorders. Their claims are wholly self-serving and speculative. It is even difficult and often impossible to show that psychiatric drugs are helpful in carefully controlled clinical trials, let alone in real-life clinical practice or on a societal scale. By contrast, the damage done by these drugs to many individuals taking them is scientifically documented by case studies, by an infinite number of controlled clinical trials, and by many larger epidemiological studies. The FDA MedWatch system is flooded with reports of psychiatric drugs causing mental and emotional turmoil, and destructive behaviors.

After studying many cases in my clinical and forensic practice, and reading and hearing communications from my colleagues, I have come to the conclusion that modern psychiatrists have misled themselves into believing that "mental illness" is difficult to treat, that many patients inevitably become worse during treatment, and that stunning improvements in the patient's quality of life are rare or even unattainable. These psychiatrists have no idea that their patients frequently grow worse, and almost never get much better, because they are poisoning their brains.

What are the alternatives to unfounded biological theories and toxic psychiatric drugs? The contest is not between drugs and psychotherapy or any other specific "mental health" approach. The potentially earthshaking contest takes place between drugs and real life, between an artificially distorted mental life and a clear mind and spirit.

How we approach life often comes down to the nature of our last resort. When we are down and out, when we can't seem to control anything or to endure our circumstances, when our thoughts and feelings have become our own worst enemies, where do we turn? Modern pseudoscience tells us we have no choice; pills must be our last resort. We are not sad, we are depressed and require antidepressants. We aren't overcome with feelings of helplessness, we have anxiety disorder and need tranquilizers. We haven't lost control over our emotions, we have bipolar disorder and need mood stabilizers. Our children aren't bored silly in school, they have ADHD and need stimulants.

In a way, the contest is between pills and people. On the one hand, we can turn to medical professionals offering mind-altering chemicals. On the other, we can dig deeper into our own personal resources and increase our willingness to reach out for help to other people and perhaps to a higher power than ourselves, whether that power is viewed as a set of principles and ideals, love, our family, or God.

In my clinical practice I deal with *all* my patients on the basis that they will become far more able to reach self-understanding and self-mastery, and to live by the best principles, when they approach life with a drug-free brain and mind.

NO WISDOM IN PSYCHIATRIC TEXTBOOKS

WHAT IS THE PREFERRED ALTERNATIVE to a psychiatric textbook? All the combined books of wisdom available to the reader. Psychiatric textbooks do not contain wisdom. They contain simplistic biological paradigms that bear no resemblance to actual human lives. Instead they promote diagnoses and treatment that undermine and shred the human spirit.

People love self-help books and many of them are genuinely useful in helping people to improve their lives. But there's no great rush to find solutions or guidance within modern psychiatric textbooks such as the American Psychiatric Publishing's *Textbook of Psychiatry* or the *Comprehensive Textbook of Psychiatry*. I don't know anyone who claims that reading a psychiatric textbook or journal personally helped him or her to lead a better, happier, or more rational life. The basic thrusts of these pseudomedical books and journals—simplistic diagnoses and absurd biological theories—are degrading to human beings. The basic function of these publications is to justify psychiatrists in what they are already doing to people—nowadays mostly drugging and shocking them.

The experts who write the drug-related sections of textbooks almost invariably have strong financial ties to the pharmaceutical industry. They are generally not much interested in how to help people by talking with them. More shocking, the most basic and relied-upon sourcebook in psychiatry, the American Psychiatric Association's *Diagnostic and Statistical Manual of Mental Disorder* (*DSM*), is also in the pocket of this huge industry. A recent study found that, without exception, *every one* of the many contributors to the all-important diagnostic sections on depression, mania, schizophrenia, and psychosis had one or more "financial associations with companies in the pharmaceutical industry."[1] Overall, similar drug-company ties were found for 95 of the 170 professionals who helped write this bible of psychiatric diagnosis. Psychiatry nowadays is all about drugs and drug company interests, and hardly at all about people and their real needs.

THE LIMITS OF PSYCHOTHERAPY

WHILE REMAINING CAUTIOUS, I feel more positive about psychotherapy and counseling than about biological psychiatry. Many people are helped by ethical therapists. But psychotherapy, while doing far less harm and offering far more hope than biological psychiatry, is not without limitations.

First and foremost, psychotherapy or counseling is no better than the personal qualities of the therapist. Psychotherapy is as fallible as the human beings who conduct it.

Second, nowadays psychotherapists work under the shadow of the psychopharmaceutical complex and tend to refer their patients to medical doctors and psychiatrists for drugs as soon as their patients start to have real feelings of any intensity.

Third, there are so many different kinds of therapists and therapies that there is no way to standardize the process or the experience for the client. Choose a psychiatrist, psychologist, social worker, or marriage counselor from the phone book, and on your first visit you may encounter a grumpy, rigid, doctrinaire authoritarian or a caring, somewhat enlightened, wise human being—all claiming to offer the same service called psychotherapy. One may be a Jungian, another a Freudian, a third a devotee of cognitive therapy, a fourth a behaviorist, yet another a Buddhist or existential therapist—you can find them all in my small town of Ithaca—and when all is said and done, the real issue may be their individual personalities and especially their individual willingness to be interested in you and your particular problems.

What is the big problem with therapy? It is conducted by people! There are no scientific tricks for getting around that.

Among the dazzling array of approaches offered by therapists, all have limitations, and there is no one best approach. What seems to help people most is a caring relationship with a thoughtful, ethical therapist who values them,[2] but nowadays these ideals are poorly embodied in what passes for mental health services.

I am a psychiatrist who practices psychotherapy and family therapy but I have no magic cure to offer. My own therapeutic approach combines building a relationship, developing understanding of the patient's life story and problems, and finding better emotional and rational approaches to living an ethical, responsible, loving life. I have written about my approach to therapy and to life in many of my books, especially in *The Heart of Being Helpful* (1997) and more academically in *Beyond Conflict* (1992). But frankly, my therapeutic approach is no better than I am on any given day. Meanwhile, psychiatrists and psychotherapists vary so much in their personal qualities and theoretical approaches, that there is no alternative other than self-reliance in selecting the kind of help you want. It is up to individual patients or clients to determine the worth of any human service that's described or offered to them.

WHAT REALLY MAKES THERAPY WORK?

PROVIDED THAT THE THERAPIST IS ETHICAL, mostly rational, and trying to be caring, the effectiveness of what he or she offers ultimately depends more on the client than on the particular therapy or therapist. A person seeking help who exercises personal responsibility and determination in facing emotional suffering will benefit from many approaches; a person who does not exercise personal responsibility and determination will not benefit from any of them. Despite these caveats, many people grow in responsibility, self-discipline, and happiness as a result of therapy, but those who bring a strong sense of self-determination to the process will always benefit the most.

It is ironic but inescapable: The people most in need of help—those who have given up taking charge of their own lives—are the least able to benefit from any form of help, whether it's economic, social, or therapeutic in nature. Being diagnosed and drugged only pushes them deeper into helplessness, further crippling them psychologically and socially.

The greatest challenge lies in helping people who lack the capacity to help themselves. Already afraid that they cannot control their lives, they fall easy prey to psychiatric theories that confirm their helplessness for them by falsely attributing their problems to biochemical imbalances and genetics. The professional group that I founded more than thirty-five years ago, the International Center for the Study of Psychiatry and Psychology (www.icspp.org), promotes the development of drug-free, voluntary havens where people in the deepest distress can benefit from genuinely helpful human services.[3] But there will always be limits to what can be offered to those who have given up responsibility for themselves.

KEEP THEM SAFE FROM PSYCHIATRY

EXCEPT FOR MASS MURDERER Joseph Wesbecker, none of the people in this book was psychotic, mad, or insane before being given psychiatric drugs. If the drugs were able to destroy the mental life and lives of these people— most of whom were relatively sound of mind—imagine how much worse it must be for truly disturbed people when their minds and spirits are bent further out of shape by psychiatric drugs.

Studies conducted by the World Health Organization (WHO) have shown that people labeled "schizophrenic" do much more poorly when treated in

Western societies than when given little or no treatment in more "primitive" cultures.[4] The drugs that are invariably forced on these disturbed people in modern societies make them more helpless and turn them into chronic patients. By contrast, the drug-free extended family relationships in the non-Western societies tend to bring people back toward effective functioning in a matter of months.

The outcome of the WHO studies challenges conventional wisdom that the most disturbed patients really need psychiatrists and their physical treatments. In reality, they really need to be *protected* from psychiatrists and their treatments. Anyone whose grip on reality is already tenuous needs more than ever to be shielded from brain-disabling, spellbinding, maddening drugs.

When not driven by drugs or genuine brain diseases, madness or psychosis is caused by a collapse of personal relationships with others. Human beings become "crazy" when they feel isolated, fearful, and distrustful in regard to everyone else in their lives. Some of the most gratifying work as a therapist involves building relationships with very disturbed individuals. In the context of a safe therapeutic relationship, these people often "come back to reality" in a relatively short time.

Modern psychiatry offers no safe havens. It bears repeating that psychiatry nowadays does more harm than good and that psychotherapy is only as good as the ethical and psychological resources of the person who provides it and the person who receives it. There are no panaceas, no magic cures anywhere in the mental health professions—or in life.

PRINCIPLED LIVING

THERAPY DOES NOT HAVE a monopoly on how to surmount or transcend human helplessness and emotional suffering, and in truth the ultimate solutions lie outside these professions within philosophy and religion. Emotional suffering has always been a part of human life and attempts to alleviate it go back to the earliest times and earliest literature. From the prophets in the Bible to Shakespeare, and from Plato to Dr. Laura and Dr. Phil, people with varying degrees of wisdom have propounded solutions to that suffering with varying degrees of success for varying people. When scanning the variety of approaches to alleviating suffering and promoting prosperity, one is struck above all by the variety.

Historically, religion as well as less-formalized spiritual approaches have offered solutions to human emotional suffering. In recent times, however, when confronted with depressed or anxious persons, even the minister, priest, or rabbi is likely to refer them to someone who gives drugs. Increasingly, there is nowhere to turn for help that does not twist its way in the direction of drugs. Variety has given way to a compulsive reliance on pseudoscience and psychoactive drugs.

Although the point has been wholly missed by psychiatry, a satisfying and potentially happy life requires sound principles of living, including the courage and determination to maintain ethical, loving relationships with the people around us. Sages have advocated the most important principles for many centuries, usually focusing on the road to becoming a more loving and responsible human being who pursues higher ideals.

Every successful approach to rehabilitating the human spirit requires giving up hateful and destructive attitudes toward oneself and others, and ultimately replacing them with positive, creative, empowering, and especially loving attitudes and values. You will find nothing about this in the training of a psychiatrist or in psychiatric textbooks.

Every rehabilitation—and we all need regular rehabilitation—requires renewed dedication to principled living and higher ideals. Happy, satisfied, and successful persons almost invariably believe that there is something going on in the universe that is beyond their individual selves. By contrast, few if any of these successful people, in my experience, believe their lives are governed by biochemical imbalances that can be somehow harmonized by drugs.

Of course, there are infinite ways to interpret what it means to become responsible and loving, and to live by sound ideals. There will always be many roads to becoming a good, successful, and potentially happy human being—but not one of them is paved with psychiatric diagnoses and drugs.

The International Center for the Study of Psychiatry and Psychology (www.icspp.org) is specifically devoted to the principles that underlie this book. Founded in 1972, by the author as a support group in his successful effort to stop the resurgence of lobotomy, it has grown into a network and educational forum for professionals and laypersons alike who are devoted to raising the ethical and scientific standards in psychiatry, psychology, and related health fields (see appendix B for more about ICSPP).

This is not the place to present my own personal philosophy in more detail than I have already done here and in earlier books such as *The Heart of Being Helpful* (1997) and *Beyond Conflict* (1992). But it may lend encouragement to conclude with my recently developed Principles of Life.[5]

PRINCIPLES OF LIFE

1.

Love is joyful awareness. Love life—people, animals, nature, gardening, art and music, sports and exercise, literature, God—anything and anyone that brings you a joyful awareness of the wonder of being a living creature in a world far greater than ourselves.

2.

Gratitude satisfies the spirit. Be grateful for all that you love and if you cannot think of anyone or anything to love, then be grateful you still have a chance to love. Be especially grateful for the opportunity to help and to serve other people.

3.

Gratitude is the antidote to self-pity. Feeling sorry for oneself is ruinous. Especially don't fall into believing that we live in the worst of times. It takes little imagination to know how much worse it has been for other people in previous ages and even now in other places. Be grateful for this life.

4.

Ethics guide the good life. Put ethics and principles above pleasure, convenience, safety, income, career, your presumed place in the world, and the way others view you. Living a principled life is the key to a satisfying life.

5.

Everything good requires courage. Find the courage to love, to be grateful, and to live by sound ethics. Especially be brave enough to speak honestly and to stand straight when you are afraid.

6.

Dare to seek romantic love. Abiding love for a partner in life is the nearest we get to heaven this time around.

7.

Make a living at something you respect and love. Many people find a way to do it. Your occupation should feel like a privilege, a pleasure, and an opportunity to serve. It should offer you the opportunity to improve the lives of others.

8.

Approach every single challenge in life with determination to master it. Otherwise, you won't handle it. Feeling helpless in the face of adversity is a prescription for failure. Deciding to take on the important challenges is a prescription for self-satisfaction and makes success more likely.

9.

Don't hide from your painful emotions. While it's often destructive to voice or act upon our negative feelings, it's important to recognize them. Feeling emotional pain signals that there is something wrong in our lives that needs immediate attention. Invite your painful emotions to tell you everything they can about what you really want out of life.

10.

Don't think of yourself as a survivor. Intending to survive guarantees little more than getting by, and ultimately leads to failure. Think of yourself as someone who intends to triumph in life.

11.

Forgiving other people liberates us from hate. You won't get even by hating, you'll get miserable, bitter, and spiritless. Take care of yourself by forgiving and, if necessary, by avoiding hurtful people, but don't waste a minute hating.

12.

Seek a worthwhile life rather than happiness. There are no shortcuts to happiness; no trick ideas or drugs that can make us happy. The search for happiness will lead you to false "cures," distract you from what matters, and even make you crazy. Much of happiness is often a matter of luck—the way we are shaped by childhood, where we happen to be born, health, and circumstance—but we increase the opportunity for happiness by remaining principled and loving in the face of adversity and disappointment.

13.

No one knows the meaning of life but it's certain that life is best lived with love, gratitude, ethics, courage, and a determination to give it your best effort. A sense of worth is guaranteed by principled living, and happiness will often tag along as well.

14.

Let your spirit be touched, and touch the spirit of others, with love. Nothing is more important than expanding our own capacity, and humanity's capacity, to love one another.

The final three principles are most specifically related to the themes of this book:

15.

You cannot solve your problems by taking psychoactive substances that impair your mind and the expression of your spirit. From illegal drugs to psychiatric medications, all drugs suppress and distort our real emotions and should be avoided, especially in time of suffering and fear when we need to know what we are feeling and to control our actions.

16.

Reject being labeled with a psychiatric diagnosis. Don't allow the sum total of your life to be reduced to phrases like clinical depression, bipolar disorder, or anxiety disorder. There are no "psychiatric disorders," only life disorders. Instead of being mangled by someone else's cookie-cutter definition of your life, seek to know the unique story of your own development and evolution as a person. Remember that all of us have to struggle, to go through hard times, and to find a way of becoming more in control of our emotions and more honorable and successful in our actions.

17.

Choose your last resort wisely. When you feel most desperate and alone, where will you go—toward psychiatry with its biological explanations and mind-altering drugs or toward improved principles of living, a more responsible and loving life, the fulfillment of your ideals, and oneness with a Meaning or Power beyond yourself? Your chosen last resort defines you as a person and gives direction to your life.

Psychiatric Medications by Category

I: THE NEWER ANTIDEPRESSANTS*

Selective Serotonin Reuptake Inhibitors (SSRIs)
Celexa (citalopram)
Lexapro (escitalopram)
Luvox (fluvoxamine)[†]
Prozac and Serafem (fluoxetine)
Paxil (paroxetine)
Zoloft (sertraline)

Other Newer Antidepressants
Cymbalta (duloxetine)
Effexor (venlafaxine)
Remeron (mirtazapine)
Symbyax (Zyprexa and Prozac combined)
Wellbutrin and Zyban (bupropion)

---

*The new FDA "black box" warnings apply to all antidepressants but in fact were developed based on the SSRIs and newer antidepressants, and not on the older ones.
[†]The brand name Luvox has been withdrawn from the market but the drug is still available in the generic form.

Older Antidepressants (partial list)★

Anafranil (clomipramine)

Asendin (loxapine)†

Elavil (amitriptyline)

Parnate (tranylcypromine)

Tofranil (imipramine)

Vivactil (protriptyline)

Surmontil (trimipramine)

II: STIMULANTS

Classic Stimulants††

Adderall, Adderall XR (amphetamine mixture)

Desoxyn (methamphetamine)§

Dexedrine (dextroamphetamine)

Focalin, Focalin XR (dexmethylphenidate)

Ritalin, Concerta, Daytrana (methylphenidate)

Vyvanse (lisdexamfetamine)

Others

Cylert (pemoline) (no longer available)

Strattera (atomoxetine)

III: TRANQUILIZERS AND SLEEPING PILLS¶

Benzodiazepine Tranquilizers

Ativan (lorazepam)

Klonopin (clonazepam)

★All the older antidepressants can cause psychiatric adverse drug reactions including mania and psychosis but they much less commonly come up in my clinical and legal experience. A more complete list can be found in various textbooks, especially *Drug Facts and Comparisons* (2007), a readily available annual publication.

†Asendin (loxapine) is metabolized into an antipsychotic (neuroleptic) drug and poses all the risks associated with antipsychotics, including tardive dyskinesia.

†† All the "classic stimulants" are Drug Enforcement Administration (DEA) Schedule II narcotics, indicating the highest risk of tolerance and dependence (addiction).

§Few people realize that doctors can prescribe methamphetamine, the deadly drug of addiction, to children for ADHD.

¶All are DEA Schedule IV narcotics, indicating a risk of tolerance and dependence (addiction), except Rozerem.

Librium (chlordiazepoxide)

Serax (oxazepam)

Tranxene (clorazepate)

Xanax (alprazolam)

Valium (diazepam)

Benzodiazepine Sleeping Pills

Dalmane (flurazepam)

Doral (quazepam)

Halcion (triazolam)

ProSom (estazolam)

Restoril (temazepam)

Non-Benzodiazepine Sleeping Pills

Ambien (zolpidem)

Lunesta (eszopiclone)

Placidyl (ethchlorvynol)

Rozerem (ramelteon)

Sonata (zaleplon)

Barbiturate Sleeping Pills

Butisol (butabarbital)

Carbrital (pentobarbital and carbromal)

Seconal (secobarbital)

IV: ANTIPSYCHOTIC DRUGS (NEUROLEPTICS)

Newer (second- or third-generation or atypical) Antipsychotics

Abilify (aripiprazole)

Geodon (ziprasidone)

Invega (paliperidone)

Risperdal (risperidone)

Seroquel (quetiapine)

Symbyax (Zyprexa and Prozac combined)

Zyprexa (olanzapine)

Older Antipsychotic Drugs

Clozaril (clozapine)

Etrafon (Trilafon and Elavil combined)

Haldol (haloperidol)

Loxitane (loxapine)

Mellaril (thioridazine)

Moban (molindone)

Navane (thiothixene)

Prolixin (fluphenazine)

Serentil (mesoridazine)

Stelazine (trifluoperazine)

Taractan (chlorprothixene)

Thorazine (chlorpromazine)

Tindal (acetophenazine)

Trilafon (perphenazine)

Vesprin (triflupromazine)

Neuroleptics Used for Other Medical Purposes

Compazine (prochlorperazine)

Inapsine (droperidol)

Orap (pimozide)

Phenergan (promethazine)★

Reglan (metoclopramide)

V. LITHIUM AND OTHER DRUGS USED AS "MOOD STABILIZERS"

Depakote (divalproex sodium) [antiepileptic drug]

Equetro (extended-release carbamazepine) [antiepileptic drug]

Lamictal (lamotrigine) [antiepileptic drug]

Lithobid, Lithotabs, Eskalith (lithium)

Off-Label or Unapproved Mood Stabilizers

Catapres (clonidine) [antihypertensive drug]

Neurontin (gabapentin) [antiepileptic drug]

★Usually classified as an antihistamine but has mild neuroleptic qualities and on rare occasion can cause or exacerbate tardive dyskinesia. All drugs in table IV are neuroleptics and can cause tardive dyskinesia.

Tegretol (carbamazepine) [antiepileptic drug]

Tenex (guanfacine) [antihypertensive drug]

Topamax (topiramate) [antiepileptic drug]

Trileptal (oxcarbazepine) [antiepileptic drug]

What Else Can You Do?

PEOPLE OFTEN WANT TO KNOW what they can do to further reform in the field of mental health. They want to help to raise the ethical and scientific standards of psychiatry, psychology, and related health professions. They want to join efforts to move psychiatry and mental health away from ill-conceived diagnoses and damaging drugs, and toward more caring, ethical human services. They also want to know how to keep up with the latest information about reform activities and independent research, and how to meet other professionals and nonprofessionals with similar interests and concerns. There is a way for professionals and nonprofessionals alike to accomplish all this by joining one organization, the International Center for the Study of Psychiatry and Psychology (www.icspp.org). Membership in ICSPP and attendance at the annual conferences are open to the public.

Benefits

Joining ICSPP helps support the reform movement. For the price of membership, you also get a discount at the annual conferences, a newsletter, and a subscription to the outstanding scientific journal, *Ethical Human Psychology and Psychiatry*. In addition, ICSPP provides feature articles, commentaries, and information on its Web site. Many find the yearly conferences a revitalizing, uplifting experience where they can meet hundreds of like-minded professionals and laypersons.

History

In the 1970s, ICSPP led a successful effort to stop the return of lobotomy and psychosurgery, and it has been a leader in opposing electroshock treatment over several decades. In the 1990s, our efforts stopped the psychiatric portion of the federal violence initiative, a racist government program that aimed at finding a violence gene and biochemical imbalances in the brains of inner-city infants and children. Also in the 1990s, ICSPP was the first to focus on the damaging effects of the newer antidepressants, including drug-induced violence and suicide, and it has also taken a leadership role in opposing the drugging of children for behavioral control. ICSPP is currently publicizing the dangers of the widespread psychiatric screening of schoolchildren with its inevitable result of even higher rates of medicating children.

I founded ICSPP in 1972, and my wife, Ginger, began adding her leadership as executive director in the mid-1980s. Several years ago, we transferred leadership of the organization to younger individuals including the current director, New York City psychotherapist Dr. Dominick Riccio. As director emeritus, I no longer take a governing role in ICSPP but I speak at the annual conferences and frequently contribute to the journal. None of the leaders of ICSPP gets paid; every one is a devoted volunteer.

Inspiring Conferences

The annual ICSPP conferences are always enlightening and entertaining. In addition to me, many of the professionals and reformers mentioned in *Medication Madness* regularly speak at our annual meetings, including international drug regulatory expert Graham Dukes, MD, JD, psychiatrists Grace Jackson, MD, and Joe Glenmullen, MD, pediatrician Karen Effrem, MD, professor of psychology Bertram Karon, psychiatric survivor David Oaks, and attorney Jim Gottstein. Jackson, Effrem, and Gottstein belong to the center's twenty-one-member board of directors. In addition, many of the other scientists and lawyers whose work I cite in this book are members of ICSPP and speak on occasion at the conferences.

If you want to help to reform psychiatry and to develop more human and ethical approaches, and if you want the pleasure of associating with people who share your concerns and values, please join the International Center for the Study of Psychiatry and Psychology. Perhaps I will meet you at an upcoming conference.

For more information, go to:

www.icspp.org

and

www.breggin.com

Notes

1. KILLING THE PAIN—AND ALMOST THE COP

1. My most detailed discussions of how to evaluate the role of a drug in causing a disorder can be found in my article "Suicidality, Violence and Mania Caused by Selective Serotonin Reuptake Inhibitors (SSRIs)" (2003), available on http://www.breggin.com and *Brain-Disabling Treatments in Psychiatry*.
2. Because the Paxil had caused such obvious agitation and maniclike behavior, in my initial evaluation and report I did not focus on this clinical phenomenon—but it deserved more attention.
3. A detailed analysis of my findings on akathisia and behavioral abnormalities in the GlaxoSmithKline sealed records can be found in my article, "How GlaxoSmithKline Suppressed Data on Paxil-Induced Akathisia: Implications for Suicide and Violence" (2006), which is available on http://www.breggin.com.
4. American Psychiatric Association, *Diagnostic and Statistical Manual of Mental Disorders (DSM-IV-TR)* 2000, page 801. Specifically, the text states: "Serotonin-specific reuptake inhibitor antidepressant medication [SSRI antidepressants like Paxil and Prozac] may produce akathisia that appears identical in phenomenology and treatment response to Neuroleptic-Induced Acute Akathisia."
5. Lipinski et al. (1989).
6. Rothschild and Locke (1991).
7. Wirshing et al. (1992).
8. Breggin, *Beyond Conflict* (1992), 89–90.

2. WHAT IS MEDICATION SPELLBINDING?

1. Marks, *The Search for the Manchurian Candidate* (1979). Before completing his book, Marks brought some of the recently declassified papers on the CIA experiments to my office for me to review with him.
2. *Physicians' Desk Reference* (2006), 2741.
3. Associated Press, "Food and Drug Administration: Watch for Behavior Change in Children Taking Tamiflu," November 14, 2006.
4. Iacuzio, "Dear Healthcare Professional: Important Prescribing Information [about Tamiflu]" November 13, 2006.
5. *Physicians' Desk Reference* (2006), 3079.
6. *Drug Facts and Comparisons* (2006), 417.
7. Richard B. Birrer and Sathya P. Vemuri, "Depression in Later Life: A Diagnostic and Therapeutic Challenge," *American Family Physician* 69 (May 15, 2004): 2375–82.
8. I took this clinical description from a Food and Drug Administration report, dated February 28, 2007.
9. Jennifer Corbett Dooren, "FDA Says Bladder Drug Needs Children Warnings," *Wall Street Journal*, April 10, 2007, D2.
10. Birrer and Vemuri, "Depression in Later Life: A Diagnostic and Therapeutic Challenge," 2004.
11. Breggin (2006a).
12. The word is derived from the Greek *nosos* for "disease" and *gnosis* for "knowledge," combined with the prefix *a*, meaning "not" or "without."
13. For discussions and research on the power of placebo, see Fisher and Greenberg, *The Limits of Biological Treatments for Psychological Distress* (1989), and Kirsch and Sapirstein, "Listening to Prozac but Hearing Placebo" (June 26, 1998).
14. Kirsch and Sapirstein, "Listening to Prozac but Hearing Placebo" (1998).
15. See my books, *Toxic Psychiatry* (1991) and *Brain-Disabling Treatments in Psychiatry* (2008) for more detailed discussions of the influence of NAMI and other drug-company-funded groups.
16. I first wrote about the psychopharmaceutical complex in *Toxic Psychiatry* (1991) and my most recent update is in *Brain-Disabling Treatments in Psychiatry* (2008).

3. THE TOOTHLESS WATCHDOG GROWLS

1. I review a variety of press reports in *Talking Back to Prozac*, coauthored with Ginger Breggin (1994).
2. The case is *Tobin v. SmithKline Beecham Pharmaceuticals.* (164 F. Supp. 2d. 1278. D. Wy. 2001.) See Josefson, "Jury Finds Drug 80% Responsible for Killings" (June 16, 2001), 1446. Andy Vickery's Web site, http://www.justiceseekers.com, provides additional information. I hadn't as yet met Andy and was not involved in the case, although since then I have worked with him.

3. Breggin, *Toxic Psychiatry* (1991), 165 ff.

4. Kapit, "Safety Review of NDA 18–936 [Prozac]" (March 28, 1986), and "Safety Update: NDA 19–936" (November 17, 1986). Kapit brought up Prozac's stimulating effects on a number of other occasions as well.

5. Kapit, "Safety Update" (November 17, 1986), 23.

6. For an analysis of conflicts of interest in the panel that approved Prozac and later whitewashed it, see Breggin and Breggin, (1994).

7. The FDA failed to mention that the three positive studies were drug-company-sponsored and conducted by drug-company drones.

8. "Antidepressant Strengthened Warnings about Pediatric Suicidality Risk Needed Immediately, Cmte. Says," February 2, 2004, http://www.FDAAdvisory Committee.com.

9. The hearing transcript is available on http://www.fda.gov.

10. Breggin, *Talking Back to Prozac* (1994), 145.

11. Emphasis added.

12. The label template can be found on http://www.fda.gov and in the *Physicians' Desk Reference* beginning in 2006. In the end, drug-company interests pressured the FDA to include the new black-box warnings in all antidepressant labels including older ones that were not reevaluated in 2004 and 2005, thus diluting the truth that only the newer, more stimulating antidepressants have been clearly associated with suicidality.

13. J. Lenzer, "FDA Accepts Weakened Antidepressant Warning," (March 19, 2005), 620.

14. Ibid.

15. T. Hammad et al., "Suicidality in Pediatric Patients Treated with Antidepressant Drugs" (2006), 332–39.

16. Ibid., 338.

17. The last-minute inclusion of the older antidepressant was probably an act of deference to the manufacturers of the newer antidepressants.

18. Officially called the Psychopharmacologic Drugs Advisory Committee (PDAC).

19. Many of the panelists have drug-company ties and even the "consumer representative" admitted to owning drug-company stock. She also described herself as struggling with depression, raising the question of whether she was a consumer of psychiatric drugs.

20. Juurlink et al., "The Risk of Suicide with Selective Reuptake Inhibitors in the Elderly" (2006), 813–21. The quotes are from the abstract, page 813.

21. The complete transcript of the December 13, 2006, PDAC meeting can be obtained at http://www.fda.gov.

22. Hammad et al., "Suicidality in Pediatric Patients Treated with Antidepressant Drugs," 338. The issue is somewhat clouded, however, by contradictory reports and by the fact that there were completed suicides, for example, in the European placebo controlled clinical trials for Paxil. See Breggin, "Court Filing Makes Public My Previously Suppressed Analysis of Paxil's Effects" (2006), 77–84.

23. Quoted in Graham, "Strong Antidepressant Warning Urged" (December 14, 2006).

24. Kirsch et al., "The Emperor's New Drugs: An Analysis of Antidepressant Medication Data Submitted to the U.S. Food and Drug Administration" (July 15,

2002). Also see Kirsch and Sapirstein, "Listening to Prozac but Hearing Placebo" (1998) and Kirsch et al. (2008).

25. Angell, *The Truth About the Drug Companies* (2005), 112 ff, and Medawar and Hardon, *Medicine Out of Control* (2004), 57.

26. Breggin and Cohen, *Your Drug May Be Your Problem* (2007). Also see the 2007 Paxil label in the *Physicians' Desk Reference* for a warning about withdrawal effects.

27. Rosack, "Congress Hammers FDA over Handling of SSRIs" (October 15, 2004), 1.

28. Harris, "Study Condemns FDA.'s Handling of Drug Safety" (September 23, 2006), 1.

29. Mathews, "FDA Plans Drug-Safety Moves" (January 31, 2007), A11.

30. Mathews, "Reports Blasts FDA's System to Track Drugs" (March 3–4, 2007), A1.

4. YOUNG GIRL MURDERERS IN THE MAKING

1. Food and Drug Administration (2000b). See chapter 3 for further discussion of the booklet

5. DOCTORS DRIVEN MAD BY MEDICATION

1. Modified from the table in American Psychiatric Association, *DSM-IV-TR* (2000), 362.

2. All of the following quotes are taken from American Psychiatric Association *DSM-IV-TR* (2000), 358–359.

3. American Psychiatric Association *DSM-IV-TR* (2000), 358–359, 361.

4. For example, pages 358–359, 361–363, and 367–368 in *DSM-IV-TR* (2000) note that antidepressants can cause mania and pages 407–8 note that they can cause mood disturbances.

5. See *DSM-IV-TR* (2000), page 316, and also footnote at the bottom of the chart, "Criteria for Manic Episode," page 362.

6. A much more expanded discussion of antidepressant-induced mania can be found in Breggin, *Brain-Disabling Treatments in Psychiatry* (2008).

7. Howland, "Induction of Mania with Serotonin Reuptake Inhibitors" (1996).

8. Ebert et al., "The Serotonin Syndrome and Psychosis-Like Side Effects of Flu-voxamine in Clinical Use—An Estimation of Incidence" (1997), 71–74.

9. Reviewed in Breggin, *Brain-Disabling Treatments in Psychiatry* (2008).

10. Emslie et al., "A Double-Blind, Randomized, Placebo-Controlled Trial of Flu-oxetine in Children and Adolescents with Depression" (1997).

11. For a more detailed discussion, including similar comments from FDA officials about why rates of adverse effects are higher in clinical practice than in con-trolled clinical trials, see Breggin, *Brain-Disabling Treatments in Psychiatry* (2008).

12. Henry et al., "Antidepressant-Induced Mania in Bipolar Patients: Identification of Risk Factors" (2001), 249–55.

13. Ghaemi et al., "Antidepressants in Bipolar Disorder: The Case for Caution" (2003), 421–33.

14. Goldberg and Truman, "Antidepressant-Induced Mania: An Overview of Current Controversies" (2003), 407–20.

15. Solvay Pharmaceuticals, Inc. sent the drug company report to the FDA concerning the toxicology report from Eric Harris' autopsy (May 14, 1999), which I obtained through the Freedom of Information Act. I have written in more detail about Eric Harris in *Reclaiming Our Children* (2000) and in the scientific literature, "Fluvoxamine as a Cause of Stimulation, Mania, and Aggression with a Critical Analysis of the FDA-Approved Label" (2002), 71–86.

16. *Physicians' Desk Reference* (1998), 2891, top of third column. The same observations appear in subsequent editions through 2002. Luvox is not contained in more recent editions.

17. Frankenfield et al., "Fluoxetine and Violent Death in Maryland" (1994), 107–17. Ninety-one cases involved the older antidepressants and twenty-three involved Prozac. Twenty-three percent of the cases taking the older drugs (tricyclic antidepressants) used violent means of suicide compared to 65 percent of the Prozac cases.

18. Serzone has since been withdrawn from the market due to liver toxicity.

19. The most up-to-date review of the literature on antidepressant-induced manic-like symptoms can be found in Breggin, *Brain-Disabling Treatments in Psychiatry* (2008).

20. ADHD is neither a valid diagnosis nor a legitimate syndrome. It's a collection of behaviors that can be caused by a wide spectrum of problems such as lack of discipline at home, anxiety, boring schools or workplaces, and real diseases like head injury and diabetes. It is a diagnosis without essential meaning or worth. In each case, the child or adult must be evaluated to see what's making him or her inattentive, impulsive, or hyperactive. See my books *Toxic Psychiatry* (1991), *Talking Back to Ritalin* (2001), *The Ritalin Fact Book* (2002), or *Brain-Disabling Treatments in Psychiatry* (2008).

21. American Psychiatric Association *DSM-IV-TR* (2000), 406.

23. Adderall is a mixture of dextroamphetamine sulfate, amphetamine sulfate, dextroamphetamine saccharate, and amphetamine aspartate.

24. In the 2007 *Physicians' Desk Reference*, in the Adverse Reactions section, under Central Nervous System.

25. Similarly, writing in Goodman and Gilman's 2001 classic textbook of pharmacology, Hoffman ("Catecholamines, Sympathomimetic Drugs, and Adrenergic Receptor Antagonists," chapter 10, pp. 215–68) noted, "The toxic dose of amphetamine varies widely. Toxic manifestations occasionally occur as an idiosyncrasy after as little as 2 mg, but are rare with doses of less than 15 mg. Severe reactions have occurred with 30 mg . . ."

26. *Physicians' Desk Reference* (2007), 208.

27. The classic stimulants such as Adderall (amphetamine) and Ritalin or Concerta (methylphenidate) are highly addictive. Because of their propensity to be abused, the Drug Enforcement Administration (DEA) places these drugs in Schedule II along with narcotics like morphine. Thus far, Strattera has escaped being labeled

as a drug of abuse, but in all other ways it possesses the same hazards as the classic stimulants, including disinhibition and mania with dangerous behavior.

28. *Physicians' Desk Reference* (2007), 1814. Bold and caps in original.
29. All of the following information about Strattera is found in the *Physicians' Desk Reference* (2007), 1815.
30. Henderson and Hartman, "Aggression, Mania, and Hypomania Induction Associated with Atomoxetine" (2004). 895.
31. Ibid.
32. Ibid.
33. Discussed in detail in Breggin, *Brain-Disabling Treatments in Psychiatry* (2008).
34. Moreno et al., "National Trends in the Outpatient Diagnosis and Treatment of Bipolar Disorder in Youth" (2007), 1032–39.

6. KILLING LOVED ONES TO SAVE THE WORLD

1. For more detailed information on dopamine-blocking drugs and their devastating effects on the brain and mind, see Breggin, *Brain-Disabling Treatments in Psychiatry* (2008).

7. DRUG-INDUCED "HAPPY FACES"

1. American Psychiatric Association *DSM-IV-TR* (2000), 359.
2. American Psychiatric Association *DSM-IV-TR* (2000), 361. Italics added. Statements linking antidepressants to mania and other mood disturbances occur remarkably frequently through the book, for example, on pages 361, 362, 365, and 368 (notes on bottom of tables), and 407.
3. S. Barancik, "Paxil Saves Him from Prison: Judge Agrees Antidepressant Was Partially Responsible for Jabil Worker Embezzling $1.8 Million" (November 20, 2006). Retrieved from http://www.tampabay.com. The defendant was Tampa, Florida executive Patrick Henry Stewart and the U.S. District Court Judge was James Moody, Jr.
4. Earl's wife made these statements under oath in a deposition in a product-liability case that Earl brought against Eli Lilly.
5. A detailed analysis of the adverse psychiatric effects of benzodiazepines can be found in Breggin, *Brain-Disabling Treatments in Psychiatry* (2008).

8. NOT QUITE TWELVE YEARS OLD

1. Carla Johnson study for the Associated Press, "Antidepressant Benefits Trump Risks for Kids," in *The Ithaca Journal* (April 18, 2007), 6A. I discuss professional resistance to the FDA warnings in Breggin, *Brain-Disabling Treatments in Psychiatry* (2008).

9. SLEEPING PILL MADNESS

1. American Psychiatric Association. *Task Force Report on Benzodiazepine Dependence, Toxicity, and Abuse* (1990), 41.
2. Attorney Michael Mosher of Paris, Texas, directed me to the significance of the Versed data.
3. A footnote disclaimer stated, "This article contains the professional views of the authors and does not constitute the official position of the Food and Drug Administration."
4. FDA (1992).
5. Breggin, P. (1992). "The President's Sleeping Pill [Halcion] and Its Maker." *New York Times*, A24.
6. Sabshin, "To Aid Understanding of Mental Disorders." Letter to *New York Times* (March 10, 1992), A24.
7. Jonas, "Dr. Jeffrey M. Jonas, Director of CNS Clinical Development at Upjohn, Replies," in *Clinical Psychiatry News* (October 1992), 5.
8. E. Benedek letter to Peter Roger Breggin, MD, as a part of a mass-mailing package, soliciting funds for the American Psychiatric Foundation (February 8, 1993).
9. The FDA undoubtedly made this broader indictment in order to defuse the economic harm that would be done to the newer drugs like Lunesta and Ambien even though these drugs are the real culprits. As stated in the *Wall Street Journal*, "When such warnings affect an entire class of drugs, they tend to damp the sales of any particular product compared with its competitors." See A. Mathews and J. Dooren, "Sleep Drugs Get Warning on Labels Sought by FDA," in *Wall Street Journal* (March 15, 2007), D9.
10. Hirshkowitz, "Neuropsychiatric Aspects of Sleep and Sleep Disorders," in *Neuropsychiatry and Clinical Neurosciences* (2002), 697–722.

10. TRANQUILIZED INTO VIOLENCE

1. *Physicians' Desk Reference* (2005), 2766. Emphases added. Beginning in 2006, the Xanax label is not reproduced in the *PDR*. The long-acting Xanax XR is included in 2006 but not in 2007.
2. For my legal case reports, I summarize the scientific reviews of benzo madness that I have published in my books such as *Toxic Psychiatry* (1991) and *Brain-Disabling Treatments in Psychiatry* (2008) and in a peer-reviewed scientific article entitled "Analysis of Adverse Behavioral Effects of Benzodiazepines with a Discussion of Drawing Scientific Conclusions from the FDA's Spontaneous Reporting System" (1998), which can be found on my Web site.
3. Rall, "Hypnotics and Sedatives; Ethanol," in *The Pharmacological Basis of Therapeutics* (1990), 355.
4. GABA stands for gamma-aminobutyric acid.
5. The materials I attached to my report in Gerry Shannon's case were (a) excerpt from DiMascio and Shader, *Clinical Handbook of Psychopharmacology* (1970);

(b) Excerpt from Shader and DiMascio, *Psychotropic Drug Side Effects* (1977); (c) Rosenbaum et al., "Emergence of Hostility During Alprazolam Treatment," in *American Journal of Psychiatry* (1984), 792–93; (d) French, "Dangerous Aggressive Behavior as a Side Effect of Alprazolam," in *American Journal of Psychiatry* 146 (1989): 276; and (e) Excerpt from Arana and Hyman, *Handbook of Psychiatric Drug Treatment* (1991).

12. A VICIOUS ADDICTION

1. Eli Lilly's use of tranquilizers in the Prozac trials was authorized by a secret in-house memo without initially informing the FDA, as required by FDA regulations, of the change in the plan (protocol) for the clinical trial. Discussed in detail in Breggin and Breggin, *Talking Back to Prozac* (1994) and in Breggin, *Brain-Disabling Treatments in Psychiatry* (2008).
2. The Xanax studies and the cover-up are discussed in Breggin, *Toxic Psychiatry* (1991) and Breggin *Brain-Disabling Treatments in Psychiatry* (2008). More recently, the FDA required Upjohn to give more indication in the label of how frequently patients are unable to stop taking the drug after short exposures in controlled clinical trials.
3. For a scientific discussion of persistent benzodiazepine-induced cognitive dysfunction, see Breggin (2008).
4. *Physicians' Desk Reference* (2005). Xanax tablets do not appear in the *PDR* after 2005 but they continue to be sold.
5. American Psychiatric Association, *Task Force Report on Benzodiazepine Dependence, Toxicity, and Abuse* (1990), 26–29.
6. Ibid., 26.
7. Studies of Xanax withdrawal reviewed in Breggin, *Toxic Psychiatry* (1991).
8. Based on American Psychiatric Association *DSM-IV* (1994), 262, and *DSM-IV-TR* (2000), 284–85.
9. *Physicians' Desk Reference* (1995).

13. HE WANTED TO DO BETTER IN SCHOOL

1. Food and Drug Administration (March 14, 2006).
2. Food and Drug Administration (June 30, 2005).
3. Food and Drug Administration (March 14, 2005).
4. Gelperin and Phelan, "Psychiatric Adverse Events Associated with Drug Treatment of ADHD" (May 3, 2006). Quotes in this section are from pages 3–4 of the FDA in-house memorandum. The Division of Drug Risk Evaluation is responsible for keeping track of adverse reports that appear after a drug has been put on the market.
5. The drugs shown to cause psychosis with positive rechallenge reports included

all those involved in treating ADHD: various preparations of amphetamine (Adderall and Dexedrine), various preparations of methylphenidate (Focalin, Concerta, Metadate, Methylin, Ritalin); Methylphenidate Transdermal System (skin patches); Strattera; and Provigil.

6. In addition to presenting this data in a verbal exchange on a panel with another expert who was minimizing the risk of stimulant-induced psychosis, I presented my analysis of the data in my published report in the Consensus Development Conference proceedings (Breggin, 1998) and in Breggin, "Psychostimulants in the Treatment of Children Diagnosed with ADHD Part II," in *Ethical Human Sciences and Services* 1 (1999), 213–42. The data is also described and tabulated in *Talking Back to Ritalin* (2001), 43–44.

7. Sherer, "FDA Panel: No Black Box Warning for ADHD Drugs," in *Psychiatric Times* (May 2006),1.

8. Cherland and Fitzpatrick, "Psychotic Side Effects of Psychostimulants," in *Canadian Journal of Psychiatry* (1999), 811–13.

9. I have reviewed the adverse effects of stimulants in some detail in three books, *Brain-Disabling Treatments in Psychiatry* (2008), *Talking Back to Ritalin* (2001), and *The Ritalin Fact Book* (2002), and a lengthy scientific review and analysis in *Ethical Human Sciences and Services* and *International Journal of Risk and Safety in Medicine* (1999).

10. In the presentation to the NIH Consensus Development Conference, in my published paper and in my books, I have marshaled abundant scientific evidence to show that, in animals and children alike, the stimulants reduce spontaneous behaviors—such as socializing, playing, exploring, and escaping—while enforcing obsessive-compulsive behaviors. See my reviews of the literature: *Brain-Disabling Treatments in Psychiatry* (2008); *Ethical Human Sciences and Services* (1999), and *International Journal of Risk and Safety in Medicine* (1999). S. Castner and P. Goldman-Rakic, "Long-Lasting Psychotomimetic Consequences of Repeated Low-Dose Amphetamine Exposure in Rhesus Monkeys" (1999).

11. Swanson et al., "Treatment of ADHD: Beyond Medication," in *Beyond Behavior* 4 (Fall 1992), 13–16 and 18–22.

12. See chapter 1 and for more details see Breggin, *Brain-Disabling Treatments in Psychiatry* (2008).

13. Whalen and Henker (1989).

14. Arnold and Jensen, "Attention-Deficit Disorders," in *Comprehensive Textbook of Psychiatry* (1995), 2307.

15. Borcherding et al., "Motor/Vocal Tics and Compulsive Behaviors on Stimulant Drugs: Is There a Common Vulnerability," in *Psychiatric Research* (1990), 83–94.

16. Solanto and Wender, "Does Methylphenidate Constrict Cognitive Functioning?" in *Journal of the American Academy of Child and Adolescent Psychiatry* (1989), 897–902.

17. The data are from Maxmen and Ward (1995, p. 366). The numbers are percentages of patients reported in studies to suffer from the adverse effect. My reviews in *Ethical Human Sciences and Services* (1999) and *International Journal of*

Risk and Safety in Medicine (1999) indicates that the rates of depression are higher for methylphenidate than indicated by Maxmen and Ward and are similar to those they cite for amphetamine.

18. For studies of persistent brain changes after stimulant treatment in animals, see Melega et al., in *Behavioural Brain Research* (1997) and Melega et al., in *Brain Research* (1997), and also my reviews in *Ethical Human Sciences and Services* (1999) and *International Journal of Risk and Safety in Medicine* (1999), and most recently in the revised book *Brain-Disabling Treatments in Psychiatry* (2008).

19. I discuss how to help so-called ADHD children without drugs in *Talking Back to Ritalin* (2001) and *The Ritalin Fact Book* (2002).

20. Breggin, *Brain-Disabling Treatments in Psychiatry* (2008).

21. C. W. Popper and R. J. Steingard, "Disorders Usually First Diagnosed in Infancy, Childhood, or Adolescence," in *The American Psychiatric Press Textbook of Psychiatry* (1994), 729–832.

22. Richters et al., "NIMH Collaborative Multisite Multimodal Treatment Study of Children with ADHD," in *Journal of the American Academy of Child and Adolescent Psychiatry* (1995), 987–1000.

23. Whalen and Henker (1997).

24. Swanson "Research Synthesis of the Effects of Stimulant Medication on Children with Attention Deficit Disorder" (circa 1993).

25. Swanson et al., "Second Evaluation of MTA 36-Month Outcomes: Propensity Score and Growth Mixture Model Analyses," in *Journal of the American Academy of Child & Adolescent Psychiatry* (2007), 989–1002.

26. Swanson et al., "Effects of Stimulant Medication on Growth Rates Across 3 Years in the MTA Follow-up," in *Journal of the American Academy of Child and Adolescent Psychiatry* (2007), 1015–27.

14. SPELLBOUND BY RITALIN ADDICTION

1. American Psychiatric Association *DSM-IV-TR* (2000); page 211 notes "Oral administration usually results in a slower progression from use to Dependence."

2. See Drug Enforcement Administration papers (October 7, 1993; October 20, 1995, October 1995, and August 7, 1995; December 10–12, 1996). A more up-to-date and available DEA source is C. Sannerud and G. Feussner, "Is Ritalin an Abused Drug? Does It Meet the Criteria of a Schedule II Substance?" in *Ritalin Theory and Practice* (2000), 27–42.

3. The chapter in Dukes's book from which the quote is taken was written by two experts in addiction, Everett Ellinwood and J. Tong (1996), 20.

4. Drug Enforcement Administration "Methylphenidate" (October 1995), 17.

5. Ibid., 19–20.

6. See, for example, Ghosh and Victor, "Suicide," in *The American Psychiatric Press Textbook of Psychiatry* (1999), 1383–1404.

7. See my reviews of the scientific literature concerning stimulant adverse effects in Breggin (2008), in *Ethical Human Sciences and Services* (1999), and in *International Journal of Risk and Safety in Medicine* (1999). For two of the scientific

studies, see Melega et al., in *Behavioural Brain Research* 84 (1997) and Melega et al., in *Brain Research* (1997).

8. Lambert, "The Contribution of Childhood ADHD, Conduct Problems, and Stimulant Treatment to Adolescent and Adult Tobacco and Psychoactive Substance Abuse," in *Ethical Human Psychology and Psychiatry* (2005), 197–221.

15. PARENTS FORCED TO DRUG THEIR CHILDREN

1. All antipsychotics disrupt frontal lobe function causing a virtual chemical lobotomy. Most produce a Parkinson's-like rigidity that also causes a chemical straitjacket. I have discussed this in more detail in *Brain-Disabling Treatments in Psychiatry* (2008).
2. Coyle, "Psychotropic drug use in very young children," in *Journal of the American Medical Association* 283 (2000), 59–60.
3. Abboud, "Treating Children for Bipolar Disorder: Doctors Try Powerful Drugs on Kids as Young as Age 4," in *Wall Street Journal* (May 25, 2005), D1.
4. Moreno et al., "National Trends in the Outpatient Diagnosis and Treatment of Bipolar Disorder in Youth" (2007). The diagnosis of bipolar disorder has continued to escalate since the survey data was collected.
5. Testimony taken from http://www.fda.com, transcripts for the 2004 hearings on antidepressant suicidality in children.
6. Effrem, "Myths and Facts about Minnesota's Plan to Screen the Mental Health of Toddlers" (May 11, 2005), and "Lame Duck Congress Will Vote on Money for Infant Mental Health Testing" (November 10, 2006).
7. The latest developments in mental health screening can be tracked on numerous Web sites including http://www.icspp.org and http://www.edwatch.org.

16. THIS IS NOT MY DAUGHTER

1. For more on deactivation, see chapter 1 in Breggin, *Brain-Disabling Treatments in Psychiatry* (2008).
2. Breggin, *Brain-Disabling Treatments in Psychiatry* (2008) reviews the latest evidence for damage to the structure of the brain and to brain cells caused by antipsychotic and mood-stabilizing drugs. The literature is extensive.
3. Zyrtec is the trade name for cetirizine.
4. I have described the drug effects and the neuroanatomy of these functions in detail in several scientific articles and textbooks, most recently Breggin, *Brain-Disabling Treatments in Psychiatry* (2008).
5. There is no controversy surrounding the 20 percent per year rate in the elderly; the American Psychiatric Association's *Diagnostic and Statistical Manual of Mental Disorders* estimates a cumulative TD rate of 25 to 30 percent in the elderly in the first year of exposure to neuroleptics, page 804. (2000). I've reviewed the actual studies in Breggin, *Brain-Disabling Treatments in Psychiatry* (2008).

6. Breggin, *Brain-Disabling Treatments in Psychiatry* (2008) examines the claim that the newer antipsychotic drugs are safer. In addition to TD, they cause a higher rate of life-threatening diabetes and pancreatitis.

7. Myslobodsky, "Anosognosia in Tardive Dyskinesia: 'Tardive Dysmentia' or 'Tardive Dementia'?" in *Schizophrenia Bulletin* (1986), 1–6.

8. Arango et al., "Relationship of Awareness of Dyskinesia in Schizophrenia to Insight into Mental Illness," in *American Journal of Psychiatry* (1999): 1097–99, found that 46 percent of tardive dyskinesia patients showed lack of awareness of their symptoms.

9. See Breggin, *Brain-Disabling Treatments in Psychiatry* (2008) for a review of studies confirming that tardive dyskinesia is associated with dementia. I have also published relevant scientific articles in *Journal of Mind and Behavior* (1990) and *Brain and Cognition* (1993) on the subject. See also Gualtieri, *Brain Injury and Mental Retardation: Psychopharmacology and Neuropsychiatry* (2002), 401. Gaultieri, one of the most experienced researchers in the field, has pointed out that every study thus far conducted has confirmed that tardive dyskinesia patients have "signs of dementia."

10. In Cade's "Lithium Salts in the Treatment of Psychotic Excitement," *Medical Journal of Australia* (1949), 349–52, he describes how he found that injections of lithium caused apathy in guinea pigs and how this led him to go immediately from the lab to the state hospital ward where he found it did the same thing to people. Hardly the birth of a "magic bullet." See my discussions in *Brain-Disabling Treatments in Psychiatry* (2008).

11. The literature on lithium effects is reviewed in Breggin, *Brain-Disabling Treatments in Psychiatry* (2008).

12. I discuss the nature of psychosis and "schizophrenia" in *Toxic Psychiatry* (1991).

13. American Psychiatric Association *DSM-IV-TR* (2000): 801.

14. See, for example, G. Chouinard and B. Jones, "Neuroleptic-induced supersensitivity psychosis: Clinical and pharmacologic characteristics," *American Journal of Psychiatry* 137 (1980), 16–21. I review the literature in *Brain-Disabling Treatments in Psychiatry* (2008).

15. Gualtieri, *Brain Injury and Mental Retardation*, 2002.

16. Breggin, "Addiction to Neuroleptics?" *American Journal of Psychiatry* 146 (1989), 560, and "Addiction to Neuroleptics: Dr. Breggin Replies," *American Journal of Psychiatry* 146 (1989), 1240.

17. Swartz, and Jones, "Hyperlithemia Correction and Persistent Delirium," in *Journal of Clinical Pharmacology* 34 (1994), 865–70. I discuss lithium withdrawal mania in *Brain-Disabling Treatments in Psychiatry* (2008).

18. DRUG COMPANIES ON TRIAL

1. Breggin, *Toxic Psychiatry* (1991), 165 ff.

2. I testified about this memo in the Wesbecker case and also discussed it in *Brain-Disabling Treatments in Psychiatry* (2008). The actual document was Exhibit 11 attached to a deposition by Fuller in 1994 in that case.

3. I describe these events in detail in *Talking Back to Prozac* (1994). Also see Medawar and Hardon, *Medicines Out of Control* (2004, p 55 ff.) analysis that's partly based on my data about the clinical trials.

4. I discuss the FDA-approval process for Prozac in great detail in *Talking Back to Prozac* (with Ginger Breggin, 1994).

5. See *Fentress et al. v Shea Communications et al.* in the bibliography.

6. No toxicology analysis was done to determine Wesbecker's blood level of Prozac. However, the half-life of Prozac and its chemically active metabolic product is approximately seven to ten days, indicating that more than half probably remained active in his body.

7. Data on suicide, violence, agitation, akathisia, and mania caused by Prozac are discussed in chapter 8 and elsewhere in this book, and in more detail in Breggin and Breggin, *Talking Back to Prozac* (1994), and Breggin, *Brain-Disabling Treatments in Psychiatry* (2008). For a detailed review and analysis of akathisia as a cause for suicide and violence, also see Glenmullen, *Prozac Backlash.* (2000).

8. Castellanos, "Kentucky Fried Verdict Up for Grabs," in *New Jersey Law Journal* (May 15, 1995), 39; Gibeaut, "Mood-Altering Verdict: Judge Suspects Prozac Settlement Though Case Went to Jury," in *ABA Journal* (August 1996), 18; Scanlon, "Secret Deal Struck at Trial Not to Appeal Prozac Verdict," *Courier-Journal* Louisville, Kentucky (April 20, 1995), B1; and most extensively, Varchaver, "Prozac Verdict Was a Sure Thing" (September 25, 1995). Also see Judge J. W. Potter's Corrected Judgment and Court's Motion Pursuant to Civil Rule 60.01 and Notice. *Fentress et al. v Shea Communications et al.* No. 90CI0633 Jefferson Circuit Court, Division Five, Louisville, Kentucky. (April 19, 1995) and the Friend of the Court investigative report from the Kentucky attorney general's office (Sheadel, "Report of the Friends of the Court. *Fentress et al. v Shea Communications et al.*" March 4, 1997).

9. Potter, Notice and Order. *Fentress et al. v Shea Communications et al.* (March 17, 1997), 1.

10. Varchaver, "Prozac Verdict Was a Sure Thing," 1995.

11. Sheadel, "Report of the Friends of the Court. *Fentress et al. v Shea Communications et al.*" (1997), 24. In addition to denying at the time that a settlement had taken place (when it had), both sides later denied the judge's recollection that they had told the judge that no money had changed hands.

12. Castellanos, "Kentucky Fried Verdict Up for Grabs," 1995.

13. Bloomberg News, "Judge Quits Prozac Case: Payout Still Sealed," in *Indianapolis Star* (April 9, 1997), C6.

14. Stevens (May 23, 1996).

15. Later on, American psychiatrist Joseph Glenmullen (*Prozac Backlash,* 2000) and Welsh psychiatrist David Healy ("Emergence of Antidepressant Induced Suicidality," in *Primary Care Psychiatry*, 2000, 23–28) would also become expert witnesses in product-liability suits involving the antidepressants.

16. The four digital folders can be found at my Web site, http://www.breggin.com, along with a detailed analysis.

17. When an increase in adverse reactions is reported in controlled clinical trials (that is, with the investigators blind to whether the reaction was caused by the

drug or a placebo), it is scientifically unethical for nonblind, company-selected consultants to rework the data to the company's advantage.

18. Parker, "The Word 'Missing' Is Misleading" (January 1, 2005), http://www.bmj.com/cgi/eletters/330/7481/7.

19. Lenzer, "FDA to Review 'Missing' Drug Company Documents." *BMJ* 330 (January 1, 2005): 7.

20. See my Web site for more details on the Lilly settlement: http://www.breggin.com.

21. Rosack, "Lilly to Pay Out Millions to Settle Lawsuits over Zyprexa," in *Psychiatric News* (February 2, 2007), 1.

22. Creswell, "Court Orders Lawyer to Return Documents about Eli Lilly Drug," in *New York Times* (December 20, 2006), C14

24. Creswell, "Court Orders Lawyer to Return Documents about Eli Lilly Drug," 2006.

25. Creswell, "Court Orders Lawyer to Return Documents about Eli Lilly Drug," (2006); Berenson, "Eli Lilly Said to Play Down Risk of Top Pill," in *New York Times* (December 17, 2006), A1; "Drug Files Show Maker Promoted Unapproved Use," in *New York Times* (December 18, 2006); A1, and "Two Views on Data Emerge from a Lilly Drug Trial," in *New York Times* (December 21, 2006), C1; and Editorial, "Playing Down the Risks of a Drug: Internal Documents Offer Persuasive Evidence that Eli Lilly Engaged in Questionable Behavior to Prop Up Its Best-selling Drug," in *New York Times* (December 19, 2006), A30.

26. Editorial, *New York Times* (December 19, 2006), A30.

27. See, for example, American Psychiatric Association *DSM-IV-TR* (2000), 800–2.

28. Breggin, *Ethical Human Sciences and Services* and *International Journal of Risk and Safety in Medicine* (2006 b, c, and d). Also available on http://www.breggin.com.

29. Ibid.

30. Food and Drug Administration, "Class Suicidality Label Language for Antidepressants" (January 26, 2005).

31. Angell, *The Truth about the Drug Companies,* 2005.

32. Abramson, *Overdosed America,* 2005.

33. Medawar and Hardon, *Medicines Out of Control*, 2004.

34. R. Smith, "Medical Journals Are an Extension of the Marketing Arm of Pharmaceutical Companies," in *PloS Med* 2 (5) (May 2005), e138

35. I have written about psychotherapy for depression in the final chapters to *Talking Back to Prozac* (1994) and *The Antidepressant Fact Book* (2001), and described my overall approach to therapy in *The Heart of Being Helpful* (1997).

19. MARKETING MYTHS AND THE TRUTH ABOUT PSYCHIATRIC MEDICATION

1. Hales and Yudofsky, *Textbook of Clinical Psychiatry* (2003), 1476. The authors cite the initial short-term compensatory shutdown of serotonin production that may "actually cause an initial decrease in the firing of serotonergic neurons" that "may be prolonged to a clinically deleterious degree."

2. Wong and Bymaster, "Subsensitivity of Serotonin Receptors after Long-Term Treatment of Rats with Fluoxetine" (1981) and Wong et al., "Chronic Effects of Fluoxetine, a Selective Inhibitor of Serotonin Uptake, on Neurotransmitter Receptors" (1985).

3. Wamsley et al., "Receptor Alterations Associated with Serotonergic Agents: An Autographic Analysis" (1987), 19–85; Wong and Bymaster, "Subsensitivity of Serotonin Receptors after Long-Term Treatment of Rats with Fluoxetine" (1981); Wong et al., "Chronic Effects of Fluoxetine, a Selective Inhibitor of Serotonin Uptake, on Neurotransmitter Receptors" (1985); de Montigny et al., "Modification of Serotonergic Neuron Properties by Long-term Treatment with Serotonin Reuptake Blockers" (1990).

4. Hales and Yudofsky, *Textbook of Clinical Psychiatry* (2003), 1059.

5. Fuller, Deposition, Volume I., in *Fentress et al. v. Shea Communications et al.*, (April 14, 1994), 266.

6. Hales and Yudofsky, *Textbook of Clinical Psychiatry* (2003), 479. The biochemical imbalance theory focuses on neurotransmitters called monoamines with familiar names like serotonin, norepinephrine, and dopamine. After reviewing evidence accumulated over more than four decades of pursuing this holy grail of biological psychiatry, the textbook concludes, "Additional experience has not confirmed the monoamine depletion hypothesis."

7. In re Paxil Products Liability Litigation" MDL No. 1574 (MRP); Master File No. CV-01-7397 (MRP), U.S. District Court, Central District of California.

8. *Physicians' Desk Reference* (2006), 1504, first column. It's buried amid a mountain of other data.

9. For discussions of neuroleptic toxicity to the brain, see Breggin, *Brain-Disabling Treatments in Psychiatry* (2008).

10. For a review of studies of persistent brain changes and damage associated with all classes of psychiatric drugs, see Breggin, *Brain-Disabling Treatments in Psychiatry* (2008). As examples of stimulant treatment effects in animals, see Melega et al., in *Behavioural Brain Research* (1997) and W. Melega et al., in *Brain Research* (1997).

11. Studies of persistent brain dysfunction and brain-damage caused by antidepressant drugs like Prozac include Wamsley et al., "Receptor Alterations Associated with Serotonergic Agents: An Autographic Analysis" (1987), who demonstrated that the overstimulated receptors of the serotonin neurons undergo a severe pruning or die back after exposure to Prozac, and Wegerer et al., "Persistently Increased Density of Serotonin Transporters in the Frontal Cortex of Rats Treated with Fluoxetine During Early Juvenile Life" (1999), 13–24, who demonstrated persisting abnormalities in frontal lobe neuronal function in young animals subjected to the drug. Because it can be so hard to believe that there is a substantial body of evidence concerning antidepressant-induced persisting brain damage and dysfunction, it's worth listing a few more studies: de Montigny et al., "Modification of Serotonergic Neuron Properties by Long-term Treatment with Serotonin Reuptake Blockers" (1990); Freo et al., "Effects of Acute and Chronic Treatment with Fluoxetine on Regional Glucose Cerebral Metabolism in Rats" (2000) 35–41; Norrholm et al., "Chronic Fluoxetine Administration to Juvenile Rats Prevents

Age-Associated Dendritic Proliferation in Hippocampus" (2000), 205–15; and Kalia et al., "Comparative Study of Fluoxetine, Sibutramine, Sertraline and Dexfenfluramine on the Morphology of Serotonergic Nerve Terminals Using Serotonin Immunohistochemistry" (2000), 92–105.

12. Gilbert et al., "Decreased Thalamic Volumes of Pediatric Patients with Obsessive-Compulsive Disorder Who Are Taking Paroxetine" (2000), 449–56.

13. Malberg et al., "Chronic Antidepressant Treatment Increases Neurogenesis in Adult Rat Hippocampus" (December 16, 2000), 9104–10. The claim for improvement through abnormal cell growth was made in a press release (Weaver, "Sustained Use of Anti-Depressants Increases Cell Growth and Protects Cells in the Brain," December 15, 2000). Also see Breggin, *Brain-Disabling Treatments in Psychiatry* (2008).

14. *Johns Hopkins Medicine*, "Popular Antidepressants Boost Brain Growth, Hopkins Scientists Report," December 19, 2005.

15. Stockton, "Recreational Use of 'Ecstasy' Causes New Brain Damage" (September 30, 2002). The scientific article is Ricaurte (2002).

16. I describe the Psych–Pharmaceutical Complex in *Toxic Psychiatry* (1991).

17. The Prozac label (*Physicians' Desk Reference,* 2007, pages 802 and 1805) states that approximately 7 percent of the population are "poor metabolizers" who have a genetic defect that leads to lower levels of activity of cytochrome P450 isoenzyme 2D6 (CYP2D6). The company believes that lack of this enzyme does not change the overall clinical effect.

18. I debunked the effectiveness of psychiatric drugs in 1991 in *Toxic Psychiatry.* For a more recent detailed examination of the scientific studies of the supposed effectiveness of these drugs, see Jackson, *Rethinking Psychiatric Drugs* (2005).

19. For details, see Breggin, *Brain-Disabling Treatments in Psychiatry* (1997). For a more in-depth analysis and an introduction into the literature on brain damage induced by antipsychotic drugs, see Breggin, "Brain Damage, Dementia and Persistent Cognitive Dysfunction Associated with Neuroleptic Drugs" (1990) and "Parallels Between Neuroleptic Effects and Lethargic Encephalitis" (1993).

20. Breggin, *Brain-Disabling Treatments in Psychiatry*" (2008).

21. I explore the issues of evil in psychiatry in *Beyond Conflict* (1991).

22. Since 1962, psychiatrist Thomas Szasz (*Myth of Mental Illness,* 1974) has been the most vocal and eloquent in opposing involuntary psychiatric treatment as an offense against humanity.

23. According to http://www.MindFreedom.org.

24. I describe my volunteer experience in *Toxic Psychiatry* (1991).

25. Frank, *The History of Electroshock* (1978), and "Electroshock: Death, Brain Damage, Memory Loss, and Brainwashing" (1990), 489–512.

21. MAKING DRUG WITHDRAWAL AS SAFE AS POSSIBLE

1. In the last few years, physicians have begun to be warned about antidepressant withdrawal problems. Shelton ("6 Safety Rules for Tapering Antidepressants," 2006) presents a similar but slightly less extensive list of "discontinuation symptoms" in a recent issue of *Current Psychiatry*, a magazine sent free to psychiatrists. Led by the drug companies, experts euphemistically call withdrawal symptoms "discontinuation symptoms." Addiction has been renamed dependence and withdrawal has been renamed discontinuation, adding considerably to the confusion of doctors and patients.
2. Cavanaugh et al., "Relapse into Mania or Depression Following Lithium Discontinuation" (2004), 91–95.

22. THE TOUGH QUESTION OF PERSONAL RESPONSIBILITY

1. In *Medication Madness*, I have only skimmed the scientific research confirming these observations. They are dealt with in much more depth in Breggin, *Brain-Disabling Treatments in Psychiatry* (2008).
2. Food and Drug Administration, "SSRIs/SNRI/Triptan and Serotonin Syndrome" (July 2006).
3. The Luvox label with this data can be found in the 2002 *Physicians' Desk Reference.* Luvox was removed from more recent editions.
4. Emslie et al., "Fluoxetine for Acute Treatment of Depression in Children and Adolescents" (2002), 1205–15.
5. There is a transcript of the debate on Bob Johnson's Web site, www://DrBob@ Truthtrustconsent.com.
6. The issue in dispute was the frequency of tardive dyskinesia in patients treated with antipsychotic drugs. I cited figures from the 1980 American Psychiatric Association *Task Force Report 18: Tardive Dyskinesia* (page 44) that at least 10 to 20 percent of patients in hospitals and at least 40 percent of long-term clinical patients will develop the disorder. I describe and quote my debate with Fink in more detail in *Toxic Psychiatry* (1991), 358–60.

23. CHOOSE YOUR LAST RESORT WISELY

1. Cosgrove et al., "Financial Ties between *DSM-IV* Panel Members and the Pharmaceutical Industry" (2006), 154–60. The investigators found that "One hundred percent of the members of the panels on 'Mood Disorders' and 'Schizophrenia and Other Psychotic Disorders' had financial ties to drug companies."
2. Breggin, Breggin, and Bemak, eds., *Dimensions of Empathic Therapy* (2002).
3. Approaches to drug-free treatment, including severely disturbed persons can be found in Breggin and Stern, eds., *Psychosocial Approaches to Deeply Disturbed*

Persons (1996); and Breggin, Breggin, and Bemak, eds., *Dimensions of Empathic Therapy* (2002, especially chapters 9 to 11).

4. de Girolamo, "WHO Studies on Schizophrenia." In *Psychosocial Approaches to Deeply Disturbed Persons* (1996), 213–31.

5. I first published a slightly different version called "The Fifteen Principles of Life" on Thanksgiving Day 2006, on my blog on http://www.huffingtonpost.com. I would like these principles to have as wide exposure as possible. Therefore, permission is granted to republish my Principles of Life from this chapter, provided that they are unmodified and provided they are attributed to the author and to *Medication Madness*.

Bibliography

Abboud, L. "Treating Children for Bipolar Disorder: Doctors Try Powerful Drugs on Kids as Young as age 4." *Wall Street Journal,* May 25, 2005, D1.

Abramson, J. *Overdosed America: The Broken Promise of American Medicine.* New York: Harper Perennial, 2005.

American Psychiatric Association. *Task Force Report on Benzodiazepine Dependence, Toxicity, and Abuse.* Washington, DC: American Psychiatric Press, 1990.

———. *Diagnostic and Statistical Manual of Mental Disorders,* fourth edition, *(DSM-IV).* Washington, DC: American Psychiatric Association, 1994.

———. *Diagnostic and Statistical Manual of Mental Disorders,* fourth edition, text revision *(DSM-IV-TR).* Washington, DC: American Psychiatric Association, 2000.

Anabolic Steroid Control Act of 2004 (H.R. 3866; S2195). An Amendment to the Controlled Substances Act, 102nd Congress, April 2, 2004.

Anello, C. (1989, September 12). Memorandum: Triazolam and temazepam comparison reporting rates. FDA Center for Drug Evaluation and Research, Office of Epidemiology and Biostatistics. Obtained through the Freedom of Information Act.

Angell, M. *The Truth about the Drug Companies: How They Deceive Us and What to Do About It.* New York: Random House, 2005.

———. "Taking Back the FDA." *Boston Globe,* February 26, 2007. Retrieved from http://www.boston.com.

Arana, G., & Hyman, S. *Handbook of Psychiatric Drug Treatment,* second ed. Boston: Little, Brown, 1991.

Arango, C., Adami, H., Sherr, J., Thaker, G., and Carpenter, W. "Relationship of Awareness of Dyskinesia in Schizophrenia to Insight into Mental Illness." *American Journal of Psychiatry,* 156 (1999): 1097–1099.

Armstrong, T. *The Myth of the A.D.D. Child.* New York: Dutton, 1995.

Arnold, L., and P. Jensen. "Attention-Deficit Disorders." In *Comprehensive Textbook of Psychiatry,* fourth ed., 2295–310, edited by H. I. Kaplan and B. Sadock. Baltimore: Williams & Wilkins, 1995.

Ashton, H. (1995). "Toxicity and Adverse Consequences of Benzodiazepine Use." *Psychiatric Annals* 25 (1995): 158–65.

Associated Press. "Food and Drug Administration: Watch for Behavior Change in Children Taking Tamiflu." *Foxnews.com,* November 14, 2006. http://www.Foxnews.com.

———. "FBI Releases Rehnquist Drug Problem Records." *MSNBC.com,* January 4, 2007. http://www.msnbc.com.

Bach, L. and A. David. "Self-awareness After Acquired and Traumatic Brain Injury." *Neuropsychological Rehabilitation* 16 (2006): 397–414.

Barancik, S. "Paxil Saves Him from Prison: Judge Agrees Antidepressant was Partially Responsible for Jabil Worker Embezzling $1.8 Million." *St. Petersburg Times,* November 20, 2006. Retrieved from http://www.tampabay.com.

Bastani, J., M. Troester, and A. Bastani. "Serotonin Syndrome and Fluvoxamine: A Case Study." *Nebraska Medical Journal* 81 (1996): 107–9.

Battaglia, G., S. Y. Yeh, E. O'Hearn, M. E. Molliver, M. J. Kuhar, and E. B. De Souza. "3,4-Methylenedioxymethamphetamine and 3,4-Methylenedioxyamphetamine Destroy Serotonin Terminals in Rat Brain.*" Journal of Pharmacology and Experimental Therapeutics* 242 (1987): 911–16.

Beer, J., O. John, D. Scabini, and R. Knight. "Orbitofrontal Cortex and Social Behavior: Integrating Self-monitoring and Emotion-Cognition Interactions." In *Journal of Cognitive Neuroscience* 18 (2006): 871–79.

Berenson, A. "Eli Lilly Said to Play Down Risk of Top Pill." *The New York Times,* December 17, 2006, A1.

———. "Drug Files Show Maker Promoted Unapproved Use." *The New York Times,* December 18, 2006, A1.

———. "Two Views on Data Emerge from a Lilly Drug Trial." *The New York Times,* December 21, 2006, C1.

Birrer, R. and S. Vemuri. "Depression in Later Life: A Diagnostic and Therapeutic Challenge." *American Family Physician* 69 (May 15, 2004): 2375–82. http://www.aafp.org/afp/20040515/2375.pdf.

Black, H. *Black's Law Dictionary.* St. Paul, Minnesota: West Publishing Company, 1979.

Bloomberg News. "Judge Quits Prozac Case: Payout Still Sealed." *Indianapolis Star,* April 9, 1997, C6.

Boerlin, H., M. Gitlin, L. Zoellner, and C. Hammen. "Bipolar Depression and Antidepressant-Induced Mania: A Naturalistic Study." *Journal of Clinical Psychiatry* 59 (1998): 374–79.

Borcherding, B., C. Keysor, J. Rapoport, J. Elia, and J. Amass. "Motor/Vocal Tics and Compulsive Behaviors on Stimulant Drugs: Is There a Common Vulnerability?" *Psychiatric Research* 33 (1990): 83–94.

Bostwick, J. and T. Lineberry. "The 'Meth' Epidemic: Acute Intoxication," *Current Psychiatry* 5(11) (November 2006): 47–62.

Breggin, P. "Iatrogenic Helplessness in Authoritarian Psychiatry." *In The Iatrogenics Handbook,* edited by R. F. Morgan. Toronto: IPI Publishing Company, 1983.

————. "Neuropathology and Cognitive Dysfunction from ECT." *Psychopharmacology Bulletin* 22 (1986): 476–79.

————. "Addiction to Neuroleptics?" *American Journal of Psychiatry* 146 (1989): 560.

————. "Addiction to Neuroleptics: Dr. Breggin Replies." *American Journal of Psychiatry* 146 (1989): 1240.

————. "Brain Damage, Dementia and Persistent Cognitive Dysfunction Associated with Neuroleptic Drugs: Evidence, Etiology, Implications." *Journal of Mind and Behavior* 11 (1990): 425–64.

————. *Toxic Psychiatry.* New York: St. Martin's Press, 1991.

————. *Beyond Conflict: From Self-Help and Psychotherapy to Peacemaking.* New York: St. Martin's Press, 1992.

————. "A Case of Fluoxetine-Induced Stimulant Side Effects with Suicidal Ideation Associated with a Possible Withdrawal Syndrome ('Crashing')." *International Journal of Risk and Safety in Medicine* 3 (1992): 325–28.

————. "The President's Sleeping Pills [Halcion] and Its Maker." *The New York Times,* February 11, 1992, A24.

————. "Parallels Between Neuroleptic Effects and Lethargic Encephalitis: The Production of Dyskinesias and Cognitive Disorders." *Brain and Cognition* 23 (1993): 8–27.

————. Testimony in *Joyce Fentress et al. vs. Shea Communications et al.* ["The Wesbecker Case"] Jefferson Circuit Court, Division One, Louisville, Kentucky. NO. 90CI06033. Volume XVI. October 17–19, 1994.

————. "Prozac 'Hazardous' to Children." *Clinical Psychiatry News* 23 (1995): 10.

————. *The Heart of Being Helpful: Empathy and the Creation of a Healing Presence.* New York: Springer Publishing Company, 1997.

————. "Analysis of Adverse Behavioral Effects of Benzodiazepines with a Discussion of Drawing Scientific Conclusions from the FDA's Spontaneous Reporting System." *Journal of Mind and Behavior* 19 (1998): 21–50.

————. "Risks and Mechanism of Action of Stimulants." *NIH Consensus Development Conference Program and Abstracts: Diagnosis and Treatment of Attention Deficit Hyperactivity Disorder.* Rockville, MD: National Institutes of Health, 1998, 105–20.

————. "Psychostimulants in the Treatment of Children Diagnosed with ADHD Part I: Acute Risks and Psychological Effects." *Ethical Human Sciences and Service* 1 (1999): 13–33.

————. "Psychostimulants in the Treatment of Children Diagnosed with ADHD Part II: Adverse Effects on Brain and Behavior." *Ethical Human Sciences and Services* 1 (1999): 213–42.

————. "Psychostimulants in the Treatment of Children Diagnosed with ADHD: Risks and Mechanism of Action," *International Journal of Risk and Safety in Medicine* 12 (1999): 3–35. Simultaneously published version of the two articles by the same name in *Ethical Human Sciences and Services.*

————. *Reclaiming our Children: A Healing Plan for a Nation in Crisis.* Cambridge, MA: Perseus Books, 2000.

————. *Talking Back to Ritalin,* revised edition. Cambridge, MA: Perseus Books, 2001.

————. *The Antidepressant Fact Book.* Cambridge, MA: Perseus Books, 2001.

————. *The Ritalin Fact Book.* Cambridge, MA: Perseus Books, 2002.

————. "Fluvoxamine as a Cause of Stimulation, Mania, and Aggression with a Critical Analysis of the FDA-Approved Label." *International Journal of Risk and Safety in Medicine* 14 (2002): 71–86.

————. "Suicidality, Violence and Mania Caused by Selective Serotonin Reuptake Inhibitors (SSRIs): A Review and Analysis." *Ethical Human Sciences and Services* 5 (2003): 225–46. Simultaneously published in the *International Journal of Risk and Safety in Medicine* 16 (2003/2004): 31–49.

————. Presentation at a Public Hearing of the Food and Drug Administration (FDA), September 13, 2004. Transcript of Meeting of the Center for Drug Evaluation and Research, pp. 353–354. Joint meeting of the CDER Psychopharmacologic Drugs Advisory Committee and the FDA Pediatric Advisory Committee. Bethesda, MD, http://www.fda.gov.

————. "Recent Regulatory Changes in Antidepressant Labels: Implications for Activation (Stimulation) in Clinical Practice." *Primary Psychiatry* 13 (2006): 57–60.

————. "Court Filing Makes Public My Previously Suppressed Analysis of Paxil's Effects." *Ethical Human Psychology and Psychiatry* 8 (2006): 77–84.

————. "How GlaxoSmithKline Suppressed Data on Paxil-Induced Akathisia: Implications for Suicide and Violence." *Ethical Human Psychology and Psychiatry* 8 (2006): 91–100.

————. "Drug Company Suppressed Data on Paroxetine-Induced Stimulation: Implications for Violence and Suicide." *Ethical Human Psychology and Psychiatry* 8 (2006): 255–63.

————. "Intoxication Anosognosia: The Spellbinding Effect of Psychiatric Drugs." *Ethical Human Psychology and Psychiatry* 8 (2006): 201–15.

————. *Brain-Disabling Treatments in Psychiatry,* second edition. New York: Springer Publishing Company, 2008.

Breggin, P. and Breggin, G. *Talking Back to Prozac.* New York: St. Martin's Press, 1994.

————. *The War Against Children of Color: Psychiatry Targets Inner City Children.* Monroe, ME: Common Courage Press, 1998. Revision of *The War Against Children.* New York: St. Martin's Press, 1994.

Breggin, P., G. Breggin, and F. Bemak, eds. *Dimensions of Empathic Therapy.* New York: Springer Publishing Company, 2002.

Breggin, P. and D. Cohen. *Your Drug May Be Your Problem.* Cambridge, MA: Perseus Books, 2007.

Breggin, P. and E. Stern, eds. *Psychosocial Approaches to Deeply Disturbed Persons.* New York: Haworth Press, 1996.

Burrai, C., A. Bocchetta, and M. Zompo. "Mania and Fluvoxamine," *American Journal of Psychiatry* 148 (1991): 1263–64.

Cade, J. "Lithium Salts in the Treatment of Psychotic Excitement." *Medical Journal of Australia* 2 (1949): 349–52.

Castellano, M. "Kentucky Fried Verdict Up for Grabs." *New Jersey Law Journal* (May 15, 1995): 39.

Castner, S., M. Al-Tikriti, R. Baldwin, J. Seibyl, R. Innis, and P. Goldman-Rakic. "Behavioral Changes and [123]IBZM Equilibrium SPECT Measurement of Amphetamine-Induced Dopamine Release in Rhesus Monkeys Exposed to Subchronic Amphetamine." *Neuropsychopharmacology* 22 (2000): 4–13.

Castner, S. and P. Goldman-Rakic. "Long-lasting Psychotomimetic Consequences of Repeated Low-Dose Amphetamine Exposure in Rhesus Monkeys." *Neuropsychopharmacology* 20 (1999): 10–28.

Cavanaugh, J., R. Smyth, and G. Goodwin. "Relapse into Mania or Depression Following Lithium Discontinuation: A 7-Year Follow-up." *Acta Psychiatrica Scandinavia* 109 (2004): 91–95.

Cherland, E., and R. Fitzpatrick. "Psychotic Side Effects of Psychostimulants: A 5-Year Review." *Canadian Journal of Psychiatry* 44 (1999): 811–13.

Chouinard, G., and B. Jones. Neuroleptic-Induced Supersensitivity Psychosis: Clinical and Pharmacologic Characteristics." *American Journal of Psychiatry* 137 (1980): 16–21.

Committee on Safety of Medicines. "Triazolam: Assessor's Report. Appeal by Upjohn Against Revocation of Product License." London, England (1991).

———. "Benzodiazepines, Dependence and Withdrawal Symptoms." *Current Problems* 21 (1998): 1–2.

Cosgrove, L., S. Krimsky, M. Vijayaraghavan, and L. Schneider. "Financial Ties between *DSM-IV* Panel Members and the Pharmaceutical Industry." *Psychotherapy and Psychosomatics* 76 (2006): 154–60.

Coyle, J. "Psychotropic Drug Use in Very Young Children." *Journal of the American Medical Association* 283 (2000): 1059–60.

Creswell, J. "Court Orders Lawyer to Return Documents about Eli Lilly Drug." *The New York Times,* December 20, 2006, C14.

de Girolamo, G. "WHO Studies on Schizophrenia: An Overview of the Results and Their Implications in Understanding the Disorder." In *Psychosocial approaches to Deeply Disturbed Persons,* edited by P. Breggin and E. Stern. New York: Haworth Press, 1996, 213–31.

DiMascio, A. and R. Shader. *Clinical Handbook of Psychopharmacology.* New York: Science House, 1970.

Dooren, J. "FDA Says Bladder Drug Needs Children Warnings." *Wall Street Journal,* April 10, 2007, D2.

Dorevitch, A., Y. Frankel, A. Bar-Halperin, R. Aronzon, and L. Zilberman. "Fluvoxamine-Associated Manic Behavior: A Case Series." *Annals of Pharmacotherapy* 27 (1993): 1455–57.

Drug Enforcement Administration (DEA). Public Affairs Press Release Concerning Aggregate Production Quota for Methylphenidate, October 7, 1993. Washington, DC: Public Affairs Section, DEA, U.S. Department of Justice.

———. Response to CH.A.D.D. Petition Concerning Ritalin, August 7, 1995. (See cover letter by Greene, 1995). Washington, DC: DEA, U.S. Department of Justice.

———. Methylphenidate (A background paper). Washington, DC: Drug and Chemical Evaluation Section, Office of Diversion Control, October 1995, DEA, U.S. Department of Justice.

———. Methylphenidate: DEA Press Release [attached to DEA, October 20, 1995]. Washington, DC: Drug and Chemical Evaluation Section, Office of Diversion Control, DEA, U.S. Department of Justice.

———. Conference Report: Stimulant Use in the Treatment of ADHD, December 10–12, 1996. Washington, DC: DEA, U.S. Department of Justice.

Drugs Facts and Comparisons. St. Louis, MO: Facts and Comparisons, 2008.

Dukes, M.N.G., ed. "The van der Kroef Syndrome." *Side Effects of Drugs Annual* 4 (Amsterdam: Elsevier, 1980): v–ix.

———. *Meyler's Side Effects of Drugs: An Encyclopedia of Adverse Reactions and Interactions,* thirteenth ed. Amsterdam: Elsevier, 1996.

Ebert, D., R. Albert, A. May, A. Merz, H. Murata, I. Stosiek, and B. Zahner. "The Serotonin Syndrome and Psychosis-like Side Effects of Fluvoxamine in Clinical Use—An Estimation of Incidence." *European Neuro-Pharmacology* 7 (1997): 71–74.

Editorial. "Playing Down the Risks of a Drug: Internal Documents Offer Persuasive Evidence that Eli Lilly Engaged in Questionable Behavior to Prop Up Its Bestselling Drug." *The New York Times,* December 19, 2006, A30.

Effrem, K. "Myths and Facts about Minnesota's Plan to Screen the Mental Health of Toddlers" (May 11, 2005). http://www.edwatch.org/updates05/051105-mhtw. htm.

———. "Lame Duck Congress Will Vote on Money for Infant Mental Health Testing" (November 10, 2006). http://www.edaction.org/2006/111006-mht.htm.

Ellenwood, E, and J. Tong. "Central Nervous System Stimulants and Anorectic Agents." In Dukes, M.N.G. ed., *Meyler's Side Effects of Drugs: An Encyclopedia of Adverse Reactions and Interactions*, thirteenth edition, chapter 1, pp. 1–30. (Amsterdam: Elsevier, 1996.)

Emslie, G., J. Heiligenstein, K. Wagner, S. Hoog, E. Ernest, E. Brown, M. Nilsson, and J. Jacobson. "Fluoxetine for Acute Treatment of Depression in Children and Adolescents: a Placebo-Controlled Randomized Clinical Trial." *Journal of the American Academy of Child and Adolescent Psychiatry* 41 (2002): 1205–15.

Emslie, G., A. Rush, W. Weinberg, R. Kowatch, C. Hughes, T. Carmody, and T. Rintelmann. "A Double-Blind, Randomized, Placebo-Controlled Trial of Fluoxetine in Children and Adolescents with Depression." *Archives of General Psychiatry* 54 (1997): 1031–37.

Fentress et al. v Shea Communications et al. [The "Wesbecker Case"] No. 90CI0633 Jefferson Circuit Court, Division One, Louisville, Kentucky.

Fisher, J. "Cognitive and Behavioral Consequences of Closed Head Injury." *Seminars in Neurology* 5 (3), September 1985.

Fisher, S., and R. Greenberg. *The Limits of Biological Treatments for Psychological Distress: Comparisons with Psychotherapy and Placebo.* Hillsdale, NJ: Erlbaum, 1989.

Food and Drug Administration (FDA). "New Halcion Labeling." *Medical Bulletin* 22 (1992): 7.

———. "FDA Issues Public Health Advisory on Cautions for Use of Antidepressants in Adults and Children," March 22, 2004. http://www.fda.gov.

———. "Transcript of Meeting of the Center for Drug Evaluation and Research. Joint meeting of the CDER Psychopharmacologic Drugs Advisory Committee and the FDA Pediatric Advisory Committee," Bethesda, Maryland, September 14, 2004. http://www.fda.gov.

———. "Class Suicidality Labeling Language for Antidepressants." Rockville, Maryland, January 26, 2005. http://www.fda.gov.

———. "Medication Guide: About Using Antidepressants in Children and Teenagers," Rockland, Maryland, January 26, 2005. Obtained from http://www.fda.gov.

———. "HHS Launches Crackdown on Products Containing Andro, March 11, 2005." Retrieved on April 20, 2005 from http://www.fda.gov.

————. "FDA Statement on Concerta and Methylphenidate for June 30 PAC (Pediatric Advisory Committee briefing information, June 29, 2005)," June 30, 2005. http://www.fda.gov.

————. "FDA Issues Public Health Advisory on Strattera (Atomoxetine) for Attention Deficit Disorder." Rockland, Maryland, September 28, 2005. Obtained from http://www.fda.gov.

————. "Summary of Psychiatric and Neurological Adverse Events from June 2005 1-year Post Pediatric Exclusivity Reviews of Concerta and Other Methylphenidate Products. Table 2: Brief Case Summaries of Psychiatric Adverse Events for Concerta, Immediate-Release Methylphenidate, and Extended Release Methylphenidate (N=52)," March 14, 2006. http://www.fda.gov.

————. "SSRIs/SNRI/Triptan and Serotonin Syndrome," July 2006. http://www.fda.gov.

————. "FDA News: FDA Approves the First Drug to Treat Irritability Associated with Autism, Risperdal," October 6, 2006. http://www.fda.gov.

————. "Summary Minutes of the Psychopharmacologic Drugs Advisory Committee [on Antidepressant-Induced Suicidality in Adults]," December 13, 2006. http://www.fda.gov.

————. "FDA News: FDA Directs ADHD Drug Manufacturers to Notify Patients about Cardiovascular Adverse Events and Psychiatric Adverse Events," February 21, 2007. http://www.fda.gov.

————. "Consultative Review and Evaluation of Clinical Data." Consult No. 10,988 by Gwen L. Zornberg, Medical Officer, on Ditropan (Oxybutynin Chloride) Adverse Effects, February 28, 2007. http://www.fda.gov.

————. "FDA News: FDA Requests Label Change for All Sleep Disorder Drug Products," March 14, 2007. http://www.fda.gov.

Frank, L., ed. *The History of Electroshock* (1978). Available from L. Frank, 2300 Webster Street, San Francisco, CA 94115. Also available on http://www.Amazon.com.

————. "Electroshock: Death, Brain Damage, Memory Loss, and Brainwashing." *Journal of Mind and Behavior* 11 (1990): 489–512.

————. "The Electroshock Quotationery." *Ethical Human Psychology and Psychiatry* 8 (2006): 157–77.

————. *Freedom.* New York: Random House, 2007.

Frankenfield, D, S. Baker, W. Lange, Y. Caplan, and J. Smialek." Fluoxetine and Violent Death in Maryland." *Forensic Science International* 64 (1994):107–17.

French, A. "Dangerous Aggressive Behavior as a Side Effect of Alprazolam." *American Journal of Psychiatry* 146 (1989): 276.

Freo, U., C. Ori, M. Dam, A. Merico, and G. Pizzolato. "Effects of Acute and Chronic Treatment with Fluoxetine on Regional Glucose Cerebral Metabolism in Rats: Implications for Clinical Therapies." *Brain Research* 854 (2000): 35–41.

Friedberg, J. *Electroshock Is Not Good for Your Brain.* San Francisco: Glide Publications, 1976.

————. "Shock Treatment, Brain Damage, and Memory Loss: A Neurological Perspective." *American Journal of Psychiatry* 134 (1977): 1010–14.

Fuller, R. Deposition, Volume I., in *Fentress, et al. v. Shea Communications et al.*, Jefferson Circuit Court, Division One, No. 90-CL-6033, April 14. 1994.

Gelperin, K. and K. Phelan. "Psychiatric Adverse Events Associated with Drug Treatment of ADHD: Review of Postmarketing Safety Data." Food and Drug Administration, Rockville, Maryland, May 3, 2006.

Ghaemi, S., D. Hsu, F. Soldani, and F. Goodwin. "Antidepressants in Bipolar Disorder: the Case for Caution." *Bipolar Disorders* 3 (2003): 421–33.

Ghosh, T., and B. Victor. "Suicide." In *The American Psychiatric Press Textbook of Psychiatry,* chapter 36, pp. 1383–1404, edited by R. Hales, S. Yudofsky, and J. Talbott. Washington, DC: American Psychiatric Press, 1999.

Gibeaut, J. "Mood-Altering Verdict: Judge Suspects Prozac Settlement Though Case Went to Jury." *ABA Journal,* August 1996, 18.

Gilbert, A., G. Moore, M. Keshavan, L. Paulson, V. Narula, P. Mac Master, C. Stewart, and D. Rosenberg. "Decreased Thalamic Volumes of Pediatric Patients with Obsessive-Compulsive Disorder Who Are Taking Paroxetine." *Archives of General Psychiatry* 57 (2000): 449–56.

GlaxoSmithKline. Important Prescribing Information (Dear Healthcare Provider Letter). [About clinical worsening and suicide in adults taking Paxil]. Philadelphia, Pennsylvania, May 2006.

Glenmullen, J. *Prozac Backlash.* New York: Simon & Schuster, 2000.

Goldberg, J. and C. Truman. "Antidepressant-Induced Mania: An Overview of Current Controversies." *Bipolar Disorders* 5 (2003): 407–20.

Graham, J. "Strong Antidepressant Warning Urged: FDA Advisory Panel Wants Labels Changed to Reflect Suicide Risk to Patients Ages 18–24." *Baltimore Sun.* http://www.baltimoresun.com (accessed December 14, 2006).

Gualtieri, C. *Brain Injury and Mental Retardation: Psychopharmacology and Neuropsychiatry.* Philadelphia: Lippincott Williams & Williams, 2002.

Hales, R. and S. Yudofsky, eds. *Textbook of Clinical Psychiatry.* Washington, DC: American Psychiatric Publishing, 2003.

Hammad, T., T. Laughren, and J. Racoosin. "Suicidality in Pediatric Patients Treated with Antidepressant Drugs." *Archives of General Psychiatry* 63 (2006): 332–39.

Harmer, C., C. Mackay, C. Reid, P. Cowen, and G. Goodwin. "Antidepressant Drug Treatment Modifies the Neural Processing of Nonconscious Threats." *Biological Psychiatry* 59 (2006): 816–20.

Harris, G. "Study Condemns F.D.A.'s Handling of Drug Safety." *The New York Times,* September 23, 2006, 1.

Hartlage, L. and G. Rattan. "Brain Injury from Motor Vehicle Accidents." In *Preventable Brain Damage,* edited by D. Templer, L. Hartlage, and W. Cannon, W. New York: Springer Publishing Company, 1992.

Hartelius, H. "Cerebral Changes Following Electrically Induced Convulsions." *Acta Psychiatrica Neurologica Scandinavica* 77(supp) (1952): 1–128.

Healy, D. "Emergence of Antidepressant Induced Suicidality." *Primary Care Psychiatry* 6 (1) (2000): 23–28.

Henderson, T. and K. Hartman. "Aggression, Mania, and Hypomania Induction Associated with Atomoxetine." *Pediatrics* 114 (2004): 895.

Henry, C., and J. Demotes-Mainard. "Avoiding Drug-Induced Switching in Patients with Bipolar Depression." *Drug Safety* 26 (2003): 337–51.

Henry, C., F. Sorbara, J. Lacoste, C. Gindre, and M. Leboyer. "Antidepressant-

Induced Mania in Bipolar Patients: Identification of Risk Factors." *Journal of Clinical Psychiatry* 62 (2001): 249–55.

Hirshkowitz, M. "Neuropsychiatric Aspects of Sleep and Sleep Disorders." In *Neuropsychiatry and Clinical Neurosciences,* fourth edition, chapter 20, 697–722, edited by S. Yudofsky and R. Hales. Washington, DC: American Psychiatric Publishing, 2002.

Hoehn-Saric, R., J. Lipsey, and D. McLeod, D. "Apathy and Indifference in Patients on Fluvoxamine and Fluoxetine." *Journal of Clinical Psychopharmacology* 10 (1990): 343–45.

Hoffman, B. "Catecholamines, Sympathomimetic Drugs, and Adrenergic Receptor Antagonists." In *Goodman & Gilman's The Pharmacological Basis of Therapeutics,* tenth edition, chapter 10, 215–68, edited by J. Hardman and L. Limbird. New York: McGraw-Hill, 2001.

Howland, R. "Induction of Mania with Serotonin Reuptake Inhibitors." *Journal of Clinical Psychopharmacology* 16 (1996): 425–27.

Iacuzio, D. "Dear Healthcare Professional: Important Prescribing Information [about Tamiflu]," Roche Laboratories, Nutley, NJ, November 13, 2006.

Jackson, G. *Rethinking Psychiatric Drugs: A Guide for Informed Consent.* Bloomington, IN: AuthorHouse Books, 2005.

———. "A Curious Consensus: Brain Scans Prove Disease." *Ethical Human Psychology and Psychiatry* 8 (2006): 55–60.

Johns Hopkins Medicine. "Popular Antidepressants Boost Brain Growth, Hopkins Scientists Report." December 19, 2005.

Johnson, C. "Study: Antidepressant Benefits Trump Risks for Kids." For the Associated Press. *The Ithaca Journal,* April 18, 2007, 6A.

Jonas, J. "Dr. Jeffrey M. Jonas, Director of CNS Clinical Development at Upjohn, Replies." *Clinical Psychiatry News* (October 1992), 5.

Josefson, D. "Jury Finds Drug 80% Responsible for Killings." *British Medical Journal* 322 (June 16, 2001): 1446.

Joseph, J. "The Genetic Theory of Schizophrenia: A Critical Review." *Ethical Human Sciences and Services* 1 (1999): 119–45.

———. *The Gene Illusion: Genetic Research in Psychiatry and Psychology Under the Microscope.* Ross-on-Wye, England: PCCS Books, 2003.

Juurlink, D., M. Mamdani, A. Kopp, and D. Redelmeier. "The Risk of Suicide with Selective Reuptake Inhibitors in the Elderly." *American Journal of Psychiatry* 163 (2006) 813–21.

Kalia, M., J. O'Callaghan, D. Miller, and M. Kramer. "Comparative Study of Fluoxetine, Sibutramine, Sertraline and Dexfenfluramine on the Morphology of Serotonergic Nerve Terminals Using Serotonin Immunohistochemistry." *Brain Research* 858 (2000): 92–105.

Kapit, R. Safety Review of NDA 18-936 [Prozac]. Internal document of the Department of Health and Human Services, Public Health Service, Food and Drug Administration, Center for Drug Evaluation and Research (March 28, 1986). Obtained through the Freedom of Information Act.

———. Safety Update. NDA 18-936. Internal document of the Department of Health and Human Services, Public Health Service, Food and Drug Administration,

Center for Drug Evaluation and Research (November 17, 1986). Obtained through the Freedom of Information Act.

Karon, B. "The Tragedy of Schizophrenia Without Psychotherapy." *Journal of the American Academy of Psychoanalysis and Dynamic Psychiatry* 31 (2003): 89–118.

Kean, B. "The Risk Society and Attention Deficit Hyperactivity Disorder (ADHD): A Critical Social Research Analysis Concerning the Development and Social Impact of the ADHD Diagnosis." *Ethical Human Psychology and Psychiatry* 7 (2005): 131–42.

———. "The Globalisation of Attention Deficit Hyperactivity Disorder and the Rights of the Child." *International Journal of Risk and Safety in Medicine* 18 (2006): 195–204

Kirsch, I., B. Deacon, T. Huedo-Medina, A. Scoboria, T. Moore, and B. Johnson. Initial severity and antidepressant benefits: A meta-analysis of data submitted to the food and drug administration. *PloS Med* 5(2): e45. doi:10.1371,/journal. pmed.0050045 (2008).

Kirsch, I. and G. Sapirstein. "Listening to Prozac but Hearing Placebo: A Meta-Analysis of Antidepressant Medication." *Prevention & Treatment* 1, Article 0002a, http://www.journals.apa.org (posted June 26, 1998).

Kirsch, I., T. Moore, A. Scoboria, and S. Nicholls, S. "The Emperor's New Drugs: An Analysis of Antidepressant Medication Data Submitted to the U.S. Food and Drug Administration." *Prevention & Treatment* 5, article 23 (posted July 15, 2002).

Kjelstrup, K., F. Tuvnes, H-A Steffenach, R. Murison, E. Moser, and M-B Moser. "Reduced Fear Expression after Lesions of the Ventral Hippocampus." *PNAS* 99 (16) (2002): 10825–30.

Lambert, N. "The Contribution of Childhood ADHD, Conduct Problems, and Stimulant Treatment to Adolescent and Adult Tobacco and Psychoactive Substance Abuse." *Ethical Human Psychology and Psychiatry* 7 (2005): 97–221.

Lenzer, J. "FDA to Review 'Missing' Drug Company Documents." *British Medical Journal* 330 (January 1, 2005): 7.

———. "Eli Lilly: Correction and apology." *British Medical Journal* 330 (January 29, 2005): 211.

———. "FDA Accepts Weakened Antidepressant Warning." *British Medical Journal* 330 (March 19, 2005): 620.

Lipinsky, J.F., Jr., G. Mallaya, P. Zimmerman, and H. Pope Jr. "Fluoxetine-Induced Akathisia: Clinical and Theoretical Implications." *Journal of Clinical Psychiatry* 50 (1989): 339–52.

Malberg, J., A. Eisch, E. Nestler, and R. Duman, R. "Chronic Antidepressant Treatment Increases Neurogenesis in Adult Rat Hippocampus." *Journal of Neuroscience* 20 (December 16, 2000): 9104–10.

Marangell, L., S. Yudofsky, and J. Silver. "Psychopharmacology and Electroconvulsive Therapy." In *The American Psychiatric Press Textbook of Psychiatry,* third edition, chapter 27, 1025–1132, by R. Hales, S. Yudofsky, and J. Talbot. Washington, DC: American Psychiatric Press, 1999.

Marks, J. *The Search for the Manchurian Candidate: The CIA and Mind Control.* New York: Times Books, 1979.

Mathews, A. "FDA Plans Drug-Safety Moves." *Wall Street Journal,* January 31, 2007, A11.

———. "Reports Blasts FDA's System to Track Drugs: Consultant Says System

Hobbled by Missteps; Agency Disputes Claims." *Wall Street Journal,* March 3–4, 2007, A1.

Mathews, A. and J. Dooren, J. "Sleep Drugs Get Warning on Labels Sought by FDA." *Wall Street Journal,* March 15, 2007, D9.

Maxmen, J. and N. Ward. *Psychotropic Drugs Fast Facts.* New York: Norton, 1995.

McClelland, R., G. Fenton, and W. Rutherford. "The Postconcussional Syndrome Revisited." *Journal of the Royal Society of Medicine* 87 (Spetember 1994): 508–10.

McGee, J. and C. DeBernardo. "The Classroom Avenger." *Forensic Examiner* (May/June 1999): 16–18.

McGuinness, D. "Attention Deficit Disorder: The Emperor's New Clothes, Animal 'Pharm,' and Other Fiction." In *The Limits of Biological Treatments for Psychological Distress,* edited by S. Fisher and R. Greenberg. Hillsdale, NJ: Lawrence Erlbaum Associates, 1989, 151–88.

Medawar, C. and A. Hardon. *Medicines Out of Control? Antidepressants and the Conspiracy of Goodwill.* London: Aksant Academic Publishers/Transaction, 2004.

MedlinePlus. "Drug Information: Ethchlorvynol. U.S. National Library of Medicine and the National Institutes of Health" (2007). http://www.nlm.nih.gov/medlineplus.

Melega, W., M. Raleigh, D. Stout, S. Huang, and M. Phelps. "Ethological and 6-[18F]fluoro-L-DOPA-PET Profiles of Long-term Vulnerability to Chronic Amphetamine." *Behavioural Brain Research* 84 (1997): 258–68.

Melega, W., M. Raleigh, D. Stout, G. Lacan, S. Huang, and M. Phelps. "Recovery of Striatal Dopamine Function After Acute Amphetamine- and Methamphetamine-Induced Neurotoxicity in the Vervet Monkey." *Brain Research* 766 (1997): 113–20.

Mender, D. *The Myth of Neuropsychiatry.* New York: Plenum, 1994.

Moncrieff, J. *The Myth of the Chemical Cure: A Critique of Psychiatric Drug Treatment.* New York: Palgrave Macmillan, 2008.

———. "Understanding Psychotropic Drug Action: The Contribution of the Brain-Disabling Theory." *Ethical Human Psychology and Psychiatry* 9 (2007): 170–79.

Moncrieff, J. and I. Kirsch. "Efficacy of Antidepressants in Adults." *British Medical Journal* 331 (2006): 155–57.

de Montigny, C., I. Chaput, and P. Blier. "Modification of Serotonergic Neuron Properties by Long-term Treatment with Serotonin Reuptake Blockers." *Journal of Clinical Psychiatry* 51 (December 1990): 12, supplement B.

Moreno, C., G. Laje, C. Blanco, H. Jiang, A. Schmidt, and M. Olfson. "National Trends in the Outpatient Diagnosis and Treatment of Bipolar Disorder in Youth." *Archives of General Psychiatry* 64 (2007): 1032–39.

Myslobodsky, M. "Anosognosia in Tardive Dyskinesia: 'Tardive Dysmentia' or 'Tardive Dementia'?" *Schizophrenia Bulletin* 12 (1986): 1–6.

Myslobodsky, M., T. Holden, and R. Sandler. "Parkinsonian Symptoms in Tardive Dyskinesia." *South African Medical Bulletin* 69 (1986): 424–26.

Norrholm, S., and C. Ouimet. "Chronic Fluoxetine Administration to Juvenile Rats Prevents Age-Associated Dendritic Proliferation in Hippocampus." *Brain Research* 883 (2000): 205–15.

Oaks, D. "Madness and the Mental Health System." *Alternatives: Resources for Cultural Creativity.* Issue 37 (Spring 2006). Available on http://www.alternativesmagazine.com/37/oaks.html.

Okada, F. and K. Okajima. "Violent Acts Associated with Fluvoxamine Treatment." *Journal of Psychiatry & Neuroscience* 26 (2001): 339–40.

O'Meara, K. *Psyched Out: How Psychiatry Sells Mental Illness and Pushes Pills That Kill.* Bloomington, IN: AuthorHouse, 2006.

Parker, J. "The Word 'Missing' Is Misleading." January 1, 2005. http://www.bmj.com/cgi/eletters/330/7481/7.

Peck, P. "FDA Says It Plans Label Changes for Concerta and Ritalin." *Medpage Today,* June 25, 2005. http://www.medpagetoday.com.

Physicians' Desk Reference (PDR). Montvale, NJ: Thomson 2006–2008.

Popper, C., and R. Steingard. "Disorders Usually First Diagnosed in Infancy, Child-hood, or Adolescence." In *The American Psychiatric Press Textbook of Psychiatry,* second edition, edited by R. Hales, S. Yudofsky, and J. Talbott. Washington, DC: American Psychiatric Press, 1994, 729–832.

Potter, J. Corrected Judgment and Court's Motion Pursuant to Civil Rule 60.01 and Notice. *Fentress et al. v Shea Communications et al.* No 90CI0633 Jefferson Circuit Court, Division Five, Louisville, Kentucky. April 19, 1995.

———. Notice and Order. *Fentress et al. v Shea Communications et al.* No 90CI0633 Jefferson Circuit Court, Division Five, Louisville, Kentucky. March 17, 1997.

Preda, A., R. MacLean, C. Mazure, and M. Bowers, M. "Antidepressant-Associated Mania and Psychosis Resulting in Psychiatric Admission." *Journal of Clinical Psychiatry* 62 (2001): 30–33.

Rall, T. "Hypnotics and Sedatives; Ethanol." In *The Pharmacological Basis of Therapeutics,* eighth edition, 345–82, edited by A. Gilman, T. Rall, A. Nies, and P. Taylor. New York: McGraw-Hill, 1990.

Review & Outlook. "Ted and Henry Camel." *Wall Street Journal,* March 13, 2007, A22.

Ricaurte, G., R. Fuller, K. Perry, and L. Seiden. "Fluoxetine Increases Long-lasting Neostriatal Dopamine Depletion After Administration of D-methamphetamine and D-amphetamine." *Neuropharmacology* 22 (1983): 1165–69.

Richters, J., L. Arnold, P. Jensen, H. Abikoff, C. Conners, L. Greenhill, L. Hechtman, S. Hinshaw, W. Pelham, and J. Swanson. "NIMH Collaborative Multisite Multimodal Treatment Study of Children with ADHD: I. Background and Rationale." *Journal of the American Academy of Child and Adolescent Psychiatry* 34 (1995): 987–1000.

Rinn, W., N. Desai, H. Rosenblatt, and D. Gastfriend. "Addiction Denial and Cognitive Dysfunction: A Preliminary Investigation." *Journal of Neuropsychiatry and Clinical Neurosciences* 14 (2002): 52–57.

Rosack, J. "Congress Hammers FDA Over Handling of SSRIs." *Psychiatric News* 39 (20) (October 15, 2004): 1.

———. "Lilly to Pay Out Millions to Settle Lawsuits over Zyprexa: Thousands of Claims Against a Pharmaceutical Giant Are Aimed at Forcing the Industry to Make Public All Data Available on the Safety and Efficacy of Medications." *Psychiatric News* (February 2, 2007): 1.

Rosenbaum, J. "Emergence of Hostility During Alprazolam Treatment." *American Journal of Psychiatry* 141 (1984):792–93.

Ross, C. and A. Pam. *The Pseudoscience in Biological Psychiatry: Blaming the Body.* New York: John Wiley, 1995.

Rothschild, A. and C. Locke. "Reexposure to Fluoxetine After Serious Suicide Attempts by Three Patients: The Role of Akathisia." *Journal of Clinical Psychiatry* 52 (1991): 491–93.

Sabshin, M. "To Aid Understanding of Mental Disorders." Letter to *The New York Times,* March 10, 1992, A24.

Sachs, G., A. Nierenberg, J. Calabrese, L. Marangell, S. Wisniewski, et al. "Effectiveness of Adjunctive Antidepressant Treatment for Bipolar Depression." *New England Journal of Medicine* (March 28, 2007). Published at http://www.nejm.org.

Sannerud, C. and Feussner, G. (2000). "Is Ritalin an Abused Drug? Does It Meet the Criteria of a Schedule II Substance?" In *Ritalin Theory and Practice,* second edition, 27–42, edited by L. Greenhill and B. Osman. New York: Mary Ann Liebert, 2000.

Scanlon, L. "Secret Deal Struck at Trial Not to Appeal Prozac Verdict. Move Halted Evidence on 2nd Drug, Judge Thinks." *Courier-Journal* (Louisville, Kentucky), April 20, 1995, B1.

Shader, A. and A. DiMascio. *Psychotropic Drug Side Effects.* Huntington, NY: Robert E. Krieber Publishing Company, 1977.

Sheadel, A. "Report of the Friends of the Court. *Fentress et al. v. Shea Communications et al.*" No. 90CI0633 Jefferson Circuit Court, Division Five, Louisville, Kentucky, March 4, 1997.

Shelton, R. "6 Safety Rules for Tapering Antidepressants." *Current Psychiatry* 5(11) (2006): 89–90.

Sherer, R. "FDA Panel: No Black Box Warning for ADHD Drugs." *Psychiatric Times* 23 (6) (May 2006):1.

Siebert, A. "Brain Disease Hypothesis for Schizophrenia Disconfirmed by All Evidence." *Ethical Human Sciences and Services* 1 (1999): 179–89.

Sim, F. "A Single Dose of Fluvoxamine Associated with an Acute Psychotic Reaction." *Canadian Journal of Psychiatry* 45 (2000): 762.

Smith, R. "Medical Journals Are an Extension of the Marketing Arm of Pharmaceutical Companies." *PloS Med* 2 (5) (May 2005): e138.

————. Editorial: "Lapses at the *New England Journal of Medicine.*" *Journal of the Royal Society of Medicine* 99 (2006): 380–82.

Solanto, M. and E. Wender. "Does Methylphenidate Constrict Cognitive Functioning?" *Journal of the American Academy of Child and Adolescent Psychiatry* 28 (1989): 897–902.

Solvay Pharmaceuticals, Inc. Adverse Event Report FLUV00299000121 to the FDA Concerning Luvox Blood Levels from an Autopsy of One of the April 20, 1999 School Shooters. Rockville, Maryland: The FDA Medical Products Reporting Program. May 14, 1999. Obtained through Freedom of Information Act.

Stevens, C. Appeal from Court of Appeals. 95-CA-1215. Opinion of the Court by Justice Wintersheimer, Reversing. Appellant Hon. John W. Potter, Judge, *Jefferson Circuit Court v. Eli Lilly and Company.* Supreme Court of Kentucky. 95-SC-580-MR, May 23, 1996.

Stockton, T. "Recreational Use of 'Ecstasy' Causes New Brain Damage." *The Johns Hopkins Gazette,* September 30, 2002. http://www.jhu.edu.

Stone, M. and M. Jones. "Clinical Review: Relationship Between Antidepressant Drigs and Suicidality in Adults." Food and Drug Administration: Rockville, Maryland, November 17, 2006.

Swanson, J. "Research Synthesis of the Effects of Stimulant Medication on Children with Attention Deficit Disorder: A Review of Reviews." *Executive Summaries of Research Syntheses and Promising Practices on the Education of Children with Attention Deficit Disorder* (circa 1993). Prepared for Division of Innovation and Development, Office of Special Education Programs, Office of Special Education and Rehabilitation Services, U.S. Department of Education, Washington DC. Prepared by the Chesapeake Institute.

Swanson, J., D. Cantwell, M. Lerner, K. McBurnett, L. Pfiffner, and R. Kotkin. "Treatment of ADHD: Beyond Medication." *Beyond Behavior* 4: No. 1 (Fall 1992): 13–16 and 18–22.

Swanson, J., G. Elliott, L. Greenhill, T. Wigal, L. Arnold, B. Vitiello, L. Hechtman, J. Epstein, W. Pelham, H. Abikoff, J. Newcorn, B. Molina, S. Hinshaw, K. Wells, B. Hoza, P. Jensen, R. Gibbons, K. Hur, A. Stehli, M. Davies, J. March, C. Conners, M. Caron, and N. Volkow. "Effects of Stimulant Medication on Growth Rates Across 3 Years in the MTA Follow-up." *Journal of the American Academy of Child and Adolescent Psychiatry* 46 (2007): 1015–27.

Swanson, J., S. Hinshaw, L. Arnold, R. Gibbons, S. Marcus, K. Hur, P. Jensen, B. Vitiello, H. Abikoff, L. Greenhill, L. Hechtman, W. Pelham, K. Wells, C. Conners, J. March, G. Elliott, J. Epstein, K. Hoagwood, B. Hoza, B. Molina, J. Newcorn, J. Severe, and T. Wigal. "Second Evaluation of MTA 36-Month Outcomes: Propensity Score and Growth Mixture Model Analyses." *Journal of the American Academy of Child & Adolescent Psychiatry* 46 (2007): 989–1002.

Swartz, M., and P. Jones. "Hyperlithemia Correction and Persistent Delirium." *Journal of Clinical Pharmacology* 34 (1994): 865–70.

Szasz, T. *The Myth of Mental Illness.* New York: Harper & Row, 1974.

Tow, P. *Personality Changes Following Frontal Leucotomy.* London: Oxford University Press, 1955.

van der Kroef, C. "Reactions to Triazolam," *Lancet* 2 (September 8, 1979): 526.

van Putten, T. "Why Do Schizophrenic Patients Refuse to Take Their Drugs?" *Archives of General Psychiatry* 31 (1974): 67–72.

———. "Why Do Patients with Manic-Depressive Illness Stop Their Lithium?" *Comprehensive Psychiatry* 16 (1975): 179–83.

———. "The Many Faces of Akathisia." *Comprehensive Psychiatry* 16 (1975): 43–47.

van Putten, T., and S. Marder, S. "Behavioral Toxicity of Antipsychotic Drugs." *Journal of Clinical Psychiatry* 48(supp) (1987): 13–19.

van Putten, T., and P. May. "Akinetic Depression in Schizophrenia." *Archives of General Psychiatry* 35 (1978): 1101–7.

van Putten, T., P. May, and S. Marder. "Subjective Responses to Thiothixene and Chlorpromazine." *Psychopharmacology Bulletin* 16(3) (1980): 36–38.

van Putten, T., L. Mutalipassi, and M. Malkin. "Phenothiazine-Induced Decompensation." *Archives of General Psychiatry* 30 (1974): 102–5.

Varchaver, M. "Prozac Verdict Was a Sure Thing." *Fulton County Daily Report* (Atlanta), September 25, 1995.

Voruganti, L, L. Cortese, L. Oyewumi, Z. Cernovsky, S. Zirul, and A. Awad. "Comparative Evaluation of Conventional and Novel Antipsychotic Drugs with Reference to Their Subjective Tolerability, Side-effect Profile and Impact on Quality of Life." *Schizophrenia Research* 43 (2000): 135–45.

Wamsley, J., W. Byerley, R. McCabe, E. McConnell, T. Dawson, and B. Grosser. "Receptor Alterations Associated with Serotonergic Agents: An Autographic Analysis." *Journal of Clinical Psychiatry* 48(3) (supp) (1987):19–85.

Weaver, J. "Sustained Use of Anti-Depressants Increases Cell Growth and Protects Cells in the Brain." From press release. New Haven, CT: Yale University, December 15, 2000.

Wegerer, V., G. Moll, M. Bagli, A. Rothenberger, F. Ruther, and G. Huether. "Persistently Increased Density of Serotonin Transporters in the Frontal Cortex of Rats Treated with Fluoxetine During Early Juvenile Life." *Journal of Child and Adolescent Psychopharmacology* 9 (1999): 13–24.

Whalen, C., B. Henker, and D. Granger. "Ratings of Medication Effects in Hyperactive Children: Viable or Vulnerable?" *Behavioral Assessment* 11 (1989): 179–99.

Wilens, T., J. Biederman, A. Kwon, R. Chase, L. Greenberg, E. Mick, and T. Spencer. "A Systematic Chart Review of the Nature of Psychiatric Adverse Events in Children and Adolescents Treated with Selective Serotonin Reuptake Inhibitors." *Journal of Child and Adolescent Psychopharmacology* 13 (2003): 143–52.

Wirshing, W., T. van Putten, J. Rosenberg, S. Marder, D. Ames, and T. Hicks-Gray. "Fluoxetine, Akathisia, and Suicidality: Is There a Connection?" *Archives of General Psychiatry* 49 (1992): 580–81.

Wise, B. "Increased Frequency Report (IFR): Alprazolam and Rage." Rockville, MD: FDA Division of Epidemiology and Surveillance, April 21, 1989. Unpublished.

———. "Reports of Hostility After Exposure to Triazolobenzodiazepines (working paper)." Rockville, MD: FDA Division of Epidemiology and Surveillance, September 19, 1989. Obtained through the Freedom of Information Act.

Wiseman, E., E. Souder, and P. O'Sullivan. "Relation of Denial of Alcohol Problems to Neurocognitive Impairment and Depression." *Psychiatric Services* 47 (1996): 306–8.

Wong, D. and F. Bymaster. "Subsensitivity of Serotonin Receptors after Long-term Treatment of Rats with Fluoxetine." *Research Communications in Chemical Pathology and Pharmacology* 32 (April 1981): 41–51.

Wong, D., L. Reid, F. Bymaster, and P. Threlkeld. "Chronic Effects of Fluoxetine, a Selective Inhibitor of Serotonin Uptake, on Neurotransmitter Receptors." *Journal of Neural Transmission* 64 (1985): 251–69.

Wysowski, D., and D. Barash. "Adverse Behavioral Reactions Attributed to Triazolam in the Food and Drug Administration's Spontaneous Reporting System." *Archives of Internal Medicine* 151 (October 1991): 2003–8.

Zhou, L., K. Huang, A. Kecojevic, A. Welsh, V. and Koliatsos. "Evidence that Serotonin Reuptake Modulators Increase the Density of Serotonin in the Forebrain." *Journal of Neurochemistry* 96 (2006): 396–406.

Index

About the Author

PETER R. BREGGIN, M.D.

Peter R. Breggin, M.D., has been called "the conscience of psychiatry" for his efforts to reform the mental-health field, including his promotion of caring psychotherapeutic approaches and his opposition to the escalating overuse of psychiatric medications, the oppressive diagnosing and drugging of children, electroshock, lobotomy, involuntary treatment, and false biological theories.

Dr. Breggin has been in the private practice of psychiatry since 1968, first in the Washington, D.C., area and now in Ithaca, New York. In his therapy practice, he treats individuals, couples, and children with their families without resorting to psychiatric drugs. As a clinical psychopharmacologist, he provides consultations and is active as a medical expert in criminal, malpractice, and product-liability lawsuits, often involving the harmful effects of psychiatric drugs. He has been an expert in landmark cases involving the rights of patients.

Since 1964, Dr. Breggin has written dozens of scientific articles and more than twenty books, including. *Toxic Psychiatry, The Heart of Being Helpful, Talking Back to Ritalin,* the *Anti-Depressant Fact Book,* and with coauthor Ginger Breggin, *Talking Back to Prozac,* and *The War Against Children of Color.*

At various stages of his career he has been decades ahead of his time in warning about the dangers of lobotomy, electroshock, and more recently antidepressant-induced suicide and violence, as well as many other recently acknowledged risks associated with psychiatric drugs. From *The New York Times* and *Wall Street Journal* to *Time* and *Newsweek,* and from *Larry King Live* and *Oprah* to *60 Minutes* and *20/20*, his views have been covered in major media throughout the world.

In 1972, Dr. Breggin founded the International Center for the Study of Psychiatry and Psychology (www.icspp.org). Originally organized to support his successful campaign to stop the resurgence of lobotomy, ICSPP has become a source of support and inspiration for reformed-minded professionals and laypersons who wish to raise ethical and scientific standards in the field of mental health. In 1999, he and his wife, Ginger, founded ICSPP's peer-reviewed scientific journal, *Ethical Human Psychology and Psychiatry.* In 2002, they selected younger professionals to take over the center and the journal, although Dr. Breggin continues to participate in ICSPP activities.

Dr. Breggin's background includes Harvard, Case Western Reserve Medical School, a teaching fellowship at Harvard Medical School, three years of residency training in psychiatry, a two-year staff assignment at the National Institute of Mental Health (NIMH), and several teaching appointments including the Johns Hopkins University Department of Counseling, and the George Mason University Institute for Conflict Analysis and Resolution.

In 2008, Dr. Breggin published two of his most comprehensive works. *Medication Madness* describes dozens of cases of adverse psychiatric-drug reactions and illustrates the principles of brain-disabling treatment and medication spellbinding. The new edition of *Brain-Disabling Treatments in Psychiatry* provides his overall critique of modern psychiatry with more than one thousand citations to the scientific literature.

Dr. Breggin's Web site is www.breggin.com.